MORNING, COME QUICKLY

Wanda Karriker

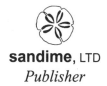

sandime, LTD
Publisher

Morning, Come Quickly is a work of fiction. Sadly, the acts of cruelty and inhumanity presented in this novel hold much truth and are similar to accounts the author has heard from her own clients and from other unwitting initiates into organized evil who have told their stories in articles and books, at survivor conferences, and on websites and Internet discussion groups.

Published in the United States of America

FIRST EDITION
First Printing

Publisher's Cataloging-in-Publication

Karriker, Wanda Wright, 1942-
    Morning, come quickly / Wanda Karriker. — 1st ed.
    p. cm.
    Includes bibliographical references.
    LCCN 2001099572
    ISBN 0-9717171-0-9

    1. Children in pornography—Fiction. 2. False memory
syndrome—Fiction. 3. Brainwashing—Fiction. 4. Ritual
abuse—Fiction. 5. Multiple personality—Fiction.
I. Title.

PS3611.A785M67 2002   813'.6
                    QBI02-701324

sandime, LTD
Publisher
8313 Long Island Road
Catawba NC 28609
www.MorningComeQuickly.com

In Honor of

All SOULS

who have been unwitting initiates

into organized evil

Crime, obviously, calls for the night; crime would not be crime without darkness, yet—were it pitch dark—this horror of night aspires to the burst of sunshine.

Georges Bataille, *The Trial of Gilles de Rais*

NOT KNOWING

Chapter 1

Startled awake.

Knowing what the face of the clock will read before she looks. Not knowing how she knows or why. Only knowing she can't go on much longer without help. She closes her eyes, coveting sleep.

Images, like meteors streaking through the deep dark cosmos, bounce around the inside of her forehead. Tonight it's the hands' show: big hands, little hands, hands that looked like witches' hands, a tiny hand on a huge penis.

Blinding bright lights. Blood-churning chills.

The little girl is scrunched in a box. It's dark as night. There's banging on metal. Painful adrenaline shoots through her body like an electrical current. She cups her ears with her hands; curls up in the soft thing at her feet.

"Are you in there?" a woman calls.

"Mommy! Mommy!"

"Wake up." Her husband places his hand on her brow. "Are you okay?"

"Just dreaming," she lies and he turns away.

More mind pictures: a naked toddler in front of a bunch of people, frosted windows, a small table holding a gold cross.

"Ah-a-a-a-a-a-a!"

"What's wrong, Hon?" Strong arms pull her close.

"A nightmare," she lies again. "Must be picking up symptoms from my clients."

Inside, outside, her worlds are spinning out of control. The office is a mess: stacks of records piled on the desk; dozens of checks to be deposited; reports overdue; plants wilting in the waiting room. At home, bizarre things have been happening: a TV turning on without remote—three times; an unset clock alarming; the answering machine activating when no one has called; light bulbs exploding all over the place; the commode in the guest bathroom flushing—over and over. But there are no guests in the house during this first week in February, 1989 . . . no mortal guests, that is.

On Wednesday night—not quite asleep, not quite awake—Emily perceives a dazzling light. Something like a wand brushes her heart, setting off an incredible ecstatic rush. Opening her eyes, she sees a glowing amorphous figure surrounded by an aura of absolute serenity. She hears a clear polished feminine voice saying: "Everything will be just fine." In less than an instant, it is gone.

Thursday morning, she's alone at the breakfast table. Ten feet across the room, a roll of paper towels spirals to the floor. Later she naps in the family room, its windows shut and outside door closed. Yet, a rousing wind swoops through the house.

Sleeping late on Saturday morning, she is awakened by a loud roaring sound, a motor at high speed. Realizing it's the central vacuum cleaner, she goes around the house checking each hose outlet. All are tightly closed. She hurries to the basement; pulls the plug.

At high speed herself, she runs upstairs to the guest room. To her amazement, but then again she's not all that surprised given everything that has been happening in her house lately, the chair in the corner is rocking. She lifts the down comforter off the queen-sized bed and curls up under it in the oversized rocker with wide, ebony armrests. In this refuge, a kind of transgenerational bridge which rocked the babies on the Lentz side of the family—first her father, next her brother and herself, and most recently her own children, Carol and Matt—she attempts to soothe away the angst.

As she teaches clients to do when stressed out, the psychologist uses self-hypnosis, willing relaxation; however, her mind, whirling like the antique carrousel at the Myrtle Beach pavilion, will not shut down:

I wanna die. I wanna die. I wanna die.

But Dr. Emily Lentz Klein does not want to die.

She sees herself in bed with a familiar-looking stranger. No, it's Jeff in bed with a nun . . . couldn't be Kate . . . is it herself dressed as a nun? . . . or a ghost?

"Is a ghost in this house?"

"Not that I've seen."

Emily opens her eyes to see Jeff—the real Jeff—standing in front of her. "Must've been dreaming again," she chuckles, nervously. Standing up, reaching for his embrace, she tells her partner about the vacuum cleaner; doesn't tell him how frightened she feels, how out of sync, how —

Revved.

Behind her the chair is still rocking.

After church services on Sunday morning, they walk into the house together. Sniffing the air around him, Jeff says nonchalantly, "Dad's been here. I smell cigar smoke."

"So do I, but didn't you just change the locks last week? By the way, did you happen to give him a new key?"

"Not on my life. You've told me a thousand times that you don't want him coming around when we're not home."

Over lunch, the couple talk about the strange things going 'bump in the night' — and day.

"Em, some of the electrical things can probably be explained logically, but not cigar smoke, and I don't see how those paper towels rolled off without your touching the holder; or that strong wind; or the commode flushing." He refills their glasses with iced tea. "Why don't you give Kate a call to see what she has to say about all this crazy crap?"

"Good idea. But you know what, the weirdest thing of all is that old chair rocking . . . just rocking by itself." Rubbing her arms with opposite hands, she adds, "Now *that* passes the goose bumps test."

"Must be your grandmother coming back to rock the babies," he smiles.

As Emily sips tea, Jeff finishes off a biscuit loaded with salty country ham. After a couple minutes pass, she pushes her chair back from the table, saying, "That sometimes happens if they're leaking."

"Babies?"

"No, silly. Commodes." She stands up and walks toward the family room, pausing to reach for a paper towel. Looking back over her shoulder, she adds a postscript: "Interesting, until something unfathomable, perhaps even supernatural, affects you directly, personally, it's easy to say it doesn't exist."

Waiting for an answer, Emily studied the sepia-toned portrait in a gilded picture frame on the rolltop desk. Against a wooden-plank wall, corn stalks had been ornamentally stacked to serve as the classic backdrop for a rustic setting. She imagined the subject's dress, made of a dark heavy fabric, as a deep-ocean green. Long puffed sleeves, a high collar and a skirt reaching to the floor, left only the hands and face exposed.

Both collar and belt were edged with crochet, creating an appearance of unaffected elegance.

A voice came over the phone. "Hello, this is Kate Stewart speaking." Kate, an ex-nun, ran a shelter for trauma survivors in Sante Fe. She was also a research subject for a group of clinical psychologists who dabbled in parapsychology on weekends.

"Hey girl. It's Emily."

"What's up? I was just about to dial your number when the phone rang. You've been on my mind all week . . . is something wrong?" Hundreds of miles away, Kate had apparently sensed that her friend was in trouble.

"Nothing much. I just need some information."

"About the shelter?"

"No, about poltergeists and ghosts and spirits and stuff like that."

"That shouldn't be too difficult. Oh Emily, someone just paged me. Can I call you back in a few minutes?"

"Sure." Emily put the phone down, focusing once more on the picture of the woman who had died giving birth to the little baby who was to grow up to become Emily's father. Hannah Lentz was seated beside a primitive-looking table with legs made from the limbs of a pine or cedar tree. It held a small book and a flowering geranium potted in a milk pail.

The hands in the picture looked like Emily's. With short stubby fingers and tiny nails, Hannah's right hand lay in the same position as Emily's usually did when sitting with clients: palm facing up with the thumb between the middle and index fingers.

Except for a much smaller waistline and long curls, the girl looked a lot like Emily did at thirteen. What the granddaughter sensed more than anything with her grandmother was an emotional connection. Hannah's eyes were hauntingly sad; her thin lips, slightly parted as if she were contemplating what needed to be said.

Emily silently asked the picture-person: "Why are you so unhappy? If you could speak, what secrets would you tell?"

She picked up the phone on the first ring.

"I'm back," Kate said. "Sorry it took so long. One of the residents was in crisis. Now what is it you wanted to know?"

Quickly, Emily rattled off some of the eerie things that had happened the previous week.

"Cool," Kate reacted. "Okay, let's start with the good part—the apparition. Of course, you could've been hallucinating, even viewing a dissociated aspect of yourself. Those who believe in discarnate beings, who believe in the supernatural, and I assume you do since you are a practicing Christian—"

"I suppose you could say that. I believe there's a God . . . most of the time I do. And I try to follow the teachings of Jesus."

"I know you do. Now back to what I was saying. If there are such things as spirits, what you perceived could've been a spirit of someone close to you, or even another type of entity hanging around to complete some unfinished business."

"Like an ancestor?"

"Uh-huh, or it could've been an angel. Lots of people, from Bible times till now, believe they've encountered angels."

"Come to think of it, as a child I pretended—probably believed—that somebody like a godmother, maybe an angel, floated over me, protecting me from big bad people like those in the fairy tales my mother read to me every evening, right along with stories from my children's Bible—some of which, I must say, were just as horrible."

"You mean like the one where God told Abraham to take his son on top of the mountain and kill him?"

"Yeah, or even Jesus hanging on that cross. But let's save religion-talk for another time, okay? Do you have any idea what's going on around here?"

"As for the things that aren't electrical, I really have no explanation. But there's a rather scientific-sounding theory for the others. From what I've read and experienced myself, poltergeist happenings may be a result of the way the unconscious works off emotional tension. Now you know from your biofeedback work that the body sends out electrical signals. All that energy could be transferring to any electrical receptors such as household appliances, say."

"Is that why a windup watch won't keep time on my wrist? Electrical interference?"

"Possibly. However there is one thing that doesn't fit your experience. From what I've learned, poltergeist phenomena usually occur around basically normal adolescent girls, those who tend to repress their feelings until they erupt through some type of unconscious workings."

"But Kate, I'm a long way from adolescence . . . although I have to admit some of my recent thoughts have been about the caliber of a thirteen-year-old's. And I've certainly had a lot of energy lately, especially sexual energy."

"Bet Jeff's happy with that."

"Haven't told him," Emily shot back, wishing the lapse into something even she didn't understand hadn't been so personal. The energy she was talking about had absolutely nothing to do with romance.

"Well friend, the good news is that the outbreaks don't usually last over a few days or weeks at the most."

"Huh?" Emily's mind—still on that unexplainable urge she remembered having felt even even as a little girl, that sense of being hung in arousal that sometimes came over her, haunted, even tortured her when she felt threatened, or when she was afraid she'd made a big mistake, or had done something terribly wrong—had temporarily strayed from the conversation at hand.

"Are you repressing anything that you know of?"

"Kate—"

They both laughed at the absurdity of the question.

"How's your practice going?" Kate tried again.

"Fine. Busy as ever, and I'm beginning to see remarkable changes in a few people who've stayed in therapy long enough to work through their traumas."

"Exactly how do you feel when you're with clients?"

"Normal. In tune. It's mostly at night when I get all revved up. Sometimes I wonder if I'm bringing their symptoms home with me."

"For example?"

"It's just that I often have trouble falling to sleep and when I eventually do, horrible nightmares have been waking me up . . . never used to have nightmares. Anyway, I'm having lots of thoughts that seem to come from . . . I don't really think them, they just like bubble up on their own. Unthought-thoughts, I call them."

"From your unconscious, of course. Speaking of—" Kate cleared her throat. "How long has it been since you've seen your therapist?"

"A few . . .well actually not since I finished my internship. Okay, I get the hint. If things don't settle down soon, I'll give her a call."

"Good idea. And you know you can call me any time."

"Thanks for listening . . . and for not being so darn neutral."

Again, Emily studied the portrait in the gilded frame. Something about Hannah seemed almost to reach out in violation of time and the distance of death to touch Emily near the core of the indefinable. Religion—always happier than science with the idea of the invisible—might have called it soul.

What would psychology have called it, she wondered—madness?

Funny, she was remembering the brightly-lit figure that had touched her so profoundly earlier in the week, and almost laughing at a new thought forming in her mind: *If I announced that I had literally been touched by, say by an angel—the world would likely open its arms and cry 'Amen'; but when a survivor of deliberately inflicted trauma seemed to be having memories of meeting something like a demon—vastly, the same would quickly close ranks against such possible recognition of evil's activities to cry <u>dementia</u> . . . <u>possessed</u> . . . <u>insane</u>.*

———————

Overhead, the moon waxed through the skylight, casting a ghostlike glow around the snores of the man in her bed. As though subliminally knowing that his wife was in distress, Jeff woke up, touching her shoulder.

"Not now." Emily pushed him away. "I need to . . . got a big day tomorrow." She was sure that he remembered they were planning to drive down to Atlanta to shop with Carol for a wedding dress. The date was set for July 29, only five months away.

"I just wanted to hold you." He rolled over to face the wall.

For a while, Emily thought about all the things a mother-of-the-bride would have to do. Finally closing her eyes, she was bombarded with bright pictures floating in the black abyss: a wall of rusty corrugated metal, big white shoes with laces, little white shoes with bows, the Red Cross—

A ringing phone startled her out of the path of the witches' hands.

Jeff sat straight up, feet hitting the floor on the second ring. "Probably some drunk with the wrong number." He fumbled with the receiver, knocking it off the nightstand, eventually getting a firm grip on it. "Hello . . . yeah, hold on." He passed his wife the phone and a disgusted look. "It's for you."

When Emily put the phone to her ear, the young man, sounding intoxicated, was already talking. "They're comin' to get me. I know they are . . . and I'd rather die . . . never shoulda blabbed last week about—"

"Who's coming?"

"Can't tell you," he whimpered. "They're comin' to get me . . . they're comin'." Then he yelled, "But not before I slit my goddamn throat and bleed to death!"

"But nobody knows you told."

"Oh yes they do. They know every word I say. They always know."

Until her client had promised to put the knife away, Emily talked to him like a mother trying to calm her own child. When it was all over, she cuddled up to her lover.

This time he pushed *her* away. "You need to get an answering ser-vice. I'm tired of that deadbeat of a man coming into our bedroom — he's not going to kill himself, and even if he were, there's no way he'd call you first. My dear wife, don't you see? You're being jerked around . . . as usual."

"What do you want me to do? Let him die?"

"Of course not. But they need to lock him away somewhere."

"He's a man who doesn't always know what he's doing."

"I rest my case." His voice had that twinge of sarcasm that always made her want to punch him hard in the belly.

"Sometimes I think you're just jealous," she jabbed.

This time there was no response.

Fed up with not being understood herself, Emily fled to the guest room where she yanked the down comforter from the foot of the bed and carried it over to the timelessness of the antique rocker.

———————

Dr. Jefferson Winslow Campbell Klein awoke before dawn: sweaty wet; muscles aching all over; feeling like someone had beaten him over the head with a two-by-four. He slipped on his running clothes and went downstairs to the kitchen. After putting on a pot of coffee, he went out to the family room and sat down on the sofa, hoping to clear his mind a bit.

Across the way was a fireplace nestled in the center of a wall made of old bricks hand-fired by slaves who'd once lived on the Campbell plantation. To his right, beside the 32-drawer rolltop desk that had been a wedding present for Emily's grandmother, stood a bookcase crafted from walnut lumber he and his daddy had cut from the Klein family farm on Slicky Rock Mountain. Wide shelves held his diverse collec-tions, including reproductions of ancient scriptures, the Foxfire series, and the complete works of Louis L'Amour.

Photographic enlargements of his favorite scenes were methodi-cally arranged on the pickled-cypress paneling behind the stairs: a sunrise over the Atlantic taken from the widow's walk on top of their beach cottage; a river in the Canadian Rockies taken from the caboose of a moving train; a lake in the Grand Tetons taken from the rental car; and an aerial view of the Campbell plantation taken from the *Pegasus*.

Lord, he was so tired of being jarred awake each morning. Heart racing. Breathing rapid. Stomach cramping. Feeling like a little boy trapped at the bottom of a hand-dug well.

Little Miss Emily wasn't the only one with problems.

When he'd reach over to touch his sweetheart, she was often gone, as if she couldn't wait to get out of bed to run to her sanctum of couches, biofeedback machines, and professional journals; or to captain hypnotic voyages to rescue the perishing from their wretched minds.

Oh dear Emmy. So many good years together and I don't understand what's happening now.

Not only was that poor boy calling at all hours of the night, but Emily was beginning to fear they were after her, whoever 'they' were.

Downright paranoid, she was. Cults, cults, cults! That's all she talked about anymore.

And, as if she were bearing the burdens of proof for her clients' struggles with pain and suffering, she'd let herself go. Gaining weight again. He didn't really know how much. Her weight was a private matter. She wanted it that way.

Had she forgotten how much he needed her?

Whether Em realized it or not, he had a life, too. He'd been offered the academic deanship but preferring teaching and writing had turned it down. As he saw it, the answers to humankind's struggle with meaning could best be found in ancient history, not by getting in touch with your inner child—whatever that meant. On the other hand, he'd give up all his material possessions if he could repress that one nightmare and the memory it rattled.

How in God's name could he have been dragged to something like that?

The grandfather clock in the corner—built by one of the Kleins who'd brought it over when the family emigrated from the Black Forest area of Germany to Pennsylvania in the 1700s—struck six times, interrupting his little private gripe session. Forgetting about the coffee, he felt his bones ready to run. Stretching, he stood up and practically skipped through the double glass doors on the south side of the house, past the indoor lap pool (the centerpiece of a huge sunroom furnished with a hot tub, classic green wicker, and filled with so many tropical plants it looked like a rain forest), and across the deck which he'd built to resemble a boat's bow. Cables below the rail allowed an unobstructed view of the water.

He headed down to the lakeside trail.

———————

"Mornin' Hon." Jeff heard Emily's voice and looked up to see her coming down the path wrapped in an aqua chenille bathrobe with a coffee mug in one hand, a sweet roll in the other. He jogged over to meet her on the pier. "Sorry about last night," she smiled.

"Me too, but I was just tired and knew I had to get up early. Dad wants me to help him clean out his basement today."

Her smile quickly changed to a grimace. "But I thought you were going to drive me to Atlanta." She balanced the mug on the rail and ate the last of the roll. "What's new? Your dear ol' daddy's always been more important than me . . . or even your own daughter."

"You know that's not true," he defended, glaring down into the dark water.

"But you always do what he tells you to do. Are you afraid of him or something?"

"Absolutely not." Jeff pressed both hands heavily into her shoulders and began a counterattack. "To tell the truth, I am afraid of what's happening to you . . . to us. Like, what's happened to all your sexual spontaneity? The way you pushed me away last night made me feel like . . . like a wound-up monster inside. And then you spent half the night talking to that—you don't want to hear what I think he is. You know, Em, we never had any problems until you started working with all those . . . people. I know you think it's your calling: to fix their headaches; to hold their hands; pick them up when they fall. Or if that doesn't work and they commit a crime, to rescue them from the law. My wife: not a woman anymore, or a mother or a daughter-in-law, but an expert witness."

"You don't have any idea what you're talking about." She pulled away from his hold on her and looked directly into his eyes, forcing intimate contact. "Sometimes I think you actually wish I'd never become a psychologist. Did you really want me to just stay good little Emily, your hoity-toity southern belle forever—is that it?"

"Settle down. You know I'm proud of you, but I do think you're too involved in the lives of your clients . . . I think you've forgotten all about being objective and neutral . . . and dammit, I don't think you see that at all!"

She seemed not to have heard what he had said.

For several minutes, they stood silent as the mist burned off the water and the eastern sky began to take on a peachy glow.

This time he was first to apologize. "I'm sorry. I shouldn't have talked to you the way I did. Really and truly, I do understand how important your work is to you. But sometimes you're just not there . . . and I never know how to react without you to hold."

"Why do you always have to bring it back to our personal sexual relationship?" Emily asked, not giving her husband a chance to answer. "I don't know what's been happening but I don't like it either. I haven't told you—"

"I know." This time it was he who interrupted. "You've been faking it some. The things you used to go wild over . . . well, now you just seem to cringe at."

"But sometimes when you touch me, I don't feel anything; nothing at all. It's as if I'm either hot or I'm cold without any kind of emotional thermostat to regulate my feelings. Maybe we could use some marriage counseling."

He looked up at the dark cloud hanging invisibly between them. Reaching over to touch her shoulders, gently this time, almost fearfully, he said, "Oh my dear sweet lady, we love each other. You know that. Always have, always will as far as I'm concerned. Let's try to work things out for ourselves. And Em, I do understand it's not all your fault."

"It's got a silver lining . . . isn't that beautifully corny?" She'd turned her eyes upward to try to see what Jeff was seeing but noticed instead a real cloud, small and puffy, between them and the just risen sun. "That edging of bright light at the bottom, it reminds me of the lace my mother used to sew on the hem of my Sunday dresses so I could get an extra year of wear out of them . . . and that's fine with me."

Over time, he'd learned that when his wife talked, she often skipped crucial bits of connecting information, leaving him to fill in the blanks. She'd been that way as far back as he could remember in their childhoods. Now, he realized, this time she was responding to his comment about counseling.

"I was thinking about a cardinal principle of therapy—"

"What's that?" he asked in private amusement, just like the old times.

"The problem—the presenting problem—is not the problem."

He was quiet and simply cradled her shoulders against him.

Some minutes later she added softly, "I wonder what the problem is."

———

Waiting for his daddy to come down and boss him around, Jeff looked around the cement-block basement. In one corner was a bin of dusty whiskey bottles of various shapes and sizes. Old magazines—about thirty years of *Playboy*—lined the walls. In the center of the floor, a wormy, dark pine table and captain's chair sat over the sump pump. Under the high point of the steps stood the forbidden gun safe.

Drawn by a whiff of cedar, he went over to the chest in the corner. Getting on his knees, he began to dig through it. Pictures of childhood, a precious few with his mother, were scattered among relics of school art and papers, blue ribbons from horse shows, a pair of flight goggles, Boy Scout merit badges, a rock collection, and certificates for this and that. Stacked near the bottom were four high school yearbooks and a chocolate-colored fake leather "Book of School Days Memories" from the sixth grade. He leafed through the latter, coming to the "My Special Pals" section displaying a photo of a smiling, curly-headed, chubby-faced Emily Lentz pasted between pictures of two other friends, both boys. Near the back on one of the autograph pages, he came across a note in Emily's youthful handwriting:

Jeff my buddy,
    It sure has been fun being with you in class this year. Too bad we got stuck with the old battle-axe. Let's you and me always stick to-gether, okay? Till the ocean has to wear rubber diapers to keep its bottom dry.
    Your friend,
    Snow Force Lentz
P. S. Please don't let Miss Jarrett see this. She might make me hold out geography books. Ha! Ha!

Snow Force. Where in the world did that name come from?
He placed the book back in the chest and picked up his sophomore yearbook, accidentally opening it to a full-page picture of Tommy Paxton wearing a football uniform. The Chestnut Ridge High School homecoming queen of 1958 was attached to his arm.

A piece of blue-lined notebook paper fell to the floor.

"Me-o-o-w!"

"What the—" Dropping the yearbook, Jeff brushed the old cat off his shoulder. The incontinent, seventeen-pound, seventeen-year-old mixed-breed his daddy had inherited from his longtime companion was just a kitten when Amanda Jarrett had uttered her last words: "Take care of Puffy Poo."

Cleat Adolphus Klein was not the type of man to break a promise.

"Way to go, girl." The old man came down the steps. Sarge, a deaf Dalmatian, was following at his heels.

"N-Not funny. That hurt. Can't you control the old p-puss any better? . . . Or did you sic her on me on p-purpose?"

"Now son. Ya know I'd never do anything to hurt ya." His daddy kicked the cat in the rear end, sending her scampering up the steps. At the top, she crouched down as if looking for her next victim.

"All right, D-Dad. What is it you w-wanted . . . wanted me to do?" Jeff picked up the notebook paper, carefully folded it twice, and stuck it in his back pocket.

Cleat eyed the magazines. "We need to get rid of those. They're full of termites."

"They're also full of n-naked women. You should call an ex-exterminator."

"Already have."

"Never knew you read that stuff."

"Ya don't read 'em, boy. Ya just look. Nothin' wrong with lookin', is there?" Cleat pointed to the chest in the corner. "And ya can have that if ya want it. It's all your junk anyways."

"Are you sure? Isn't it the one b-brought over from Germany by one of our ancestors?"

"That's what my daddy said."

"S-Speaking of Germany, Emily and I'll be leaving on the eighth of March for the Black Forest. Still time for you to get reservations if you want to come along."

"Ya gotta be kiddin'." The old man's sickly grin spread wide open. "That woman of yours would never stand for it. Anyhow, I ain't lost nothin' over there no ways." Cleat held up his left hand. "Unlessen you count the pinkie. Never kept me from doin' what I had to do, though." He reached around Jeff and slammed the lid closed. "Get it out of here. It's all yours."

For the rest of the morning, Jeff was the obedient child. Following Daddy's orders: Do this. Do that. Don't do that.

After carrying out the last stack of magazines, he loaded the cedar chest onto a hand truck. Pulling it up the steps, as there was no ground-level door to the outside, his foot slipped, causing him to turn loose of the side handle. The chest tumbled down the steps barely missing Cleat who'd jumped out of the way just in time.

Face red, eyes enraged, Cleat bellowed, "Ya stupid—"

"W-Will you please shut up. It w-was an accident, Dad. I couldn't help it." Remembering the times his daddy had belittled him as a child, Jeff pointed his left index finger at Cleat and threatened, stutter-free, at the top of his voice, "Don't you ever call me stupid again or I'll— " He took a deep breath and lowered the volume. "You get on upstairs. I'll do it myself."

"Whatever ya say." Cleat slid past the chest and gingerly climbed the steps.

As if trying to console a brother, Sarge stayed at Jeff's side.

Sitting on the grimy bottom step, groping for the energy and motivation to complete the task, Jeff scratched Sarge behind the ears saying sadly, hopelessly, "Wish the old man loved me as much as he does you. I can never . . . could never . . . do anything to please him."

Sarge was unable to hear what his master's son was saying but, appearing to sense his anguish, licked the younger Klein across the hand. Jeff hardly noticed. In his mind,

—he was seeing a redheaded kid streaking through the woods.

—he was hearing raucous laughter, ribald hoots, and feigned recriminations. *Ya little sissy.*

—he was seeing a teenager who, hoping to surprise his daddy, had painted the trim work on the outside of the duplex. Arriving home from a week-long fishing trip, Cleat had looked all around, deadpan, before pointing to a corner of the eaves, ridiculing, "Ya missed a spot."

How many times had the daddy made the kid feel like a whipped pup?

The boy, the man, was inevitably coming up short.

To hell with it!

Em was right—as always. Jeff was going to have to quit trying.

———————

The basement job finished, father and son sat across from each other on the kitchen bar stools: talking, eating doughnut holes, and drinking coffee. Puffy Poo, as if begging for forgiveness, brushed around Jeff's legs.

"D-Dad, what ever happened to Blinkers?"

"Blinkers who?"

"The cat. My cat when I was little."

"Don't know what you're talkin' about, son. Puffy's the only cat we . . . I ever had."

They drank some more coffee. Cleat dropped a few crumbs on the floor for Sarge then lit a cigar.

"There's s-something . . . there's something I've been meaning to talk with you about," Jeff said.

"Go ahead. Ya know ya can talk to me about anything."

Yeah sure, Jeff thought before asking, "Have you ever heard of any groups around here that have s-secret r-rituals where they—"

"Ya mean like the Masons. Don't know nothin' about 'em. Ya could ask Phil. He's big in that. Nobody ever asked me to join. Let's see now," Cleat took a long puff on the cigar and blew the smoke toward Jeff's face, "there's the Klan, of course. But here in this part of the country, it's not really all that secret. Been around a long time. Got a bad rap really. Casey Paxton'll tell ya it had a noble purpose when it first got started. Runnin' the damn Yankees out of town who bankrupted the folks around here and took their land and always seein' that justice gets . . . got done."

"I don't want to hear it."

"Hear what?"

"How the K-K-Klan justifies their actions. Their message of hate. People who gravitate to the Klan have to believe they are better than someone else and that requires hating, doesn't it? And frankly Dad, I don't give a damn why anyone felt they were justified in wearing the robe or the sheet or whatever else it was they used to cover their hypocrisy. I was wondering more about . . . have you ever heard of any d-d-devil worshipers around here?"

"Where did ya hear such a thing?"

"Well, I've heard kids over at the college talking about some wild parties where they deflower virgins and stuff like that." Jeff wasn't about to mention the work Emily was doing.

The phone rang and Cleat went back to his bedroom to answer it. Remembering the note in his pocket, Jeff took it out to read:

> Ah! These nights that besiege me
> That fill with bitterness.
> There is no one to appease me,
> Alone in my loneliness.
> Ah! These nights that plague me
> When all my kinfolk sleep.
> There is no one to save me.
> I lie here lonely and weep.
> But someday when all is well,
> And with this I remind,
> I will defeat the demons that dwell
> Within my wretched mind.
>
> (J.W.C.K. 1958)

Strange.

The writing of a severely depressed teenager. The adult had no memory of having composed the poem. Jeff had never been depressed — not that he recalled. Angry. That's it. He must have been angry at Emily because she was dating that son of a bitch, Tommy Paxton.

I'm a most fortunate fellow, Jeff thought, trying to repress the perturbing experience from earlier in the day. Here I am a thousand feet off the ground, the wind whipping in my face and a sweet running engine purring along as though it has a spirit of its own.

He was high above his homeland on what they call a bluebird day: no overcast, no crosswinds, no turbulence.

"Flying is an art," the instructor had said a few years earlier when he'd handed Jeff a license to fly. "It never forgives poor judgment."

The new air school graduate had prided himself on being a responsible person, optimistic, looking toward unknown destinations and unknowable adventures, not at all like a man named Cleat who was always expecting the crash.

Pegasus, he'd christened the YMF. She was gorgeous: a 1935 canary-yellow vintage biplane outfitted with a state-of-the-art instrument panel. It included everything except radar which would've been too heavy. Instead, he'd installed a gadget called a TCAD (Traffic Collision Avoidance Detection) to let him know when another plane was near. Because it didn't give a direction, Jeff would have to continually look all around making certain he could see and be seen. Using an extra fuel tank, he could stay up four hours give or take a few minutes, or about 400 miles depending on the wind. It was possible to fly to and from the beach cottage or his dad's cabin in the mountains without refueling.

Running his fingers over the white satiny scarf around his neck, he remembered the first time his family had seen him dressed in proper flight attire: jumpsuit, scarf, leather helmet, and goggles. Emily had said he looked like one of the flyboys in an old John Wayne movie. Carol had called him Snoopy. Matt had asked if he'd chased down the Red Baron yet.

God, how he wished his wife was sitting in the front seat right now instead of on her way to Atlanta. Flying solo was not his preference. He guided the plane through a loop, almost hearing Emily scream. Whether with delight or horror, he couldn't really tell.

Trying not to think about the lonely night ahead, as he often tried not to think about things that he couldn't change, he scanned the landscape below. Purely peaceful. Just like the replica covering a large table in the local Historic Museum.

Flying over the land of his ancestors, Jeff was euphoric. Feeling free. He was thinking about all the people down there living simple uncomplicated God-fearing lives, working hard five days a week and practicing their religion on weekends: cheering at the high school football game on Friday night and praying at church on Sunday morning.

Directly over the old courthouse, he was barely able to make out two tiny flags flying on the spring-greening lawn. The monument to the "Southern Dead of the Lost Cause" was much easier to see.

Every building, every institution, every piece of real estate in Campbell County had its own story to tell: Olde Town Cemetery, Acadia, the old cotton mill that had been developed into a modern factory shipping synthetic materials all over the world, Mt. Hermon Lutheran Church.

The pilot veered toward the college campus. "Naw, I'd better not," he grinned, speaking aloud since no one was listening anyway. "Man, if I buzzed them right now, I could give the brothers something to discuss over lunch in the 'Slop Shop.' But the Dean might not consider it proper for his tenured professor to rattle the cafeteria windows and his students' brains . . . it would be a lot of fun, though."

Beep . . . beep . . . beep. He swiveled his head around to see a military helicopter hovering over what had once been the old air school for World War II fighter pilots.

With the town itself slipping beneath the plane's double wings, Jeff headed toward the plantation and its natural grassy airstrip in a meadow behind Winslow Manor. Passing over the water reservoir, he carefully maintained enough altitude to safely cross over the spokes of high tension wires jutting out from the power plant.

Smoothly setting the *Pegasus* down on the hard ground of reality, he pined—

Ah! To be back in the days before the patina covering the sins of our quiet little town in the Bible Belt began to peel away.

Chapter 2

Feeling like a first-day imposter, the newly-licensed psychologist stared at the black rotary phone, waiting for someone to call.

"Hello. Is this the biofeedback place? I seen y'all's ad in the paper that ya treat headaches. And I . . . I mean my grandbaby needs help." The woman sounded desperate.

"Yes, it is. This is Dr. Klein speaking." *Doctor* Klein. Was she really ready to be a professional helper, or was she only masquerading as one in the restored cottage which had served as a servants' quarters for her great-grandparents, and later as a honeymoon cottage for her grandparents, Peter and Hannah Lentz?

"Well ma'am, Freddie's almost eighteen. Already quit school . . . couldn't make it at the academy. And they even paid his way 'cause I wuz cookin' there at the time. Poor lad, he can't keep a job. Smart as a whip ya know, but gets them terrible migraine headaches what knocks him out. Do ya think you might could help him any?"

"I'll be glad to see him. Let me check my appointment book." It wasn't necessary. Everything was still open. "How about three o'clock?"

"Today?"

"Yes, of course."

"Much appreciation, ma'am."

And on that cool brisk autumn afternoon, the clinical interview began: "Tell me about yourself."

"Whacha wanna know?" Wearing cutoffs and a black shirt stamped with a Confederate flag, Fred Crabtree peeped through the long, scraggly, sandy-colored hair draping over his dull green eyes.

"Whatever you want to tell me." Emily noticed scars on both of his arms, making them look as if they'd been grazed with a handsaw.

"Well, I reckon ya could say this ol' dude wuz raised in the pit o' hell by Mr. and Mrs. Satan." He looked down at his dirty sneakers.

Conditioned to be neutral, the therapist acted as if he'd said something like: The sky is blue.

"Are your parents living?"

"Have no clue who my daddy wuz. Never seen my mama." His right leg began to shake like a wind-torn limb on a sycamore tree. "They say she run off with a bunch of hippies when I wuz just a little feller. Grandmaw and Grandpaw, they raised me. Ain't give 'em nothin' but trouble. Least that's what they say, so I guess it's so. They put me in one of them insane asylums a couple times . . . once't overheard my shrink talkin' to my grandmaw. Claimed I wuz makin' up crazy stories. Called me a schizophreniac or somethin' like that. Then they went and put me in the military school acrost town. Grandmaw thought they could straighten me out, but I got kicked out so I reckon I wuz a lot of trouble."

"Why did you get kicked out?"

"Smokin' pot." Now both legs were shaking. "And maybe 'cause this little brat down the hall claimed I bu—claimed I messed with him in the john, but that wuz a lie . . . leastways I don't recall doin' nothin'."

"Where did you go after that?"

"From there to trainin' school. Ain't been out too long."

"Your grandmother mentioned that you have bad headaches?"

"No shit. Said . . . in the paper . . . she told me the paper said somethin' about bio-somethin'. What the hell's that?"

"Biofeedback. Let's go back to another room and I'll show you."

Once in the lab, the street-wise teen checked out his surroundings. "What's all them black boxes for?"

"They give you information about your body." Emily motioned for him to sit in the recliner. "Feedback from the machines helps you know what it feels like to relax. And if it's muscle tension causing your headaches, and if you can learn to consciously relax, to relax when you want to, you may be able to prevent them."

When the psychologist reached for the wires, Fred, looking like a frightened child in a dentist's chair, asked, "Is it gonna hurt?"

"I promise it won't. These are sensors which will record electrical activity on your skin surface and send it to the machine—"

"The box?"

"Yes that's right . . . which will convert it into microvolts and feed it back to you in numbers and beeps or tones."

Fred's body visibly tensed as she cleaned the placement sites on his arm and forehead with alcohol, then attached the electrodes.

Immediately, he lunged from the chair, yanking them off his head. "Keep those goddamn wires away from me!" From a compliant, soft-spoken young man, he had changed into a raving maniac and trampled through the lab, stopping only to beat his fists on the pale blue wall. After settling down a bit, he looked around the room; looked at the therapist and declared in a bold assertive tone, "No one will ever hurt the kid again!"

And then, big husky bearded Fred crawled under the table. He pulled his knees to his chin and crammed a thumb into his mouth.

There it was! Right before her eyes. What, in 1979, was supposedly the rarest of mental disorders. Her very first client had switched from his personification of an out-of-control teenager, to a protective adult, to a terrified child.

"Who are you?" At the time, Emily thought it was the right thing to ask because the person on the floor genuinely looked different from the person who had walked through the front door.

"I'm Stupid," a fragile voice trembled.

"You're not stupid."

"I *am* Stupid. That's my name."

"Okay. How can I help you, Stupid?" If he were playing games, so could she.

"I am *not* stupid." His manner changed to deep and gruff. "Who're you?"

"I'm Dr. Klein. Who're you?"

"Dino. What's it to ya?" Looking up at the bottom of the table, his facial expression changed to bewilderment. "I'm Fred Crabtree. Who do ya think I am?" The crass teenager had come back to himself. "What am I doin' under this damn table?" Not giving the therapist a chance to answer, the client crawled to the middle of the room and stood up, asking, "When we gonna to do the bio-thing?"

"What about next week? That is, if you decide you want to give it a try."

Fred looked surprised. "Next week? I just got here." He glanced at the small clock on the table at the doctor's side. "My gosh! Ya mean I been here that long?"

All alone in her sporty red Probe, Emily sat at the railroad crossing, waiting for a long train to pass. Her thoughts were running with the clack of heavy metal wheels.

In less than an hour the burgeoning professional had forgotten everything she had not learned about multiple personality disorder (MPD) in graduate school. In the seventies, behaviorism, the principle that a person's behavior can be conditioned by systematic rewards and punishments, was the thing. The possibility that a person could have two or more personality states which are capable of taking over one's life was mostly Hollywood stuff. It was 1980 before this condition became an official diagnosis in the *Diagnostic and Statistical Manual of Mental Disorders*.

Dr. Klein's studies had not prepared her for the raw realities of the kinds of wounds a Fred Crabtree had apparently lived through, somehow defending himself without Freud, without Jung, and without all the analysts and behaviorists who were to follow them. Real wounds are never as cut-and-dried as the clinical descriptions created by those who arbitrarily codify diagnoses.

The child-man had been horrified at the sight of boxes and wires. His spontaneous age regression had not been faked to try to please the therapist. And she had not created his alters or ego states or personified defenses or dissociated aspects of himself—whatever one chooses to call those parts who answered to the names: Dino and Stupid.

The caboose wobbled by, the barricade flipped up, and just as Emily stepped on the accelerator, she glanced at the rearview mirror, easily reading backwards the glossy new Chamber of Commerce billboard:

> WELCOME TO CHESTNUT RIDGE
> AMERICA'S BEST KEPT SECRET

Chapter 3

J eff opened the unlocked door.

"Dad, it's me." Excited as a kid just named MVP for his Little League team, he was looking forward to what should turn out to be one of the happiest nights of his life: February 14, 1989.

"Hey, boy," the old man called out. "Come on in if your nose is clean."

Well, it was before I got a whiff of cat pee, the younger man thought.

Stepping into the stale-smelling front room, Jeff flipped off his baseball cap and finger-combed his wavy hair, now much darker than the strawberry-blond of youth. Thankfully, his signature freckles had blended into a year-round tan or were concealed by the neatly trimmed beard he'd first grown in the '60s, not so much to snub a clean-shaven society, more to rankle an authoritarian father: Cleat Klein, founder of *CK Custom Furniture* and town drunk.

Mr. Klein had lived in the brick duplex since coming home from World War II with a medical leave and a Krieghoft 1942 Luber Auto Pistol, supposedly pilfered from the German soldier who'd shot off the little finger on his left hand. He'd garnered a civilian job as gate keeper at the flying school and had stayed on during 1944 and 1945 when the town rented the property to the Federal Government for a German POW camp. A few years later, a group of local investors had bought the property and converted it into a private prep school for boys, a military academy of sorts, hiring Cleat as grounds superintendent. In the late '70s, rather than admit women and Blacks, the school had shut down. As if to look respectably employed, Cleat built a small woodworking shop in his backyard, probably imagining that he would be crafting future heirlooms for the town's elite.

Pickled by a steady diet of alcohol, the septuagenarian's gangly body reminded Jeff of a comic-strip villain. His hair, dyed as black as a roof rat's, was greasily pasted to an elongated head. Unshaven, wearing multicolored-striped boxer shorts and a dingy ribbed undershirt, the old man was sprawled out on a run-down vinyl recliner, chewing on an unlit cigar. His eyes were fixed on a semi-nude couple cavorting across the television screen. Sarge was dozing at his feet.

Jeff pulled the tuxedo out of the bag and hung it on a spoke of the dusty wagon-wheel light fixture in the center of the room.

"Surely ya don't expect me to wear that fuckin' faggot's costume, do ya?"

"Th-That's your decision." Jeff had always tried to treat his dad with the respect he seemed to think he deserved.

"Just kiddin' boy. Maybe it'll attract some horny young broad. By the way, where's your ol' lady?" He pushed the chair into the upright position and slowly stood up. "Wanna drink?"

"Good grief, D-Dad. It's not even nine o'clock yet, and to answer your first question, my lovely wife is seeing clients this morning, as usual."

"For the life of me, I don't understand why ya let her work . . . you've give her all she needs." Cleat staggered over to the bar separating the kitchen from the sitting area and poured a couple shots of bourbon into a plastic cup.

"Emily's a grown person and I've never tried to control her life . . . will you turn that b-blasted TV down a little?"

"No, I will not. The reason I gotta keep it so high is 'cause of the racket those gals make next door playin' that loud music and gigglin' all the time. Should've left the damn thing empty."

Jeff pointed toward the tuxedo. "You'd better go ahead and try that on to make sure it fits in case I need to find another one. B-By the way, did I tell you I'm planning to pass on the story of Acadia tonight?"

"Naw, but I'm tellin' *you*, ya better do it right. Wouldn't want for ya to get history wrong in front of that crowd of ancestor worshipers."

The sarcastic bite cut deep. Jeff still coveted the praise Cleat had never seemed able to give, daring to fantasize that, for once, the father would express pride in what the son was doing for the community. Tonight Jeff would be serving as Master of Ceremonies at the genealogical society's annual charity ball. Proceeds this year were designated for the new heart wing at Campbell Memorial Hospital.

Forty-seven years old and Jeff was still intimidated by his father. He could lecture to a class full of students or a couple hundred people at a professional conference; read scripture lessons at First Lutheran Church; talk to small groups, individuals, anybody else without a glitch; but around his daddy, he stuttered like a kid caught passing a class-mate one of those little Popeye porno books popular with pubescent boys in the '50s.

"Gr-Grandmother and I have a little sa-sa-surprise for tonight."

Snubbing Jeff's comment, Cleat bent over the coffee table and picked up a sweat-stained, frayed-around-the-edges wallet. "I been meanin' to give ya this." He took out a yellowed card engraved with the name of his now defunct business and pushed it into Jeff's palm. "Turn it over," he ordered in the mode of a drill sergeant.

"What is it?"

"Can't ya see? It's a combination . . . goes to my old gun safe in the basement. You-a be needin' it someday, so ya better put it in a secure place."

Jeff pulled out his billfold and stuffed the card behind his driver's license.

"Do ya think ya could ever help me get mine back?" Cleat asked, almost humbly.

"Wh-What?"

"My license." His bloodshot eyes became teary. "I'm tired of ridin' around town on that dad-blame 'likker sickle.'"

"W-We'll see." But Jeff had no intention of abetting a dangerous man on the road. "N-n-now you better try on this suit," he repeated. "That is, if you still want to g-g-go."

"All right . . . all right boy, ya should slow down before ya have a nervous breakdown. I'm gonna go, but before I drape those fancy duds on my dirty body I oughta take a shower." Eyes now clear, Cleat gave his only son one of those don't-you-know-anything looks. He clicked off the TV and went back to the bedroom.

Sarge didn't budge.

Picking at a crack in the armrest, Jeff sat in the recliner trying to stifle the stage fright mobilizing around his diaphragm. Even with fore-thought, he couldn't have planned a better fiasco. Before the charges against Dr. Bill had come out in the paper in January, he'd already asked Margaret Rucker and her gospel choir to provide a short musical pro-gram for the occasion. Making a mental note to put the big announcement before the choir's last number, he gazed across the room at the intricately-carved oak mantelpiece.

On one side of the centered table-clock was a portrait of a stern looking Amanda Jarrett. The public school teacher, having moved down from Charlotte about a year before Jeff's mother died, had rented the adjacent apartment which had always been easily accessible through the shared basement. Jeff suspected that after his mother's death, he'd often been shipped across the river to Grandmother's house while the young widower was 'visiting' his neighbor.

On the other side was a plaque, a community service award given by the YMCA. It was engraved: "To Cleat Klein. In Appreciation for Your Generosity in Helping Children." For years, the man had collected used bicycles to fix up for needy children at Christmas time.

In a small dime-store frame about to fall off the edge of the shelf was a black-and-white photograph of the young Klein family: Mother wearing a tailored two-piece suit and open-toed high-heels, her long wavy hair blowing in the wind; Daddy in a soldier's uniform sitting next to Mother in a wooden swing on the veranda at Winslow Manor; Baby Jeff propped on Daddy's knee.

Perhaps things would have been different if . . .

She was in the bathroom with blood dripping from her wrist.

"Daddy, come here!"

His daddy had come in and wiped her clean. "Son, your mother was very sick. She's gone to heaven now."

Little Jeff couldn't comprehend why a mommy would prefer God to her own son. He looked up at the ceiling but there was no hole. How did she get to heaven? Or had she not really left? Just sleeping, he'd wanted to believe.

This was his first experience with human death. Pets had died or disappeared. Something had happened to his cat, Blinkers. Calves had died while being born and hounds had drowned while running the coons. A horse was shot when it broke a leg. He knew these things; had heard people talking about them. But this was different. She was his mother.

Death is not easy for anyone to grasp, especially a little child. The different ways people react can be confusing. Hired hands were quiet. Strangers would come to view the woman sleeping in that box in Grandmother's parlor. They would look sad and moments later be in the dining room eating from a well-stocked table, laughing, talking in loud boisterous voices. A few women cried. No men cried. What his daddy had told him was true: "We have to be strong. We have to show everyone we can handle things. Big boys . . . we men don't cry."

Men don't cry.

The little boy had wanted to cry then—and many times after that. But he never did. Not around the mighty Cleat Klein.

Jeff never understood why—even with what is called a photographic memory, able to retain almost anything he'd ever read, and having little patience with students who couldn't call up dates and facts for their examinations—he held only one image of his mother alive, one that never allowed him to hear her voice, smell her perfume, or feel her hand holding his. He shut his eyes, bringing her as close as he could.

Dressed in a navy sailor suit, the three-year-old boy covers his ears with both hands trying to muffle the roaring of biplanes flying overhead doing their aerobatics—rolls, loops, dipping low. Mommy sits beside him on the hood of a shiny black 1944 Buick. The beautiful young woman, wearing shorts the color of her fiery-orange hair and a starched white off-the-shoulder blouse, protectively swats flies and mosquitos away from his freckles. A pilot in a jumpsuit with a white satiny scarf around his neck walks by carrying a leather helmet and goggles. The little sailor hops off the car, positions himself at attention in the broiling hot sun and salutes. The man smiles and presents the goggles to his admirer.

Sarge barked.

Jeff opened his eyes to see his daddy prancing through the door like an over-aged model coming down a runway. Rubbing his palms across the ruffled shirt, Cleat asked, "How do I look?" before stopping by the bar to pour himself another drink.

"You look f-fine," Jeff said as Cleat took a big gulp. "B-But that's enough, mister." The son took the cup from the father's hand and set it on the coffee table. "Be ready about six and I'll pick you up."

As Jeff was going out the door, Sarge stood up, stretched, then ambled across the room to lap up the last few drops of *Country Gentleman.*

The light caught him at the intersection, near the point where power lines had gone underground and gas lamps brightened the brick sidewalks. Sitting high in his old pickup truck, wearing comfortably faded jeans and a Wesley College T-shirt, Jeff looked more like a lanky pulpwood worker than a professor and a son of both the Revolution and the Confederacy. Fortunately, as a daily runner his tall lean body, even with its ever-present, long-standing aches and pains, had been conditioned to withstand the burden of heritage.

Ahead was a long block of antique and speciality stores, restaurants, and coffee shops, anchored at one end by the five-story First Bank of Campbell; at the other, by the three-story Acadia Hotel. Façade grants were being used to refurbish the original exteriors of the downtown buildings, one of which, surviving Sherman's rampage through the South, had served as a commissary during the Civil War.

On its surface, the town, laid out on a sandy hill above the curve in the river, had changed its face; however, the monument on the courthouse lawn was a reminder that its roots ran deep with resentment.

One of Jeff's family trees had been grafted back to a William Campbell who had migrated to Virginia in 1640 to escape religious and political struggles in Ireland. William's great-grandson, Josephus Winslow Campbell, had moved to Charleston in 1751 when he was twenty-one to work at a mercantile firm. In 1753, he'd come to this area halfway between the beach and the mountains and homesteaded on land granted to the colonists by King George II. A farmer, businessman, and legislator, Josephus was a catalyst in the development of Chestnut Ridge, a village which he had died protecting during the Revolutionary War. His work and influence had continued all the way down to Jeff's grandfather, Winslow Campbell, a World War I army officer.

After the war, Winslow had married the little lady he called "the prettiest maiden of the ball," linking two of the wealthiest families in the state. His bride, Mary Katherine, was from aristocratic Delacroix ancestors: French Protestants, dissenters not satisfied with Catholicism and the monarchy who had formed an organization which came to be called Huguenots. Because they were bound by a secret oath, they were also known as *Eid Genossen*, or oath fellows. When Louis XIV deprived them of their civil and religious liberties, many, including one of Jeff's forefathers, had left France, reportedly bringing a ghost along with them all the way to North America.

Papa Campbell, known as 'the Colonel' around town, had fit the stereotype of the Scotch-Irish who kept the Ten Commandments and everything else they could get their hands on. He farmed the land, planting cotton and corn, raising horses, cattle, sheep, and hogs. During World War II, with the help of German POW's rented from the local camp, he sold pulpwood and replanted the forests. After his death in the early

'50s, Mrs. Campbell, living in Winslow Manor, the Greek renaissance-style house they'd built when setting up housekeeping in the '20s, continued his ventures—and making money.

How the Campbell and Klein families got connected was a marvel. Cleat Klein—coming from hard-working farmers, common people who'd worked the fertile Carolina soils without the help of slaves and didn't care pea turkey what their German ancestors did or didn't do—had somehow attracted the attention of Katherine, the only Campbell heir.

Why his parents got married was a foregone conclusion. From Jeff's calculations, he was conceived in 1941 shortly after Cleat, a recent high school graduate, had been drafted into military service. Upon coming home from basic training, the soldier had probably found out that his girlfriend was pregnant and, as they used to say, the couple had to get married. There was a hasty wedding by a justice of the peace in another county. The next morning, the young groom was shipped off to Germany.

What a shock that must've been to the mother of the bride. The Klein boy had denied her the pleasure of seeing young Katherine walk down the aisle, as she herself had done, wearing an antebellum wedding gown and the Delacroix family's jeweled headpiece.

Five years later, Mary Katherine's daughter was gone. Although Grandmother Campbell had never come right out and admitted it, Jeff believed that she had always blamed her son-in-law for the untimely death.

Little Jefferson had grown up in two different worlds: with his grandmother on the plantation where everything was safe, where he'd been treated like an heir to the throne; and in town with a man who had often been bitterly cruel to his own flesh and blood.

Almost a half-century later, Mary Katherine Delacroix Campbell was still grieving for her child. Every morning after breakfast, she'd enter Katherine's room—preserved as it was the day the couple had eloped—to meditate; always sitting on the edge of the mahogany four-poster bed that was covered with an elegant spread and canopy, ninety yards of rose-colored imported satin.

To Grandmother Campbell—no question about it—family was the most important thing in the world. If her precious daughter had to die, fortunately there was Jefferson to carry on the bloodline.

A horn blared from behind, nudging Jeff's wandering mind away from history. On the opposite corner in front of the bank, a digital sign, anachronistic in its historical setting, alternated between 72° and 9:15, giving him just enough time to stop by and water the daisy pot.

He turned left on Church Street and drove a few blocks before pulling into the parking lot next to his wife's office building. After grabbing a bottle of water from under the seat, he jiggled the loose handle, got out of the truck, and darted across the busy street toward the graveyard.

Olde Town Cemetery. Ironically, it was one of his favorite places. In their own way, dead men—and women—do tell tales, he believed. And his way of hearing them was through research. Scraping the mosses and lichens from slowly disintegrating monuments and deciphering their faded inscriptions had led him to learn a lot about local history: about Revolutionary War soldiers who'd fought for freedom from England and Confederate generals who'd fought for states' rights; about Negro slaves who couldn't fight for themselves; about doctors, shopkeepers, ministers, lawyers and laymen; and about all the men, women, and children who'd brought this frontier settlement into the ages of industry, technology, and information.

In front of the Campbell monument, Jeff tipped the beak of his cap and stooped to water the flowers at the base of Katherine Campbell Klein's marker. To his surprise, he suddenly remembered a little freckle-faced boy and a pretty young woman down by the river playing the daisy game: *Loves me . . . loves me not . . . loves me.*

A repressed memory, Emily would say. Now he had two of his mother alive.

Usually, Cricket Cassidy gave perms on Tuesday, but today was special. Already ten shampoos and sets; one left to go.

After finishing cosmetology school, the young self-proclaimed hillbilly had moved to the Midlands to take a job in one of those ritzy beauty shops she'd only heard about where she came from in the 'Georgie' mountains. Chestnut Ridge was a good place to live, she thought, with a lot of good people *and* a lot of good tippers.

The last few weeks had been wonderful because her partner had moved to town. The couple were together again, at last. Sure, today she felt like Cinderella not invited to the ball, but was genuinely happy for Danny who'd be covering the event for *The Gazette.*

Hearing the door buzzer, Cricket walked up front to meet her last appointment for the day. Dr. Klein, who'd said she preferred to be called by her first name, didn't act at all like the other rich women in town who were so picky about appearance; those always complaining about the way she styled their hair. The woman was a quiet, private person to whom Cricket had revealed more about herself than she'd ever told anyone. And the psychiatrist—or was it psychologist? she didn't know the difference—had only listened; had not judged at all.

"I feel kinda wild this afternoon," the customer said, handing Cricket a sparkling headpiece. "Could you do something with this?"

"Such as?" Cricket asked, helping Dr. Emily get her head settled in the deep porcelain sink.

"Why don't you surprise me?"

Under brittle limbs of live oaks drooping over the north section of Main Street, the muscular, middle-aged man accelerated to sixty in the thirty-five miles per hour speed zone. Who's gonna stop me? he grinned to himself. The way he always did. The way he'd been grinning at them all since first figuring out how a young man with no pedigree could make it in this town. So what if he'd flunked out of Carolina after the first football season. He'd joined the Air Force before the inevitable draft and served his country in Vietnam. Because he had influence and because of his daddy's friends in high places, he had come back home and made it.

Yep, he was a card-carrying member of the good ol' boy network.

Chief Thomas Paxton parked in the no-parking zone in front of Acadia Hotel. Across the street, that crazy-woman, China Doll, was preaching to a few winos lolling on the corner. On the sidewalk in front of the entrance, J. D. Reid Jr., dressed up in a white polyester '70s-style leisure suit, spit a wad of snuff through the rusty grate. Smiling a toothless grin, he threw up his huge weathered hand at the chief. Paxton, struck by a silly feeling of discomfort, ignored the gesture and picked up a note pad, pretending to write. Nothing needed to be said to that poor retarded boy. And he hoped that J. D. would never want to talk with him either, especially about that long ago night in the woods.

It had been sometime around Halloween because most of the leaves had fallen to the ground. J. D. and that other kid had cowered in the back of a pickup truck, but he had stayed there right in the middle of things.

That night Thomas Paxton became a man.

The other daddy was yelling at his son, "Ya see that? He's not scared of what a man's gotta do." Then looking at Tommy's daddy, the man said in a soft deep voice, "Ya got yourself a real one here, Sheriff."

The face of Paxton, the elder, seemed to glow in the dark. Accepting the compliment. Wallowing in the praise.

And the son of the other daddy must have begun the torturous journey into manhood filled with the assumption that he might never make it; that he was weak and detestable in the eyes of his own daddy; that he was a Nobody while Tommy Paxton was already a Somebody.

He belonged.

A false spring, that's what the Colonel would've called it. Amidst prematurely budding dogwoods, Acadia was lighting up for its final night of glory. Buckled in the back seat of a long two-toned grey and green Cadillac with classic '50s-style fins, Mary Katherine Delacroix Campbell, waiting for Henry Kiser to open the door, smiled at the photographer on the sidewalk. Mr. Kiser had been one of the German POW's the Campbells had rented from the local camp during World War II. After the war, they'd sponsored him to come back to the States, taking him on as a gardener. In recent years, he'd given up physical labor but had stayed on as a chauffeur.

Mrs. Campbell, a tiny woman who often joked that at ninety-five her age had finally caught up with her weight, placed her left hand under Henry's right arm. They walked through the revolving door into the Victorian foyer and up three steps into the lobby. "Thank you very much, Mr. Kiser. You can go now. My grandson's meeting me here."

She sat on a faded red velvet sofa looking around the expansive room. A registration desk and cubbyhole mailboxes on the back wall were reminders of the years when Acadia had offered the only guest rooms in town.

"Good evening, son," she greeted when Jefferson came over. "You look so handsome tonight. Wish your mother were here to see what a fine man you've become."

He kissed her on the forehead.

Patting the cushion at her side, she motioned for him to sit down. "Well sir, I can't see that much has changed since the last renovation. Let me see . . . that was in 1929 just before the stock market crash. My, my . . . those were the days. The 'Roarin' Twenties.' Parties galore, whiskey and gin, dancing the Charleston and more romantic activity than anyone in my generation would've ever cared to admit." Her hands, knotted and twisted with blue veins embossed on finely transparent skin, clasped the broach over her heart. "Have I ever told you before? Your grandfather presented this to me the night he proposed under the arbor of wisteria vines out back."

"A couple times, maybe. I'll bet you were a knockout."

"The Colonel thought so." She closed her eyes, basking in a few more moments of memory, then opened them to look at her watch. "We'd better get along."

Jeff offered his arm, helping her stand. Slowly they walked across the speckled marble floor toward the elevators.

"Let's take the one you have to crank," she smiled.

Her face brightened by cakes of rouge on her cheeks and orange-red lipstick, the grande dame looked at her reflection in the mirrored sliding door of the older elevator. She straightened the skirt of her royal blue satin gown, an outfit which had served well for the last twenty or so charity benefits. "Jefferson, do you suppose the old lady is still wandering around these halls?"

"Strange you should ask, Grandmother. I was just thinking what a treat it'd be if you'd tell her story tonight. There might be a few people here, the newcomers of course, who've never heard it. Would you do it? Please?"

"Oh Honey Child, I'd love to," she answered, fluffing the cottony ball of hair on the back of her head.

———————

The elevator door opened and they stepped into the antiquated contraption where J. D. Reid, Jr. was sitting on the stool next to the controls.

"Up please," Mrs. Campbell gently ordered in a high-pitched creaking voice.

J. D. pushed the outside wooden door closed, then unfolded the metal accordion door and locked it. He flipped off the safety switch and turned the crank to the right.

"How long have you been doing this?" Jeff asked.

"Since I wuz jus' a wittle chap. Use to wide up and down wit' my pappy."

"The elevator stops at the third floor, isn't that right, Mr. Reid?" asked Mrs. Campbell.

"Yes ma'am, it do."

"And you have to take the stairs to get to the attic. Right, Mr. Reid?"

"Yes ma'am, dat's wight."

"Did anyone ever tell you that you look just like your grandpa did?"

"Yes ma'am. Dat's what my mama say."

"He was such a good worker for the Colonel."

Junior, his family called him, was the only son of Nina Belle and literally a part of the Campbell family; in fact, a very distant cousin of Jefferson: one of those tidbits of information no one ever talked about. Nina Belle's grandfather, a slave until freed when he was about twelve, was a bastard son of General Campbell. According to family lore, the slave boy had the reputation of being the plantation owner's 'pet' of which the African-American descendants were quite proud; of which Jeff was deeply ashamed.

J. D., Tommy Paxton, and Jefferson had been together in the woods on that night J. D. had supposedly fallen and hit his head on a rock. It was a long time afterwards before he could say a word. When he began to talk again, his speech was difficult to understand. The principal and teacher at the white-framed school for Negroes in Campbell County had called him a moron, telling Nina Belle it wouldn't do any good to keep him in school because the boy would never be anything but a field hand anyway. By becoming an excellent maintenance man for the city of Chestnut Ridge, Junior had proved them all wrong.

"Why ya always workin' for de honkies?" Jeff had overheard a friend of J. D.'s ask when the old cotton mill shut down and Syn-Tec moved to town in the late '50s to get away from the unions up North. "You be makin' scads more money over at de new plant. And I hear dey're hirin' coloreds."

J. D. had answered, "I don't care for nobody puttin' de white folk down. Dey've always done me wight, even dough some of my own kind make fun 'cause of how I talks and 'cause dey tink I be beholden to de Whites."

The elevator stopped.

"Much obliged, Mr. Reid." Mrs. Campbell squeezed a five-dollar bill into the operator's palm.

J. D. slid the doors open and offered his hand. "Wat chur tep, ma'am."

Emily was on the mezzanine talking with Carol, Matt, and the Weavers. Jeff nodded to their children, then walked over and kissed his wife on the cheek. "I thought you were going to be late," he said.

From somewhere a flashbulb went off. Emily stiffened like a scared raccoon caught in a hunter's spotlight.

"You're gorgeous tonight, my little princess," he whispered in her ear, patting her thick, naturally-frosting hair that was uncharacteristically piled on top of her head. "Thanks for wearing my mother's jewels."

As if embarrassed by her husband's public show of affection, Emily pulled away.

Sue Weaver, who looked like anybody's plump silver-haired grandmother, commented, "The girl's never late for anything, is she Dick?"

"Nope." With a GI crew cut and fat-free body, Dick looked much younger than his wife and his World War II vintage. The Weavers had been Emily's back door neighbors when she was growing up on Main Street.

Dick extended his hand to Jeff. "You're a lucky man, Mr. Klein. And my little bride and I will have to take some of the credit for that. We practically raised her, you know. 'Emma Wee Wentz'—that's how she introduced herself the day we moved into our first little home, when she came bringing a basket of cookies hot out of her mother's oven." Glancing at Emily, he asked, "How old were you then, Honey? It was right after the war."

"I would've been three. Thank heavens I can talk a little plainer now. Mr. Weaver, Mrs. Weaver, I really do appreciate everything you folks did for me," Emily said politely, then addressed Mrs. Campbell: "How are you tonight?"

"Can't complain. Doesn't help a' tall. I just thank the good Lord for letting me be here one more year."

"Where's Granddaddy?" Matt asked. Luckily the boy took after his mother and had never been required to put up with red hair or freckles. He'd be graduating from college in May and was trying to make up his mind which medical school to attend, having been accepted at every one to which he'd applied.

"Out wandering around somewhere," Jeff answered.

"I'm sure he'll come in when it's time to eat," quipped Carol, almost as tall as her father, stunning in a sleek black gown. After graduating from college, she'd passed the CPA exam on the first try. Much to the dismay of Grandmother Gladys, she and Brad Amato, a corporate attorney, were already living together in Atlanta. Surprisingly, Cleat had been delighted with Carol's choice of a partner. At the engagement dinner, the elder Klein had said, "What this family needs is a good law-yer."

"Is Granddaddy sick?" Matt asked, using the family's standard eu-phemism. "Should I go try to find him?"

No one responded.

Looking at Emily, Mrs. Campbell said, "You look stunning tonight. More like Miss Hannah every day."

"Oh Grandmother, you think everybody looks like someone else," Matt joked, apparently forgetting that Granddaddy Cleat might be in distress.

"Wish y'all could've known her. Maybe I've told you before . . . she was my first grade teacher, Miss Hannah . . . I was just a little girl and it was the saddest thing I'd ever seen . . . that fine lady, she never even got to rock the baby . . . that would've been Emily's daddy . . . poor little Jacob growing up without a mother . . . everybody in town came to the funeral. Pardon me, I shouldn't be rambling like this. It's supposed to be a happy occasion."

A photographer came by and broke into the conversation. "Hi, I'm Danny Evans from *The Gazette*. Just got a nice shot of your little group here and was wondering if it'd be all right to use it with tomorrow's story about the gala."

"That'd be fine," Mrs. Campbell answered for everyone. "How about getting a few of me with my great-grandchildren here?"

"Y'all go ahead and take pictures," Jeff said. "I'm gonna go check to make sure everything's ready."

Scattered around the ballroom were a several dozen round tables cov-ered with white linen, each centered with a red rose and surrounded by eight straight-back chairs upholstered with well-worn black leather. Crowding each place setting were carefully folded napkins, too many pieces of silverware, a cup and saucer, both a water and a wine glass, and keeping with tradition, an archaic finger bowl.

On one end of the long food bar, salad and dinner plates mono-grammed with *A*'s were stacked up like old 45 and 78 rpm phonograph records. At the other end was a three-tiered, heart-shaped cake. Gold brocade drapes with dingy sheers hanging over floor-to-ceiling windows on the north side, and artificial palmettos stationed in the corners, made the room feel cold and hard.

Hanging over the fireplace, a Rotary Club banner questioned, "Is it the truth?"

Jeff would've rather been hosting an oyster roast at the beach.

Stomping on the platform to make sure it was sturdy enough to hold fifteen singers, he heard Emily's mother talking. "Let's just stay in here. I don't like watching people drink and make fools of themselves." Apparently the couple had come in through the back entrance. Gladys was saying, "Phil, just look at all these red roses. We'll be lucky if Emily doesn't have one of those sneezing fits."

Her family had not been 'old money,' but by virtue of her position as a preacher's daughter, Gladys had always moved around in the higher circles of Chestnut Ridge society. After her young husband died, she had taken Phil's advice and sold the slaughterhouse business. Profits were invested in the local Food King which had grown into a regional chain of supermarkets. The company's recent acquisition by a Belgian company had made Gladys Keller Lentz 'new money.'

Not at all like her only daughter, looks and material things seemed very important to Gladys. Every tooth in her head was crowned; her nails, always professionally manicured. In public, she wore a reddish-brown wig to cover thinning gray hair and globs of makeup to mask the unstoppable effects of age. In spite of the attention given her body, the woman looked unhealthily thin.

Phil Owens, a man of short-stature and tall ideas, had always been involved in about everything in town. Coming to Chestnut Ridge during World War II, he served as the Army Air Corps coordinator at the flying school. At one of the officers' parties at Acadia, he met Gladys' sister, Luella. After the war, he went back to Ohio State and finished law school, later returning to marry Luella and open a private practice. A major stockholder with Chestnut Mills, the company made him chief legal counsel when it was sold to Syn-Tec. In the '70s, Phil entered politics and served several terms as mayor.

According to Emily, Phil was around to help Gladys when Jake passed away, and Gladys was there to help Phil when Luella was dying of lung cancer. For years, Phil had wanted to get married and move in with his sister-in-law, but recently Gladys had decided to move to the plush Whispering Pines Retirement Center while she could still read the Bible and play bridge.

After speaking briefly with the couple, Jeff went through the swinging doors into the kitchen, right past his daddy who was examining the label on a bottle of champagne, over to the stainless steel counter where the caterers had laid out several time-honored southern dishes. Some had been prepared according to directions in the classic *Charleston Receipts:* She-Crab Soup, Low-Country Oysters with Mushrooms, Fillet of Veal, Hampton Polonaise, and Jeff's favorite, Shrimp Royal.

Behind him a cork popped, releasing the unmistakable spew of a man out of control. Reflexively, Jeff turned around and tried to grab the bottle. The old man held on, putting it to his mouth.

"D-Don't Dad . . . please don't. N-No telling what might happen, mixing it with whiskey—"

"Young man, why don't ya mind ya own business? You just take care of yourself; I'll take care of me. That is if ya ain't too ashamed for me to be sittin' at ya table."

"Let's go, Dad. It's time to eat."

With a somewhat pathetic complicity, Cleat traipsed behind Jeff into the dining area. At one of the front tables, Emily was already seated between Gladys and Mrs. Campbell; Phil beside Gladys; then Sue and Dick, leaving two seats vacant. Cleat chose to sit next to Dick. Jeff sat between his daddy and grandmother. Carol and Matt were at a table with the younger crowd.

When everyone in the large room had settled down, Jeff went to the microphone to deliver a welcome and direct the serving. "We'll have the choir go first, then start with the table back there in the right corner. Everybody . . . help yourselves."

"We shoulda been goin' first," Cleat griped.

It was difficult for Jeff to focus on the mostly banal conversation of those around him. He noticed Emily staring at something and turned to follow her line of vision, just in time to catch Tommy Paxton who was sitting at the next table, boldly winking at his wife.

She turned her head downward, saying. "I feel so conspicuous in this low-cut dress. All this fat hanging out the top."

Jeff wanted to tell her that she *was* conspicuous, making eyes with that s.o.b., but decided on a different approach. In a voice so low no one else could hear, he said, "Let's just call it cleavage. You've heard what the Klein men have always said, 'We like a little meat on our women.'" He put his hand under the table, rubbing it across her thigh. As if it were a stun gun, she brushed it away. Obviously he'd touched a nerve, along with a few of the extra twenty or thirty pounds she'd gained since their wedding day.

When it was their turn to go to the buffet, Cleat was first in line. He stacked his plate with a little bit of everything. Not hungry at all, Jeff chose a handful of shrimp and a few vegetables.

"Phil, what do you think is going to happen to the old slaughterhouse building?" Dick Weaver asked after everyone was back at the table.

"Looks like they'll get that permit to make it a topless bar after all," Cleat answered for Phil. "Hear they plan to name it *The Mona Lisa Bar and Grill.* Such a classy name, don't ya think?"

"The town council should be able to do something to keep it out," Gladys said. "First thing you know, they'll have gambling and prostitution moving right in and making this place a regular Sodom and Gomorrah."

"We can't ban them," added Phil, a member of the zoning board. "The ordinance says you can only keep them from opening within a thousand feet of a church, school, home, or playground."

"Used to be a church across the road but it burned down before my husband died," Gladys said.

Emily responded, "I remember that Mama. I was in the third grade, maybe fourth, and Daddy took me out there to watch it burn." Then speaking softly so only Jeff could hear, "I'm beginning to feel sick . . . thinking about those bloody carcasses hanging from the rafters in the basement . . . I can almost smell them."

Jeff felt a slap on his shoulder. "Well my friend, is this some kind of joke? Having that nigger and those singers here tonight." He turned his head to see Casey Paxton. "When that little black bitch went an' accused our ol' buddy Bill of molestin' her . . . it's a wonder she ain't give him a heart attack, well . . . I'll jus' say times wuz a lot simpler when they knew their places."

One thing about Casey, having ridden in on the Republican landslide and elected county sheriff during the 'racial wars' in the '60s because of his power in the Klan, he made no bones about where he stood; never trying to defend his loathing of the black race. Retiring in the mid '70s, the tall big-boned man had made sure his son was appointed the city's police chief.

"Phil, do you think he'll fight it?" Casey asked.

"If he wants my opinion, I'd advise him to cop a plea as well as quietly surrender his license. With that woman being an attorney and all, she wouldn't have made the charges if there wasn't a case."

"But honest, ya gotta admit, those people sure can sing." Cleat probably considered the remark complimentary.

"The colored have come a long way," Mrs. Campbell added. "Why, before they got their civil rights, the darkies were considered to be like children and in a class of their own. I can remember when right there on the society page of the town paper, they had their own place under the section, 'Negro News and Activities.'"

"Well, they sure did know how to cook." Characteristically, Gladys was trying to smooth things over. "I just don't know how I'd have managed without my Lossie Mae. That woman always put in a whole day's work for a day's pay. Don't get me wrong, we were good to our colored help, weren't we?" She looked to her daughter for the expected automatic agreement.

Emily ignored her.

"Have y'all seen the moon yet?" Casey pulled up a chair and sat down. "It'd shore be a good night to go huntin', what with a cold front movin' in and all."

"We always enjoyed goin' coon huntin', didn't we son?" Cleat paused long enough to burp. "Excuse me . . . for the four-legged kind, of course . . . durin' the time of the full moon . . . sometimes the sky wuz so bright we didn't even have to use a flashlight."

"D-dad, can't you say anything w-without using epithets?"

"What's an epithet?"

"F-forget it."

Casey took over the story. "Yep, six or eight of us would hike into the back country and build a campfire. Sometimes start a stew a-cookin' in that big ol' black cauldron we carried out there. We'd turn the hounds loose, pass around a jug of rotgut an' listen for those long bayin' sounds to change to sharp barks, then we'd know they'd done treed 'em a coon. Well, we'd all jump up like we wuz on fire an' take off to find them dogs. It wuz a hoot. Us big boys playin' hide-and-seek with them dogs . . . plowin' through bushes and briars, jumpin' over dead trees. No tellin' how far the run might go . . . till we found that poor critter high up on some tree limb. An' watchin' them dogs go to circlin' and barkin' and leapin' way up . . . scarin' the ya know what outta the ol' coon."

"Did you shoot it?" Emily asked. "I certainly hope you put it out of its misery."

"Nah. Didn't wanna kill it," Casey answered. "Only wanted to see it squirm. We'd jus' laugh, call the dogs off an' let it loose so we could chase it another time. The chase was the fun of it, don't ya see?"

"I have vague memories of some of that. What did you guys do with us kids when we went along?" Jeff didn't really care who answered.

"Sometimes ya ran with us." It was Cleat talking as if he were sober enough to know what he was saying. "But mostly, we'd leave ya by the fire playin' around or if ya wuz already sleepin', we'd take ya back to the truck. Next mornin' we'd all go home, sometimes limpin', always worn out and red-eyed. Plum covered with chiggers and mosquito bites. Those were some good times and—"

"My daddy used to take me coon hunting," Emily interrupted rather timidly. "That's actually one of my only preschool memories."

"We took ya with us a bunch, Mizriz Klein," Cleat smirked. "Donchu 'member our families campin' and goin' on trips with each other?"

"Not at all."

"Me either," Jeff said. "No wonder we don't recall much about it. Must've scared us senseless: the dark night, animals howling."

"Your daddy was a hell of a character, *Mizriz* Klein," Casey also smirked. "Shore could hold his liquor. You can bet all of us shore appreciated havin' him around. Providin' a little one-stop slaughterin' . . . from field-to-freezer . . . no hassles."

The other men at the table laughed.

"You fellows are talking nonsense. My Jake rarely took a drink." It was Gladys defending her long-dead husband.

Scanning the room, noting that about everyone had finished eating, Jeff stood up, pushing his chair under the table. He walked up to the podium and after making several recognitions, reported that more than $100,000 had been raised for the new heart wing. Next he introduced the entertainment for the evening: "Tonight we are pleased to have with us Ms. Margaret Rucker and the Happy Hollow—or as my friend J. D. Reid and some of the other singers affectionately call it, the 'Happy Holler'—Gospel Choir. Ms. Rucker, better known to many of us as Maggie, is a native of Campbell County. Currently she's Director of Legal Services which most of you know is a nonprofit agency that serves the poor. With all her accomplishments, she's made quite a name for herself in our community—"

"Well that's the God's truth," mumbled someone in the audience.

Jeff cleared his throat and continued, "As a leader in the professional and business communities, Ms. Rucker is on the City School Board and active in the Chamber of Commerce. In addition to serving as music director at her church, she organized the gospel chorus . . . Ms. Rucker."

After a few seconds of cordial applause, the choir members, dressed in white suits overlaid with colorful kente sashes signifying African-American pride, arranged themselves on the platform. Their director rolled her motorized scooter down front, poised to take the mostly Caucasian audience to a place of pure soul.

Before long, all the diners including unabashed racists, Cleat Klein and Casey Paxton, were clapping their hands on the offbeat, tapping their toes and rocking back and forth to the tunes of Negro spirituals, many of which had been passed down from slaves who'd worked the cotton fields of Campbell County.

When the choir had finished singing "He's Got the Whole World in His Hands," Jeff addressed the audience again. "Before the final number and before I turn the program over to the disk jockey who'll be playing music for all ages: big band, beach music, and," he looked toward the table where Carol and Matt were sitting, "whatever it is you young folks do, I've asked my dear grandmother, Mary Katherine Delacroix Campbell, to introduce a very famous lady in this town. For those who've heard the story, I ask your indulgence; for those who haven't, please enjoy."

———————

Her back hunched over, the oldest woman in the room slowly walked to the podium. Jeff helped her onto a footstool, allowing the audience to see all of her shining face. Smiling at the photographer, Mrs. Campbell began. "As you folks know, about every old house around here has a resident ghost and Acadia, which has been in my family since before the Civil War, is no exception. My mother told me this story handed down from her grandmother.

"It goes like this: In southern France in the early 1500s, there was a Jeanette Delacroix born to strict Catholic parents. As a teenager, she told her father about being in love with a young Huguenot. Now he was most upset because his daughter was going to marry a Protestant, so he sent her away to a convent in Germany. Soon afterwards, Jeanette became sick with the cholera. Now in case you don't know what that is, it's a really bad case of diarrhea.

"Well sir, she got feverish and went out of her head, putting a curse on her father and all his descendants. They say though, that just before dying she repented for hexing her family and I'm sure the good Lord forgave her.

"After Jeanette's death, her mother died of a broken heart and her father, who was surely grieving for his precious baby girl, stabbed himself in the heart. On his deathbed, he told his two sons that the spirit of Jeanette had come and ordered him to kill himself and that he was just doing what she'd told him to do.

"Well sir, several years later, the brothers converted over to being Protestants and moved to Paris. And on the night before the big Huguenot Massacre in 1572, I think it was, they say the spirit of Jeanette, dressed in a gray nun's habit showed up.

"Next morning, one of her brothers was killed and the other got away by wearing a monk's clothes that the ghost had left. So this brother disappeared and from then on we don't know anything at all about the Delacroix family until the early 1800s when a gentleman named Louis was exiled from Acadia—that was a French settlement in Canada—and found his way to Charleston.

"Down here he became successful in the rice, indigo, and cotton trades and built a house on this very spot and named it Acadia. Some people around here believe the ghost tagged along after them. A couple folks saw her just before Sherman came through and with just about everything else around here burned the big house to the ground. They say the lady ghost was seen out a few times right before other bad things in the family like murders and suicides happened.

"Well sir, the house was rebuilt and the family got into the castor oil business where they made a fortune off a couple hundred acres of the castor oil plant. 'One hundred and fifty gallons from each acre,' so my grandmother told me, 'and it was every bit effective in cleaning out your innards as the imported medicine.' I always wondered if the ghost . . . remember now, I told you she had bowel trouble . . . had anything to do with them getting into that business . . . maybe not though, because I'm not sure if ghosts can have diarrhea."

Laughter rippled through the hall, giving the speaker time to pause and take a sip of water. "Maybe y'all don't believe in ghosts. I sure do." She set the glass down. "And it's part of the story I've never told anyone . . . but the night before my beautiful daughter Katherine died back in 1946—"

She set her glass on the podium, inadvertently pushing the microphone off its stand making it likely no one else except those at the front tables could hear the rest of the secret. Staring at her son-in-law, as if her eyes were the tips of red-hot pokers ready to puncture the bubble of booze which had prevented him from accepting any responsibility for her daughter's unhappiness, the old woman announced with conviction: "I saw . . . I saw some kind of apparition in my bedroom. A long time later, it dawned on me that it must have been her . . . the Gray Nun."

Afraid the woman was going to fall, Jeff went to the podium and helped his grandmother to her seat. He stepped back in front of the audience. "Well folks, to make a long story short, the hotel was deserted during Reconstruction. It's been said that when the carpetbaggers came down here trying to tell people how to run their businesses or take them over, the ghost showed up and ran them clear out of town. Legend has it, they were having a party in this very ballroom one evening when the Gray Nun came wafting through the window and one of the revelers had a heart attack and died on the spot and—"

"Serves him right."

Casting Cleat a harsh look, Jeff went on talking.

"In the 1880s, about the time the Chestnut trees were getting wiped out by the blight, the reigning Delacroix added two more stories and developed the homeplace as a hotel for wealthy Northerners who turned our town's southern hospitality, golf courses, and stables into a winter playground."

"Right on boy. This time the damn Yankees had to pay their way."

Restraining himself from rushing over to his old man and stuffing a napkin down his throat, Jeff, skipping about fifty years of Acadia's history, continued. "When the Depression came along, it was closed down for a while because of financial difficulties. During World War II, the government leased it to use as an officers' quarters for the flying school."

There was a commotion at the family table. Jeff looked down to see that Cleat's head had fallen smack-dab into the middle of a plate of Hampton Polonaise. It was all he could do to stay composed as Phil and Dick, wiping the citron and frosting off the drunken man's flushed face, stood him up and hustled him through the swinging doors to the kitchen.

Trying to disguise his anger, embarrassment, whatever it is when one's father makes an ass of himself in public, Jeff hurriedly finished the speech. "As many of you know, when the interstate highway was completed and all the new motels were built around the interchange, none of the visitors to town wanted to stay here anymore so our suites became useless. Because my grandmother believes this is such a waste, tonight she's donating this property to the county for use as a home for our less fortunate citizens."

On cue, the chairperson of the County Commission came forward to accept the deed, after which the choir began to sing their final number.

Not even thinking to say anything to his wife, the humiliated son slipped out of the room. He found his dead-drunk daddy on his knees under the wisteria arbor. When the heaving stopped and Cleat was too weak to open his big acerbic mouth, Jeff pulled him to his feet and dragged him through the alley to the truck.

Drifting through the open windows of the banquet hall, J. D.'s clear tenor voice was calling out a melodic statement from the Negro spiritual, *'Tis the Old Ship of Zion*:

> It will take you home to Glory . . .

And the choir responded:

> Ain't no danger, danger, danger,
> Danger in de water.
> Ain't no danger in de water.
> Git on bo-o-o-ard, git on board.

The woman is not me, Emily was thinking; looking at, but not really seeing her partner. Shuffling around the hardwood floor, mindlessly following his rendition of the shag, a classic Carolina beach dance, an existential question reverberated in her mind like an echo in an unexplored cave.

Who am I?

Proud mother of Carol and Matt. For sure.

Devoted wife of Jeff. Right this minute, not sure. Lately she'd stayed angry at him a lot. Mostly because of the way he kowtowed to his daddy. Cleat was a 33rd degree hypocrite. Always oozing with respect for women and children, moms and flags, and apple pie. But behind that mask, he was rougher than a sawmill plank. Oh, how she despised— no, hated—her father-in-law and really couldn't understand the intensity of those feelings. The lush had never done anything to deliberately hurt her. Not that she remembered.

Who am I?

A therapist. It was her calling. Rewarding. But there were some constraints. Being a therapist in a small community limits participation in community activities; otherwise, you'd run the risk of becoming involved in dual relationships. Being a therapist anywhere affects relationships. Your kids don't want you to 'play' psychologist with them; your spouse doesn't want you to get overly involved with clients; your mother wonders why you're working with all those 'crazy' people.

In reality, the therapist/client relationship is mostly time-limited to the session hour. Don't get too close. Detach. Be neutral. And whatever happens, don't let them know what you believe about God and the Devil, heaven and hell, ghosts, spirits, and all those other unscientific things that can't be proved in a laboratory.

Who am I?

Somebody's old girlfriend. Was the man across from her also remembering the junior-senior prom? Together in this very room, slow dancing to "In the Still of the Night," he'd asked her to go steady. She: a measly sophomore. He: the best-looking guy in the senior class, captain of the football team, no less. The only boy in the party crowd she'd ever dated wanted plain-looking Emily Lentz to be his girl. Afterwards, they'd driven out to the reservoir 'to park' meaning, in those days, to 'make-out.' He'd rolled back the top of his snazzy '57 black and white Ford Fairlane convertible suggesting they climb into the backseat 'to get a better view of the full moon' meaning, in those days, to 'pet.'

Cuddling up, he had asked, "Are you a virgin?"

"Of course, I am. Are you?"

"I'll show you," he said, cramming her down on the seat, clawing till he found the zipper of her strapless baby-blue, net-over-taffeta gown. The hoop supporting several layers of crushy-crinoline lopped over her face. Next thing Emily knew, she was pushing him away demanding, "Take me home."

Turning the ignition key, revving the motor, he dug out of the gravel parking lot leaving a trail of gray dust to settle in the town's deep clear water supply.

Tommy Paxton never called again, making their going-steady time about three hours long.

The virginity part was a lie. Her brother got that in 1949. Emily was seven years old. At the time, she'd believed, had to believe, all kids did those things. In the seventh grade, she'd figured out what it was all about from reading a rudimentary facts-of-life book.

Who am I?

Somebody's sister. Jimmy is five years older than Emily and nobody knows if he's dead or living on the streets somewhere. According to their mother, "He was a perfect son before the government messed him up. Served his country, but what does he have to show for it?"

Her brother had always been unusually quiet about his experiences in Vietnam. Drinking heavily one night, he'd described to Emily how he and five comrades had fallen into a deep pit and gotten skewered with poison bamboo sticks. After admitting to himself that he felt guilty because he was the only one who'd survived, he broke down, howling like a wolf in beastly pain.

Leaving college after his GI benefits ran out, Jimmy had taken off to only God knows where. Last time she'd heard from him was in eighty-two or three. Sounding happy, her brother had called to say he was in a VA hospital in Arizona. "Sis, the government's given it a name: post-traumatic stress disorder or PTSD. Now I can get the benefits I deserve and get well. Hope to see you and Mama soon."

Once Emily had tried to explain PTSD to her mother. "It's the same thing the World War II vets called battle fatigue or shell shock. Symptoms are similar to those of my clients who withstood trauma as children: nightmares and flashbacks of horrible things that happened, afraid all the time, insomnia, not being able to control emotional reactions. I believe Jimmy has tried to drown the bad memories with alcohol and that he'll have to face them before he can get well."

"Who should know better than my daughter, the doctor?" Gladys had asked. "That's your job, isn't it? To help people who aren't quite right. Well, there's one thing I know for certain: it's not my fault he turned out like he did. Why, when you and Jimbo were little, everybody called you the best behaved children in church," she defended, then preached, "If he could just 'get right with God' again, everything else would take care of itself."

Who am I?

Daughter of Jacob and Gladys Keller Lentz.

Anyone in town would tell you that Mrs. Lentz is a fine Christian woman who cooks delicious nutritious meals, takes food and flowers to shut-ins, and gives to the church and various charities. Her house is a showpiece filled with antiques and plants she's nurtured for years. A yard full of azaleas, rhododendron, and two huge magnolia trees have always shielded her from what was going on up and down busy Main Street.

Emily's mother had taught her the social graces, things such as putting on a dinner: how you'd go to the kitchen and bring out all the dishes of food on a serving cart and one at a time pass them around the table, a throwback to the days when servants waited on the master and his family. When you had company, you were counted on to bring out the sterling silver, the dinner china and fine crystal. Already, she'd passed on the linen Madeira tablecloth and napkins inherited from her own mother.

From a long line of Lutheran preachers, Gladys, trained in classical piano and organ, had served as organist at First Lutheran Church for fifty-some years. She'd also taught Emily about God and Jesus and the Devil and heaven and hell; had made her memorize dozens, maybe hundreds of Bible verses; had taught her to play hymns on the piano; and, each year come December, had taken her to practice for the Nativity play at church.

Interestingly, Emily didn't actually remember having been in a single play. Seems as though she'd always been sick around Christmas time.

Emily had only a few memories of her father. He taught her to play poker when she was in the fourth grade; sometimes called her 'Twisty Tail.' And he drowned on June 4, 1955, her thirteenth birthday. Those were in the days when Ronald Reagan was starring in western movies; during the Cold War era when everyone was afraid Communism would take over the world.

The music stopped.

"Thanks for the dance, Miss Emily." Tom pulled her close. "Let's get together soon. We can talk about old times."

One side of Emily felt the butterflies of a teenager who'd just been asked for a date by the most popular boy in school. Another side felt too close to his firm muscular physique and sinfully guilty for fantasying about doing unspeakable things with her husband's nemesis. A midlife crisis? Not a good excuse. But at this point in life, it was stimulating to think that a man other than Jeff might find her attractive.

Chief Tom Paxton led Emily back to her seat, then wandered off to find another partner.

Sometime after midnight, Danny Evans and Cricket Cassidy were cuddling under the covers in the tiny bedroom of the duplex they'd rented two weeks earlier.

"I felt invisible much of the night," Danny said. "For the most part, no one seemed to notice me or the camera. Except maybe the wife of Mr. Klein, the Master of Ceremonies. When she'd see me coming, she'd duck behind her husband like I was trying to get a shot of her in the nude or something. Don't know why she was so skittish. The woman looked exquisite. Must've been wearing a couple thousand dollars worth of diamonds in her hair."

"Sounds like you're talkin' about Dr. Emily Klein, one of my customers. In fact, I styled her hair this afternoon, diamonds and all. Till today, I never seen her wear any jewelry at all 'cept a gold weddin' band."

"So she's a doctor. Maybe that's why she didn't seem to fit in at all with that gaggle of society gals sashaying across the floor."

"She knows about us," Cricket said sheepishly.

"What?"

"She won't tell anyone."

"Well she better not. I don't want to lose another job because—"

"Oh Danny, it's too bad we can't come out—"

"But sweetie, from what I saw tonight, we should fit in just fine in this little Bible-thumpin' town. As long as we mind our own business, I'm sure we'll be ignored."

"How can ya mind your own business if you're a reporter?"

"You know what I mean—our personal business. Tonight I had this gut feeling that I was meandering around in a stable of hypocrisy; that this town itself is some kind of stage and a lot of those people on the top tier are playing like—"

"Dr. Klein's anything but phony."

"You're probably right. Her husband appears to be a good guy too, but I feel sorry for the way he has to put up with his old man who, I learned tonight, just happens to be our dearly beloved landlord."

"No joke?"

Danny spent several minutes recapping the evening's events and they laughed for a long time at the image of Cleat Klein with his head facedown in a plate of Hampton Polonaise. "I don't think anybody suspects anything about me. I know the police chief doesn't. After shagging with Dr. Klein, he came over to the bar and asked me to dance."

"He danced with Dr. Klein?"

"At an affair like that, I'm sure everybody dances with everybody."

"Did ya do it? Did you dance with a man?"

"Come on, you're not getting jealous, are you my little Cricket?" Danny teasingly caressed her lover's tiny breasts.

"Turn out the light," Cricket said softly.

———

In the dark hours of the morning, Jeff looked out over Lentz Mill Pond — a lake really: fifty acres, fifty-five when it rained a lot. Yes, the previous night should have been one of the happiest of his life. But it had been a fiasco and not only because he had invited Maggie Rucker's group to sing. He felt terrible for having left Emily in the ballroom sitting on her hands while he took care of his old man.

Dear Em. He'd loved her all his life, it seemed, as though long ago they'd melded at their souls. He couldn't help but ponder how pitifully empty and lonely life would be without his wife. He admired her independence, her ability to bounce away from adversity. Why, if the Devil himself ever knocked on their door, she'd probably tell the joker where to go.

They'd played in the same sandbox, so he was told; were sweethearts in first grade; best friends through elementary school. He'd always believed cute little Emily Lentz with the sparkling brown eyes would be his princess and they'd marry and live happily ever after. That is until high school when she started dating Mr. Paxton. The jealousy when Emily no longer had time to do things with him because of forever running around with that dumb jock was awful. Luckily, the Paxton-Lentz fling hadn't lasted very long. By their senior year, Jeff and Emily were a couple.

Not the cheerleader type, when friends were teasing their hair, curling their eyelashes, and experimenting with cigarettes and alcohol, Emily was playing competitive tennis and lifeguarding at the public pool. Probably as a reaction to the mother's always-present-yourself-in-your-best-light-in-public mentality, the daughter eschewed heavy makeup, coiffured hair, and holes in her earlobes. To this day, Emily's hair was in the same pageboy style worn since she was thirteen and declared: "No more prissy curls."

As sophomores in college, they'd decided to get married. When first told of their wedding plans, Cleat had admonished, "You're making the biggest mistake of your life," immediately before breaking down and weeping like a man just sentenced to die. Emily's mother, slightly more supportive, had warned, "If you make a hard bed you have to lie in it."

Mostly, they'd enjoyed that bed.

So what if they hung out on different poles of life's spectrum. At the ice-cream shop he usually chose vanilla; she, chocolate. On a day-to-day basis, he was neat and orderly; she, rather messy at times. He went to bed early; she stayed up late. He turned the thermostat down; she turned it up. He was compulsive; she, obsessive. When making decisions, he mostly relied on feelings. Trained as a scientist, she tended to intellectualize, usually making decisions based on cold hard facts—but not always.

Strange as it was, after he'd completed a Ph.D. in religious history at Duke and had taken a position at the local Wesley College, a small predominately black liberal arts school established a few years after the Civil War to educate Negroes for the Methodist ministry, Emily had been drawn back to the deserted farm inherited from her father. Grandmother Campbell had wanted them on the plantation; however, the young couple had agreed that the red clay hills with hardwoods in the western part of the county were much prettier than the flat fields and pines on the Campbell land further east.

They'd torn down the dilapidated homeplace where Emily's grandmother, Hannah, had grown up, building in its stead a modest two-story eclectic-style house, "a cross between a mountain lodge and a beach cottage," they jokingly called it. With dark cedar shakes on the outside, the inside was bright and airy. A setting perfect for bringing up Carol and Matt. Safe. Secluded. Not pretentious. Unless you considered the massive sunroom and lap pool. Em was the swimmer in the family. A mile a day was her rule, whether in the pool or lake. 'Legally dissociating,' she called it. A way to lose herself, he thought.

When Matt entered school, Emily gave up bridge, most of her volunteer work, and enrolled as a doctoral candidate at Carolina. Following a postdoc internship at the VA hospital in Columbia, she'd established a private practice which was quite successful, although he feared that her continued overinvolvement with her very first client, who he deduced was a sociopath beyond rehabilitation, was going to wreck their marriage.

Jeff turned and looked toward the house where Emily was sleeping peacefully, he hoped. For some reason, he thought of a story Nina Belle had passed along, a story handed down by her grandmother: A few years before the big war, she'd said, several slave families picnicking around the pond had decided to take a cruise on a flatboat. When it struck a snag, twenty or twenty-five panic-stricken passengers jumped overboard and drowned.

As the sky began to brighten, his thoughts began to rustle with the noise of wildlife all around: doves mourning; carp splashing in the shallows; night birds twittering in the thickets; and the resident owl calling out questions from the top of a centuries-old chestnut oak whose gnarled roots were desperately clinging to the edge of the bank.

Chapter 4

As if trying to rip his head off, Fred Crabtree was pulling viciously at his long pigtail. "This clamorin' in my head . . . it's comin' . . . can't stop it . . . they're doin' somethin' . . . but don't feel nothin'. I'm . . . I'm helpless."

"I'm here with you," Emily supported. "It's 1989, almost spring. And you're safe in my office now. Do you want to go on?"

Through his hypnotic state, the young man nodded, aware of both time realities at once. "I'm tied down . . . on a box . . . a cold box . . . there's a fence around . . . all rusted . . . I'm holdin' my knees together . . . they pry them open . . . a masked man hits me between my legs . . . they take a black stick . . . no, it's a candle . . . the torch is near my head . . . so scared . . . singed . . . my hair stinks . . . scorched hair . . . hot wax . . . drippin' on my face. They roll me over . . . push somethin' in. . . . oh no . . . it hurts . . . back over . . . black box . . . wire . . . here it comes . . . no . . . don't." His body was convulsing all over.

"Fred." Feeling a throbbing pain between her own buttocks, Emily stood up and crossed the room. "Fred, it's over now." She touched his shoulder. "Time to come back . . . Fred."

He put his left hand on his crotch and went limp. The voice plunged a full octave: "His terror is as cold as the stone they laid him on." Then returned to its feminine range. "I faint . . . when I come to, I hear chantin' . . . risin' louder . . . and faster . . . louder and faster, and —"

"What are they saying?" the therapist interrupted quietly to renew Fred's subliminal awareness and connectedness to the present.

"Don't know . . . I just don't know . . . they cut me loose . . . hold me up as an offerin' . . . a sacrifice . . . let me down . . . my insides are shakin'." With his right hand, he covered his eyes. "Bright lights all around. Whirrin' . . . I hear whirrin'. Somebody sez, 'One more time.' Have to get it right . . . touch me with the wire . . . awful . . . awful. Can't scream. Can't cry."

He was shaking all over again and the voice went back down. "The child is as hot as smoldering embers, yet shivering with chills."

Taking his hand away from his face and opening his eyes, Fred spoke for himself. "Clappin'. I heard clappin'. They were clappin' for me." Glancing down at his left hand, apparently embarrassed or ashamed, he quickly drew it up and placed it over his wide-open mouth. "They were takin' pictures. Bloody pictures. The goddamn cock-suckin' fuckers! Dirty pictures of the shit they were doin' to me. And if I didn't get it right, they'd pour the juice to my pecker. Make me do it again."

"It's over Fred. They can't ever hurt you again."

"The hell they can't!"

Intent on helping him in the moment, Emily let the comment slip by. "Take some really deep breaths. Begin to relax." The words sounded shallow, reflecting a numbing shock at being a once-removed witness to the torture. If what her client had just abreacted, had relived emotionally, represented a real event, it was more than just child abuse. No wonder he'd been frightened at the sight of the biofeedback wires on that day a decade earlier when he'd first come to her office.

Still fidgeting, Fred stood up and fled to the waiting room. Standing at the window, he pointed toward the cemetery. "Over there. It happened over there. A voice in my head says it was some type of ancestor worship ritual, but I don't know. Have you ever heard of anything like that?"

"It could've been. In some of the primitive cultures, they do perform sadistic rituals trying to gain power from ancestor spirits."

"But do they film it? . . . And do they electrocute you? Oh Dr. Klein. I gotta finish the memory. I gotta go back. Over there. I know exactly where they laid me."

"Do you want me to go with you?"

"Oh yes, please."

As if this were a normal therapy happening, which it wasn't, Emily followed Fred across Church Street through the gates of Olde Towne Cemetery to the plot of a Rheinhart family. Standing in horrified fixation, she watched as he shambled through the dry leaves which carpeted the sandy soil; as he circled a primitive unfinished concrete box covering one of the graves; as he suddenly spit out words in singular staccato—

"Amen. Forever. Glory. The. And. Power. The. And. Kingdom. The. Is. Thine. For—"

He appeared to have no realization at all that he was reciting "The Lord's Prayer" backwards. Halfway through, she'd recognized it.

Like a marionette with strings controlling its limbs, he lay on the symbolic altar and rolled over on his stomach. Writhing and grunting, Fred finally dropped into submission, becoming still, as if he'd drifted to another plane of existence.

After two or three minutes, he leaned forward, lifting both arms toward the sky. Screams of molten rage, like lava spewing from a volcano, erupted from a deep cavity somewhere inside the receptacle he presented to the world.

Not sure what to do or say, Emily stood by his side till the flow had ceased.

From the opening day of her career, Emily had suffered the ironic disadvantage of having a person with multiple personality disorder be the first client to walk through the clinic door. Fred, on the other hand, had suffered the equal disadvantage of having been her first client.

"I feel diabolically opposed," he'd casually remarked one day during his first year in therapy.

"What do you mean?"

"Hell, if I know." He looked puzzled. "It just came out."

The malapropism began to take on significant meaning as later, Fred recalled things done to him by what appeared to be an organized group of pedophiles that used satanic trappings in their pseudo-religious rituals. Her client had called it a satanic cult.

With Fred's florid switching from one behavioral or mental state to another—which few professionals had dealt with or knew anything about at the time—it had been easy for Emily to get hooked into his private belief system that the alters, those fractured bits of his psyche, were distinct persons. Sessions routinely ran overtime because he would re-enact what could have been a memory, or switch to another persona at the end of the therapy hour, and Emily would never have allowed him to leave the office in a hysterical or regressed state.

Several parts were capable of taking full control of his behavior while some didn't know about the others, so isolated had they been from conscious awareness. One described himself as a male prostitute. That part—clearly imbued with his own version of ethics—had never revealed, even in the confidential therapy setting (or reportedly to the host personality, the one who had most control of the body) who his consorts were. Amazingly, Fred had acted appalled when another of his alters first described his having been ravished at the hands of his tormentors as deliriously enjoyable.

Emily had walked with Fred into and out of his past; had listened to the separated cries of a childhood in which experiences—of some kind, surely—had ultimately accumulated to such an unbearably confusing degree, that consciousness could no longer integrate experience with meaning and so had to put experience away. It was as though his memories—too revealing to wear—had been stored in a mental closet until it was safe to bring them out, see and hear them, touch, taste, and feel them, embrace them, and move on to something else. Such an operation may have effectively disallowed what should have been the normal integrative psychological process, simplistically referred to as "growing up."

She'd heard cries of the inner children who had been so damaged they'd never been allowed to grow up; had sat with the host as he described other mental constructs: censors, guardians, protectors, self-therapists, self-mutilators, perpetrators, programmers, gay men and lesbians, demons, mythical gods, angels, psychics—and even animals.

"Animals. Fred, why do you think you created animal alters?" she'd asked.

"The purpose of animals is to reject humanity," he'd answered, devoid of emotion.

Why did the young man have such a dire need to reject humanity?

The answer was simple: because humanity had rejected him; had treated him as a mere object of pleasure and possession.

Once Fred had appeared to change from his human-self to a so-called robot speaking in a slow monotone. "I'm spinning . . . splitting. The code is 6-13-8-15-42. Awaken core . . . unlock core . . . initialize . . . flood." In a rapid-paced staccato, he named-off a string of images: "bell, chanting, dagger, babies, grave, box, cage, coffin, pit, snakes, blood, robes, bats, candles, cats, knives, hearts." The voice returned to the empty monotone, instructing, "Distribute . . . self-destruct . . . reconfigure core for now."

"Why did you come?" she asked the robot-man.

"Because of impending system shutdown," he replied concisely: a businesslike answer to a businesslike question.

"How can I help you?"

"Reprogram me to have feelings." Again so direct: an objective statement. Simple.

Not knowing how to respond to it—the statement, the speaker, the unfathomable request itself—Emily stalled for time, asking, "What else?"

"Delete the screams of the children." A poignant but, for the therapist's part, an unfulfillable request.

Fred lived in confusion, never knowing where he might find himself. "It's like I'm livin' in a time-share condo," he'd once commented. Often, even in what looked like a physical adulthood, he escaped to fantasy worlds created when the real world was intolerable. Some of the inner worlds he described as fixed and horrible; others, beautiful and changeable. The latter, Emily perceived as hope. Hope that Fred Crabtree could one day function as a normal human being. Find peace. Reclaim his soul, his identity as a human being.

As a therapist, an interesting thing happened. Through interacting with Fred's alters, Emily had become aware of different aspects of her own self, of the different roles she played in the life of the real world which Fred, self-protectively, had sought to escape.

The mother part had been unavoidably charmed by the child personalities. Once Freddie who believed he was seven had convinced the 'big lady' to watch the Christmas parade with him. Because it would pass in front of the office window, there didn't seem to be a problem. The problem came later when he'd ask her to drive him up to Jim and Tammy Faye Bakker's Heritage Village to look at the seasonal lights and displays. The request was refused and Fred, acting like a spoiled kid, pouted himself into a full-blown temper tantrum.

It had taken the therapist years to learn that even though treating child alters like they were real children sometimes makes a client feel better for a while, in therapy, the 'littles' are most helpful to the whole self in working through the trauma, not reliving a childhood the person missed.

A therapist is a teacher.

Emily tried to learn everything possible about MPD in order to teach Fred to cope with life. None of the articles that had slowly begun to filter out through the literature in the early eighties addressed the severity of Fred's alleged maltreatment, or the complexity of his defenses. Her methods of treatment and teaching were—of necessity—mostly instinctive, not data-based.

The client had also been a teacher, introducing his student to an unmistakable phenomenon of deliberately inflicted trauma and to some of the brainwashing techniques used by its executors. Emily hadn't wanted to believe that the separated psychological evidence—the pain, terror, and rage presented by Fred's dissociated states—was actually rooted in something; she'd wanted to believe that everything he said was a product of his exceptionally creative imagination.

Yet, as a human being as well as a therapist, an interesting thing happened. In trying to face the clear inferences of what Fred's extreme dissociation had attempted to hold at bay, Emily was forced to realize that any initial revulsion or immediate tendency to disbelieve was grounded on the fact that for her, all ritual was associated with the deep sense of goodness of a happy childhood and strong church-upbringing. All religious ceremony, supporting the liturgical practices of her Lutheran church worship, was associated with her concept of God. Undeniably there were other concepts, other religious rites supporting the cult-beliefs and worship-rituals of a theology in exact opposition to good: a glorification of evil.

One evening, hysterical because he believed two men in a black Mercedes had been following him all day, Fred had showed up at the Kleins' house. Emily was out of town, so Jeff, seeing Fred's distress and being a gracious host, invited him in. Perhaps because Jeff was such a good empathic listener, Fred dumped his life's story into their family room.

It was a gift, what he did, freeing Emily—so she rationalized—to openly discuss the case with Jeff, to share the impact this unfortunate man was having on her at a personal level.

Over the years, the family had put up with many of Fred's calls during dinner, in the middle of the night, and even when they were trying to relax at the beach cottage. Jeff had always listened as his wife poured out details of crimes which defied understanding, offering comfort, especially as she grappled with the 'god thing.'

Why? Why, if there's a God, does he or she let little children suffer? Sometimes her husband had tried to explain things from a historical viewpoint. And that helped. It really did.

Fred had wanted his therapist to be a friend. One of the counselors at the training school had been, in fact, both friend and lover, she later found out. Her client never completely understood the difference between therapist and friend. Perhaps she should've refused the small gifts he brought, but she hadn't wanted to hurt his feelings.

With the extra sessions, Fred's insurance benefits had quickly run out. And with what Emily later realized was the grandiose notion that no one else could help him, instead of referring her client back to the mental health center where he'd been misdiagnosed, she continued to treat him without charge.

As with some people who've been severely damaged, Fred, because of his prolonged suffering, had developed a sense of entitlement and had come to believe society owed him recompense, including free treatment and pity. He often blamed others for his faults and had never learned to take any responsibility for his own behavior in the here-and-now of life.

Taking on the social worker's role, Emily had once helped him get a job with a local construction company. The man worked one day and quit. He couldn't stand the weather. "Too hot," he whined. Later, she'd persuaded a local charity to provide funds for his prescriptions and medical bills. Upon learning that he'd received the insurance refund and had used it to go to the beach for a big weekend, Emily was extremely disappointed—but whether in him or herself, she rather refused to ask at the time.

When Fred was arrested for writing bad checks, Emily was subpoenaed to court for the non-jury trial. His court-appointed attorney wanted to show that because the man suffered from MPD, he wasn't responsible for his actions. The judge qualified Dr. Klein as an expert witness, even after she'd tried to explain that her relation to the defendant was as a therapist.

She certainly didn't feel like an expert and wondered if she were really helping Fred by telling the judge that the accused didn't know what he was doing when he wrote the checks. Also there was that nagging question: Had Fred really coveted what he bought with the bad checks and, consciously or unconsciously, sent a sociopathic alter to commit the crime?

Fred wasn't called to the stand which was probably just as well. Emily noticed he'd reverted to a child's demeanor when he saw the judge enter and, wearing a long judicial black robe, come to roost above the courtroom.

"Klein. Are you related to Cleat Klein?" the judge had inappropriately asked the witness. "We were together in basic training, he and I."

"Mr. Klein is my father-in-law," she answered, wondering what that had to do with the achieving of justice or the accused.

"How's ol' Cleat getting along?" he asked. "Haven't seen him in a long time. You be sure an tell him I said howdy, won't ya?"

Treating multiple personality virtually as a joke, the judge didn't seem to understand or make any attempt to understand the therapist's explanation of Fred's behavior as she had observed it for several years.

On the stand for more than an hour, Emily used the opportunity to educate the district attorney and a few courtroom observers about the relationship between childhood trauma and dissociative defenses.

The judge didn't believe an alter had written the checks. Finding Fred guilty, he reluctantly accorded MPD as a mitigating circumstance and gave the defendant a suspended sentence.

During the court appearance, Emily had realized that Fred couldn't get better until he took full responsibility for his actions. Leaving the building with him, she'd admonished, "If you get arrested again for anything, I won't be your advocate. You're accountable for your own behavior . . . and the behavior of your parts."

This therapist—who early on had been emotionally seduced by a desperate adult personality who wanted only understanding and rescue; by child personalities longing for a nurturing mother-figure; and by worldly personalities needing something resembling normal friendship—couldn't meet Fred's insatiable needs. She'd learned the hard way that an enmeshed, overinvolved therapist does not empower clients. Her new goal was to guide Fred toward becoming a more integrated person so that he could better manage his life. He had to decide to accept or reject the offer. Taking steps to gain control of the therapy venture, Emily established limits on the number and length of sessions and telephone calls.

Making superficial cuts on his wrists, Fred balked. Lashing out at the therapist, he yelled, "You don't care about me! You're like all the other shrinks!"

And like a child, he continued to test the limits. Three months after the court appearance, a policeman called. "I have a man named Fred Crabtree in custody. Picked him up for drug possession. He's crying like a baby and wants you to come down here."

Emily didn't go.

Fred dropped out of therapy for a while but in late 1988 had come back saying that he was remembering the names of a few people who had messed with him and was ready to work through 'some things.'

Chapter 5

Ilt is one thing to sit with an adult who is telling a story of having been assaulted, shamed, and humiliated in the distant past; quite another to sit with a five-year-old child whose wounds are still raw, who you just know is likely to be severely harmed again as soon as you let her out of your sight, and there's nothing you can do about it.

"She does peculiar things in class," the kindergarten teacher said when Emily had gone to the school to evaluate Kelley Reynolds the previous Friday. "A few days ago, she announced in class that a bunch of people had come to her house and put a bomb in her tummy. The other kids laughed because they didn't believe her. They know she lies all the time and sometimes they're really afraid of her. She's big for her age and I've seen her push them around. They get scared when she has seizures and I have to say, I do too."

"What does she do?" Emily asked.

"Acts crazy. Her eyes cross. Starts wringing her hands and sometimes falls to the floor crawling around like a baby. . . . and uh . . . I forgot to tell you, she has a crooked arm. The medical report said a broken bone wasn't set, but nobody seems to know when she broke it."

"Is she on any medication?"

"Not that I know of. There's a note in her file from a neurologist who said he'd terminated treatment because Kelley's mother wouldn't follow his recommendations. Ms. Reynolds seems mentally slow. Records show that she was only sixteen when Kelley was born. Technically, Social Services has custody, but they're letting the child live with her mother, trying to teach the young woman better parenting skills, they claim. And there's one more thing: sometimes the child's so sweet and docile and then, just like flicking a switch, she starts beating on anything she can find."

Rocking back and forth in her chair, quietly talking to herself, Kelley was easy to spot. The teacher called the child to the door, introducing her to the woman who would be 'playing some games.'

On the way to the testing room, the sad-eyed, poorly dressed little girl with stringy blond hair and dirty fingernails bitten to the quick, reached for Emily's hand. "What's your name?" she asked.

"Doctor . . . just call me Dr. K."

In an attempt to gain good rapport, the psychologist asked Kelley to draw a picture of a person. The output was a crude sketch of a woman with three heads, each having big lips and dangling earrings. About where the stomach should've been, Kelley, tightly gripping the crayon, furiously scribbled a red glob. "That's a baby," she explained spontaneously. Next she drew a dozen other figures, all unrecognizable as humans, placing them around the woman.

"Tell me about your picture."

Not appearing to understand the request, Kelley responded, "Guess what Dr. K, I have a boyfriend named Cow. And guess what," she grinned, "he takes me out on dates, real dates. Guess what, last night he picked me up and took me to a dance."

"You're such a little girl to be going to a dance. Did your mother go with you?"

"No, but Cow gave her some money to buy something pretty for us."

"Where was the dance?"

Her eyes darting around the room like those of a secret service agent protecting the President, Kelley whispered, "I not 'posed to tell. But it was in that place where dead people live. That's what Cow said. But he said dead people don't bite." She wadded up the paper and pushed it across the table. "They do what you can't say."

This can't be.

Although Emily never routinely recorded testing sessions, she took the mini-recorder from her briefcase and showed it to the little girl. "Is it okay if I make a tape of what you say?" Therapists are so often accused of asking leading questions in assessing the likelihood of abuse, and this examiner wanted an unassailable record of the interview. Either the child had a very vivid imagination or was about to disclose that she'd been a victim of crime.

"Can I listen to it?"

"Sure, sometime."

Kelley stood up, walked over to the chalkboard, and drew a round head, topping it off with a cone-shaped hat. Next to that, she drew a stick-figure lying flat on its back. "That's me. I had on a party dress," she explained.

"What color was it?"

But Emily had known before she asked.

"White. White as snow. She was pretty. Making love. Jamie was her name. And Cow took a bunch of pictures of her because he said she was his pitty pie."

Evidently, little Kelley had mentally created Jamie to do—or endure—what she herself couldn't do and remain aware at the same time.

After the session, Emily met with the teacher to show her Kelley's picture. "Something's bothering this child and we need to know what it is. I'd like to do a more comprehensive evaluation. Since it might take several meetings before she'll feel safe enough to open up, if she will at all, would you ask the social worker to bring her to my office where it'd be more comfortable for both of us?"

"Sure, I'll give her a call."

The next day Emily received a fax from the protective services supervisor, authorizing five additional hours of evaluation time and requesting that the sessions be videotaped. Very concerned about the child's safety, Emily asked to see Kelley the following week, everyday for an hour at a time.

Near the end of the first session in Emily's office, Kelley went to the toy box. She picked out a heart, a snake, a doctor and nurse, a policeman, pigs and goats, and a sword. There wasn't time to play, but the disturbed child had obviously seen the tools for telling.

In the second and third sessions, the little girl seemed to become comfortable using toys to depict horrors that defied verbal expression, acting out scenes that would require an X-rating if they were shown in movie theaters. Observing the child's play allowed the psychologist to witness dissociated aspects as they were still being cultured in the seemingly unprotected environment in which little Kelley was being forced to live. Apparently, monitoring by a caseworker had not been sufficient to assure that Kelley was not being exploited by a group of pedophiles.

In the last authorized session, the child carefully laid a tiny baby doll on a rectangular wooden block, undressed it, then slowly and deliberately searched through the toy box until she found a plastic sword.

Kelley held the weapon, which was a little larger than the doll, over her head, and—

Oh no! Oh no! Don't! Emily screamed without making a sound.

As Kelley pretended to stab the doll in the heart, Emily's professional ability to detach vanished for the moment.

Could it be that at some time in her brief life, Kelley had been forced to murder a baby? Or at least had been made to believe she had done so? For a child, it wouldn't have made any difference if it had actually happened, or if the suggestion had been implanted in her mind. The horrible guilt of believing that she had been a perpetrator herself could possibly tie her to a destructive cult for the rest of her life.

When the van driver from Social Services came to get Kelley, Emily spoke privately with him. "I believe this child's in imminent danger and should remain in protective custody at all times. Please don't take her home to her mother who is undoubtedly not competent to care for her."

"Ma'am. You'll have to take that up with the department. I'm paid to do my job and I've come to take the little girl home."

"But you can't—"

Ignoring Emily's request, the driver went to the playroom where Kelley was drawing on the dry-erase board. "C'mon sweetie. It's time to go."

"Bye, bye, Dr. K," Kelley waved as she was led away, "I love you."

After canceling the remaining appointments for the day, Emily put the videocassette in her briefcase and sped over to the Department of Social Services to speak with the protective services supervisor. "It's my gut feeling that Ms. Reynolds has offered her daughter up to some type of organized crime group, possibly child pornographers, where she's routinely being sexually assaulted—"

"Do you have any evidence?"

"The first time I saw her she claimed a man took her out on a date— in a cemetery of all places—and claimed he made her do things 'what you can't talk about.' And in today's session, she played like she was stabbing a baby."

"Get serious, Dr. Klein. 'Played like' does not constitute evidence."

"Well, if you have a video recorder, I can show you what she did."

The supervisor called his secretary into his office to set up the tape.

Watching the video, at the point when Kelley brought the knife down, the man actually laughed. "Surely you don't believe in such garbage, do you?" He shut it off. "The kid's nuts. I've met her mother. She's a kid herself and crazy, too."

"But where do you think she would've seen something like that?"

"Could've seen it on TV . . . or some porno flick . . . wouldn't put it past her mother and the lowlifes she hangs out with to have them around. And anyway, if Kelley is this easily able—and willing—to 'tell and draw,' would the people she's talking about even be letting her come to school at all?"

"Perhaps they're certain she's too scared to tell." Emily didn't believe it would do any good to attempt to explain the concept of dissociation as she defined it—the defense of mentally and/or emotionally separating from a traumatic event as it is occurring, and blocking the memory of that event from conscious awareness—to this insensitive bureaucrat. "What I'm asking you now, though, is to keep her safe."

"With all due respect, Dr. Klein, we're doing everything we can. Like trying to help the mother learn better parenting skills. It'll take a lot more than a videotape of her playing with dolls for us to go after parental rights."

Doesn't the child deserve to grow up without the cloak of murder hanging in one of her closets? Emily refrained from asking. Rather, she questioned, "Is there anything else I can do?"

"Not unless you want to file a complaint with the police department," replied the man who had been charged with protecting children.

Incomprehensible!

"How could anyone murder babies?" Sitting at the rolltop desk organizing her notes on Kelley Reynolds, Emily called to Jeff who was in his study grading mid-semester exams.

"Been going on since time began," he called back.

This was an unlikely exchange between middle-aged married folks on a Saturday afternoon, four days before they'd be leaving for Germany to run down the Klein ancestors, as her husband had punned.

Jeff ambled into the family room and over to the walnut shelves. He picked out a small book from the section on alternative scriptures. "Have you ever heard of the book, *Enoch*? It's part of the pseudepigrapha."

"The pseudo-what? Sounds like a disease."

"They're ancient writings named after well-known Biblical figures, but probably not written by them." He put one foot on the bay window seat, continuing to speak as if he were lecturing in front of a class. "Since Enoch was called a wise man, he was probably a scribe and a priest. In his day, wise men also knew about magic and astrology. It was usually part-and-parcel of what was meant by the word wisdom. Supposedly, Enoch walked with God and didn't die and—"

"I believe anybody can walk with God in his or her own way." Emily looked past Jeff toward the ancient chestnut oak down by the lake that was budding with the promise of spring. "And I doubt if it matters whether you're dead or alive when you get to heaven."

He laughed politely, then continued with the lecture. "In fact, this book may be where a lot of the mythology associated with witchcraft comes from. *Enoch* gives a different way to look at the origin of evil than the myth in *Genesis* which talks about original sin. Enoch's, as theologians refer to it, is a different myth entirely, detailing horrible things that can happen when people use scientific knowledge and power without moral restraint . . . and there's another thing you might be interested in: Some of the ideas and behaviors are similar to the things that survivors of satanic ritual abuse describe. Listen." He read chapters six through eight, a narrative about the fall of angels and the corruption of mankind.

"Okay professor, exactly what does that mean?" Emily grinned.

"Okay doc," he grinned back, "I'll try to paraphrase in today's language: A long time ago when the earth first got populated, there was a revolt in heaven. Some two hundred angels led by a guy named Semihazah looked down from heaven at the beautiful voluptuous daughters of men. Like a gang of teenagers with a vendetta, they'd rebelled against the authority of their father and asked their leader to take them to this place called earth where they could get all the sex they wanted, where they didn't have to abide by the home rules—"

"Not unlike a lot of the kids whose parents drag them to see me."

"Exactly. 'So,' the leader said, 'okay. I'll go. I'll take you there. But I'm afraid you'll all cop out and leave me standing with my pants down. And I'll be stuck there and have to take the consequences.' And they said, 'No. That could never happen. Let's all swear on an oath and bind ourselves by mutual imprecations or curses to do what we've set out to do.'"

"Interesting," Emily said. "A sort of prototype oath for all the secret societies to come."

"Ah, but there's more. So they land on this high mountain at the top of the known, populated part of earth, and they all swear the oath, but to this day no one knows exactly what the oath was. They call the place Mt. Hermon, which means 'forbidden place.'"

He interrupted the story to answer the question in her eyes: "Em, I doubt our ancestors knew where the name came from. As I was about to say, they set out to become gods, to gain power and control over the creation before them. According to this translation, they literally raped women and fathered children who were considered demons. Later, so the story goes, those children turned against their parents and devoured mankind. You see, in heaven before the angels fell, they had been given the gift of divine wisdom, the knowledge of heavenly secrets. That wasn't so bad in itself but they used it for evil purposes to oppress human beings, especially women. For their own gratification, they took advantage of the power it brought."

"So what were the secrets?"

"Several, including how to make and use weapons, which obviously had never been used by man for anything but damage and murder. Also, how to use medicine and astrology to control other people. They taught sorcery and witchcraft and exorcism; showed women how to decorate their eyelids and use makeup and jewelry to make themselves more seductive; taught them charms and enchantments, the cutting of roots, and how to tell fortunes. Listen to this from the seventh chapter: 'And they began to sin against birds, and beasts, and reptiles, and fish, and to devour one another's flesh, and drink the blood.'"

Emily took a big gulp of air.

"There's more. Over in chapter 69, it talks about the task of one of the fallen angels: 'This is he who showed the children of all men all the wicked smitings of spirits and demons, and the smitings of the embryo in the womb—'"

"Incredible."

"I'm not through yet." He finished the verse: "'—that it may pass away, and [the smitings of the soul] the bites of the serpent.'"

"Good grief, Jeff. In the parables of Enoch, the Satanists could have found a pattern to justify their behavior."

"But there's another side if you read the whole book."

"What's that?"

"It's the apocalyptic belief that good will triumph over the forces of evil; the message of hope that God's going to make things right in the end."

"Sometimes I wonder about that," Emily said, stuffing her notes about the little girl who had been forced to do things 'what you can't say' back into her briefcase.

"I knew you'd call." The voice was smooth, seductive, confident.

Without having made a conscious decision to dial the phone, Emily heard herself talking to Tom Paxton. "There's something I want to discuss with you. Could we get together?"

"Your time, your place," he answered without hesitation.

Imagining her recent dance partner sitting behind his desk, she felt her heart speed up. "What about today? I could be at your office by three."

"Terrific dahlin. See ya after while."

Thirty minutes after making the call, she was sitting beside the police chief on the sofa in his private office in the new Justice Center, wishing she'd taken the time to put on a little makeup.

"Sure was fun the other night at Acadia." He placed his hand heavily on her thigh. "Us out there shaggin' like a couple o' beach bums. Brought back a lot of memories, wouldn't ya say?"

Faintly aware of some long ago feeling, not yet ready to take it away—the hand or the feeling—she just smiled.

"My dear Dr. Lentz—I meant Klein—I'm probably the reason you became a shrink. Do you reckon you could tell me what's goin' on in my head?"

"I don't want to know." She lifted the huge hand and placed it back on his lap.

"Let me try again." He licked his upper lip. "Emily, dahlin, I've been under a lot of stress lately. Do you think you might could help me any?"

"I'll be happy to refer you to one of my colleagues." Feigning naivete, the psychologist got on with business, telling him all about little Kelley, even the way she'd acted out a child sacrifice. When finished with the case history, Emily asked, "What kind of investigation do you guys do when you find evidence of satanic activity?"

"Satanic? Surely you don't think the devil-worshipers got to her."

"You sound like you believe they're around here."

"No doubt about it. We're always havin' to clean up their messes and just hope the paper doesn't find out. If they did, it'd scare all the holy-rollers around here off their pews. Sorry bunch of kids, they are.

Mostly seem to hit the country churches, especially that old Lutheran one at the edge of town. Matter of fact, just a couple days ago we got a call from one of the neighbors—as you probably know, they don't hold regular services out there any more—sayin' somebody had turned over a whole row of tombstones."

"Mt. Hermon? Do you have any idea who did it?"

"Nah, but we pretty much know some of the wild kids around here who're dabblin' in that bullshit. Pardon my French."

"How's that?"

"Lots of times you can tell by the clothes they wear, their tattoos and stuff."

"But Tom, I can't agree with you there. Some of my son's friends have tattoos. And I'm sure they're not dabblers."

"To finish answerin' your question, sometimes we go to the public library to see who's checked out books on black magic, witchcraft, and Dungeons and Dragons and other stuff like that."

"Gosh, am I on your list? I bet I've checked out every book in the library related to Satanism and demonology; ordering more on interlibrary loans. Doesn't make me a Satanist, though. And the types of criminals a few of my clients have talked about would never leave any signs of having been there because important people, even some community leaders, appear to be involved."

"And just how do ya know that?"

"Because I've been working on and off with a man for ten years and Fred—" Emily put her hand over her mouth, realizing she'd almost breached confidentiality. Thank heavens, she hadn't said his last name. "I meant to say a man I'll call Fred."

"Don't worry. Down at the station, we all know Fred Crabtree. He's been tellin' everybody around town who'll listen that a satanic cult used him in makin' porno flicks when he was a kid. And it's common knowledge in the locker room out at the country club that he services the closet queers around these parts. But nobody I know believes much of anything he says. Everybody down here at the station knows he's a mental case, and . . . we do see him goin' in and out of your office a lot."

"You've been staking out my office?"

"Not really. We were just keeping an eye on that boy."

Afraid to say any more about her client, she changed the subject. "What about the little girl? Can I file a complaint?"

"Do you have any idea what cemetery she was talking about? Or when she was there, if she was, or who all was involved?"

"Unfortunately, no. She's too young to realize where she was taken or when, exactly. The only name she ever mentioned was Cow."

"Cow? Never heard that name before? Tell you what, let me make a few calls first and then we can ride out to the old Lutheran cemetery to see if there's any signs out there of what she was tellin' you about."

In her heart, Emily could hear something foreboding about the offer, but her body was saying *go, go, go.* Or was it her mind talking? And she *did* need to find out if there was anything to link the place with Kelley. Amazed at how easy it was to rationalize the propriety of going out to a deserted cemetery with the town's number one lawman, she accepted his offer.

They pulled into the grassy parking area. Quickly, Tom got out of the police car and went around to open her door.

Walking past the little brick church, he put his right arm around his old girlfriend's shoulders. In a little more than a blink, she ducked her head, scooting out in front of him. "Did you just hear a train whistle?"

"Hell no. We're a long way from any tracks."

"But Tom, don't you remember when we were kids and came to their big Vacation Bible School out here, we used to sneak off down there to throw rocks at train cars as they went by?"

"Sorry dahlin. I have no idea what you're talkin' about."

They stepped over the low rock wall bounding the cemetery and walked down to a section of old graves where several narrow granite monuments had been turned over, scattered like toy blocks a frustrated child had pushed aside. Someone had scratched a crude swastika on one, probably with a jagged rock; on another, a pentagram with "NIVLAC orders" was scrawled in red paint.

Reversing the letters in her mind, Emily asked nonchalantly, "Wonder who Calvin is?"

"Calvin who? What the devil are you talkin' about?"

"Look." She pointed to each letter from right to left, "C-A-L-V-I-N. "Cow-vin. Oh no! Kelley Reynolds said the boyfriend's name was Cow . . . Calvin." She stomped her foot on the tombstone. "Well Mr. Police Chief, here's your proof."

"It's not proof of a damn thing, dahlin. Not unless we can find some blood out here somewhere . . . or some baby's body."

"What's that over there?" Emily pointed toward a brittle, broken down chinaberry tree spread out like an oversized umbrella. Under it, four poles held a slab of marble about a yard square. Stepping closer, she saw where several fieldstones had been neatly arranged in a circle. "It's some kind of al—"

Without warning, he grabbed her from behind, forcing her hands to her sides. "Who're you kiddin', dahlin? This trip's not about the little girl." He was breathing hard. "It's about you and me and some unfinished business . . . we both know that."

"Don't—" She tried to pull away.

"Just stay calm." He swirled her around, clamping his lips on hers, cramming his tongue into her mouth.

She grunted her rejection.

He pulled back. "Come on dahlin. You let me do it once. Why not now?"

Squiggling her head out from under his big hairy arm, she asked, "What in the world are you talking about?"

"So-o, my little-miss-perfect. Forgotten about that night at the reservoir, have you? It's awful easy to forget what you don't want to remember, ain't it?"

Suddenly, Emily came back to herself, realized the dangerous position she'd let herself get into, and for the first time clearly remembered their last date.

They'd gone all the way.

He'd raped her all the way *before* she'd pushed him off.

"Nobody's a virgin but once, Tom."

"Well, it wasn't me."

Was he telling her that what she'd just remembered didn't happen? Or had he, himself, simply chosen denial?

"Wish it would've been—but wasn't." He turned around and headed back toward the car mumbling barely loud enough for Emily to hear, "I never did figure what you saw in ol' Jefferson anyway."

Chapter 6

The morning after.

Skies were gray with a forecast for afternoon thundershowers. Emily had come to the office to check the mail, get caught up on insurance claims, return a few phone calls, water the plants, complete the report of Kelley Reynold's evaluation . . . to do everything that had to be done before leaving for Germany.

Unlocking the office door, the psychologist suddenly realized that her life could have been ruined in five minutes at Mt. Hermon Cemetery, and even entertained the thought that she might have unconsciously led the man on.

To heck with Tom Paxton! May she never have to face that bastard again.

Sitting at the computer twenty minutes later, she heard someone coming through the front door.

"Hey Dr. Klein It's me. Got a few minutes?"

"Fred, I'm really busy—"

"I have to talk to ya. It's very important. Can't wait."

"Okay, come on back then."

So much for your ability to set limits, Emily scolded herself as they both got situated: Emily in the recliner; Fred on the couch. Today'll be a good time to confront him about the suicide threat, she thought. "About that call—"

"Sorry, Doctor. Don't know what came over me. Ya know me, I'm too skeerd to die. What I come here to tell ya today is that I wuz layin' on the bed last night . . . couldn't get to sleep and somethin' very important came back to me and made me think what happened a long time ago might be what made me want to take the knife and stab myself, and I feel like I gotta tell ya what it wuz . . . I 'member seein'—"

"Hold it a minute. Would you mind if I record what you have to say? I don't have much time right now and we may need to come back to it later."

"Whatever. Ya know I've always trusted ya to do what's best with what I tell ya."

The therapist stepped across the hall to her office. She came back with a recorder, placed it on the floor, and pushed 'record.'

Fred began to speak: "I saw one man's face . . . .."

When he finished with what he'd come to say, he reached down and pressed 'off.' Looking directly into the eyes of his therapist he said, "And that's what happened Dr. K. That's the God's truth. I ain't makin' it up."

"I believe you," Emily validated. *That's not very neutral*, her professional conscience said.

For ten or fifteen minutes, they discussed what the recovered memory meant to the client. No way could Emily tell Fred, or anybody, what it meant to her.

The therapist could tell nobody nothing.

Alone at home, Emily went to Matt's room to get his old boombox. She took it into the family room and sat on the floor in front of the fireplace with her legs crossed over each other. Inserting the tape, she had the eerie feeling that she was being watched — and she was. Looking up at the picture on the rolltop desk, she saw the eternal eyes of young Hannah Lentz looking down.

For the second time, she listened to Fred's robotic voice telling her what she never would have chosen to hear:

I saw one man's face — one time. Usually they wuz covered with masks or hoods. My grandpaw wuz an important man, but he wuzn't the leader. The leader wuz a short fat man. The man who coached me wuz very tall. They called him Casey. His job wuz to teach one of me to learn to cut.

As part of my practice time, Mr. Casey would ask me to perform for him. He expected me to do these technical-like exercises but I wuz never good enough. I could never please him. I'd always pick up the knife careful-like and move it as clean as I could across the flesh, but sometimes I slipped and made a tag somewhere. He taught me to make scars of identification, to do what they call 'pattern tissue.' Now this required cuttin' and shavin' through different layers of skin.

One time I done a piece and thought it wuz perfect, the best I'd ever did. The leader looked at it, winked at me, and walked over to the next student. But then, Mr. Casey came over and looked at the job and looked at me with such a mean look in his eye, I wuz afraid he wuz gonna stab me with my own knife. Instead, he grabbed my jaw and squeezed the shit out of my mouth. I wuz only ten or eleven and didn't understand what I done wrong.

Once't I asked Grandpaw why Mr. Casey hated kids, and he said it wuz 'cause he wuz disappointed in his own boy—for some reason. The last thing I ever recall Mr. Casey tellin' me wuz, if I ever ran when I wuz supposed to perform or if I ever told anybody what my job wuz, he said there would be the devil to pay and the payment would be my life—me. And he said to me if I ever 'member what they done to me, I'll have to kill myself. And that I oughta keep the knife with me always in case I had to die.

Emily knew only one person named Casey and he was a very tall man.

There was no way Tom Paxton would ever believe Fred Crabtree's words about his daddy.

She took the cassette out of the boombox and labeled it: "Crabtree: March 7, 1989." Planning to put it in her office safe when she got back from Germany, she pushed the tape into the back corner under a pile of unreconciled bank statements and rolled the top closed.

Outside, rain was pouring down. A bolt of lightning grounded near the chestnut oak, threatening its tenuous balance on the shoreline.

Startled by an almost simultaneous thunderclap, Emily began to feel as if she were below decks in a small yacht, whirling inside a tornado out over the dark ocean, unable to step outside to see what was happening.

Chapter 7

"**S**o what goes on during the lost time?"

"Huh?" Jeff looked up from his book. "What did you say?"

"Oh, nothing." Waiting for takeoff, Emily had typed a note into her new laptop computer:

> Flying from here to Frankfurt, you lose time. Example: Trip takes about 12 hours. A whole plane load of passengers leaves on March 8 at 3:00 p.m. 12 hours of flying time later, it's 3:00 a.m. in the States, but 9:00 a.m. in Germany. They lose a whole night?

The plane began its ascent. She closed the computer and reached over to touch Jeff's arm, smiling at him as if they were the only two people in this space and for the moment nothing else counted. "What are you reading now?" she asked.

"It's an old German book which gives accounts of parochial visitations in the Rhineland."

"Gotta be a best seller. Who visited whom?"

"Church officials. As early as the sixth century, they'd go into local parishes and do a job evaluation of the preacher and inspect the buildings and discipline errant members and preachers. Genealogists believe the parish registers form a connection to the passengers' lists of those coming to America in the 1700s. If we can find the old church and a record of Johanne Kleinreich . . . just think, Em . . . I could set foot on the very land my ancestors actually walked on; the trip of a lifetime . . . like finding myself at last."

He began to read aloud, translating and paraphrasing as he went: "In some of the minutes, the pastor was openly condemning the younger generation because they didn't follow the Lenten tradition of asking forgiveness for their sins. Instead of being solemn and introspective, they were eating, drinking, and making merry—and Jane and Lucy and all the rest of the young maidens—"

To let him know she was listening, she chuckled at the old joke.

Grinning, he continued, "There were also rumors of black magic being used to cure diseases, tell fortunes, and call up spirits by making gestures and muttering cabalistic words—"

Emily put her right hand in front of her face, studying the scars on the palm and fingertips. "Something like that went on when I was little. Supposedly, my daddy took me to an old man down in Black Bottom, you know the one I'm talking about—Mr. Wilbur Lee . . .Wilbur Lee Jackson—when my hand got burned. I think they called it 'using' to get rid of the fire. I still don't know for sure how it happened. Mama said I was about ten months old, just walking a few steps, and I fell against the coal stove, but I've always had the feeling I was pushed—maybe by Jimmy. Seems like I do remember her rocking me in our big rocker. They say you can't remember things that early, so I don't know if it's true or not."

"How could you know one way or another?" Jeff asked. Without waiting for her answer, he moved on. "Traces of occultism have lingered in our culture. Farmers around home still plant by the signs . . . probably handed down by our German ancestors just like the folklore brought over from Africa. One time I went with J. D. Reid to see Mr. Jackson who counted the warts on his hands, chanted some mumbo jumbo—"

"Did they go away?" Emily asked.

"He said they did."

"I don't have trouble believing that. In my opinion, what Wilbur Lee did was a type of hypnosis. I suppose he got J. D. in a relaxed state and used the power of suggestion to—"

"Think I'll relax a little myself." Jeff leaned back into his own space, closed the old book and carefully placed it in his briefcase. Fiddling with the headset, he finally got it turned on and tuned into the classical music channel.

The flight attendant was making her way down the aisle, passing out small pillows and asking who wanted a blanket, while trying not to unduly disturb those watching the movie screen and listening through their headphones. A good bit of sign language and smiling was going on.

Part of her job, Emily thought, as they both accepted pillows and the young woman said she'd be right back with a blanket. "What does one do on a twelve-hour transoceanic flight if you can't dissociate?" she asked her husband.

"How about making small talk with the person next to you? Or playing possum so you won't be bothered?"

Getting the hint, Emily shut her mouth and peered out into the darkness moving with them, moving at the same speed, keeping pace with the big silver whale in which they were passing through the night. Reopening the computer, she typed:

> Flying at night, to me, is surreal. Not asleep but not awake. Dream quality. Closed in the cabin—overhearing bits and pieces of conversations. Hear the cry of a child somewhere off in the distance.

> Now I think I know why the down comforter was so important and maybe still is. Aunt Luella had a comforter like the one I used as a child, but since I wet the bed, by the time I grew up all the feathers had floated out the seams because it had been washed so much. When she died, it's the only thing I asked for and that comforter of hers is the one I use to cuddle under when . . . when I need comforting.

Closing the computer again, she looked out into the boundless unknown universe stretching in all directions. The water below was too black to see and indistinguishable from the rest of the night. "I'm going to try to stay awake to see the sun slip up—"

"Hmm?"

"—through the water. Remember, Jeff? The first time?"

Looking at her best friend, she saw he was in another state of mind and chose not to disturb him further. Smoothing out the gray cotton blanket, she craved transportation to the place she was moving further and further away from:

—the good side of her childhood: running a lemonade stand on the sidewalk in the front yard of her house on Main Street; catching lightning bugs on hot summer nights and putting them in a blue Mason jar; making homemade peach ice cream with the Weavers and her bottom getting colder and colder, numb, sitting on top of the freezer to hold it down while Jimmy cranked; cliff-hanger serials at the Saturday picture-show; pajama parties and band trips and basketball tournaments; tennis matches and horseback riding; Bible School picnics; water skiing and hikes in the mountains.

Strapped in the seat, Emily felt a cold draft and opened her eyes; at first, disoriented, then cognizant that they were on their way to a place she didn't want to go. Not really caring where the Kleins came from, to appease Jeff she'd agreed to go, taking off almost two weeks from work even though she was uneasy about leaving some of her clients that long, especially Fred Crabtree. He appeared to need her like a child needs his mother, although there was no way she could ever protect him from the demons he faced on a daily basis.

A woman was standing over her with a tray of food. It wasn't appetizing, but she ate it anyway because Jeff was still asleep and there was nothing else to do.

The child was crying again.

The woman came back with hot towels so Emily could get cleaned up; so she could walk away from the night looking as if nothing had happened.

———————

Guards were walking around with machine guns. American soldiers and their families were coming and going. Posters of nude women advertising fine wines greeted visitors to a cocktail lounge.

After picking up the prearranged rental car at the Frankfurt airport, they headed south to the Black Forest. For over a week, they crisscrossed the countryside, stopping often to act touristy, spending nights in quaint inns, hiking on snow-covered trails to the top of a waterfall, browsing in clock shops, touring a castle, cruising down the Rhine. They strolled through well-kept cemeteries looking for German versions of familiar American names of which they found an abundance, even some Kellers and Lentzes.

On the second Sunday morning, they stopped in a village of little houses stuck together like a Gingerbread montage and parked in front of a Lutheran church. "Service starts at eleven," Jeff translated from the sign out front. "Want to go in?"

"All right with me, if that's what you want to do."

They walked into the sanctuary. It could've been a Lutheran church in the States: the altar, the focal point; the pulpit to the side; purple paraments for Lent.

Often in the same place, at the same time, during the same religious service, Jeff and Emily reacted differently. Here, thousands of miles from home was no exception. He participated in the liturgy, sang the familiar hymns in German and understood the pastor's sermon. Comfortable in that setting, he patted his foot to the familiar Bach and Handel soaring from the organ pipes in the balcony.

Wearing jeans and a wool sweater set, Emily felt out of place, but not because she wasn't dressed in her Sunday best. When she glanced around at the stoic Germans, they looked the other way.

Did some of them or their fathers and mothers look the other way during World War II? she wondered. Because if they had seen the mutilations and murders, they would've had to do something. Did they not see evil in their land? Did they get all revved up and reach states of ecstasy when Hitler spoke?

They were probably just ordinary people following orders.

But what about the Nazi doctors? How in the world can anybody who uses humans as expendables live with themselves? Perhaps the Nazis were able to separate from work. Living under the chimneys of the camps, they were a million miles away. The real separation was in their minds. The wives kept things going for them—rocked the babies and stoked the fires of denial. Fed and nurtured the children. Made them believe their fathers were good men. The same men could kill Jewish babies at work and play with their own children when they got home at night.

Did they see Jews as less than human? If so, they could've sacrificed them and felt no compunction. Emily had read somewhere that a half dozen psychiatrists had certified Adolf Eichmann as normal. But Holocaust survivors who experience nightmares and flashbacks of atrocities and other posttraumatic stress symptoms are considered abnormal—mentally ill.

Did some of the people in this church or their fathers and mothers hide and feed the outcasts? Help them escape? Or, like the presumed caregivers of so many of her clients, simply look the other way—just close their eyes and go to sleep.

———

When they were on the road again, Jeff commented on the experience: "I felt right at home. Even found myself thinking in German, something I haven't done since language classes in college. If the service had been in English, it wouldn't have been much different from First Lutheran's."

"I agree. Think about it. The leader gets the group focused and suggestible to his, or in this case, her authority. Liturgy or any repetitive thing like singing gets people in trance. Surprised me they had a woman pastor. When we were kids, girls weren't even allowed to be acolytes, and if that church were still Catholic, the preacher would be a nun . . . that would be a cold day in hell."

"In my opinion," he quickly responded, "the warmup to the sermon is not necessarily bad."

"Didn't say it was. I like the liturgy, the music. But I often daydream during the sermon. From the bulletin, I could tell her text was *Psalm* 23. What did she say about the valley of the shadow of death? That we should fear no evil? I felt so out-of-place and almost paranoid. No one even spoke to me."

"They're just country folk, Em. Probably don't have many visitors, let alone foreigners in their little village. They could've been thinking: 'What are those Americans doing here? They killed our sons. Destroyed our cities.'"

"Yeah, and they probably thought God was on their side. Like Americans thought he was on ours."

"You're right," Jeff agreed, "but you could tell by their actions that they're loyal to God."

All day the skies wavered between winter and spring: snowing a little, raining a little, with the sun peaking out now and then. Late in the afternoon they came to Schiltach. After finding a place to park, they walked on a street made of cobbles worn smooth by the years, stopping at the top of a hill in front of the town hall where frescoes on the sixteenth-century building told the history of the town. Above the dates *1510, 1533,* and *1590* was a picture of a man with two horns protruding from his head. He was clutching the waist of a maiden who was slinging a torch.

"The Bull," Emily whispered.

"What did you say?"

"Oh nothing."

Not pressing for further explanation, Jeff pulled out his trusty guidebook and read a description of how the maiden had allegedly burned the city three times, blaming the Devil for making her do it.

After a restful night in a small inn, the Kleins sat in a quaint dining room with beamed ceilings at a wooden table covered with a white linen cloth. Eating smoked ham and cheese and hard rolls with a softboiled egg on the side, they watched the locals across the street standing in line to purchase cigarettes from a vending machine that was attached to the outside wall of the building.

"Better keep that Philip Morris stock your mother gave us for Christmas," Jeff said. "If they go busted in the States, they'll still sell their poison over here."

When they'd finished eating, he pulled out a local map. "Should be able to make it by nightfall. Looks like it's just off the old Roman highway."

"One of the most beautiful places in the world and they call it Hell," Emily remarked as they were driving though Hell Valley, nearing their final destination. The sun was shining as they passed well-kept farms and pasturelands with placid streams. Oaks and beeches budded with the promise of spring. Scatter rugs of wild yellow crocuses dotted verdant meadows. Across the hillsides, workers were pruning ancient vineyards, some of which were planted when Charlemagne and his troops had come through in the eighth century. "This must have been unspoiled land and unspoiled people in pagan times before the 'good Christians' came through to change things," she said.

"Can't you imagine our ancestors fleeing their homes?" Jeff was in history-heaven. "Marching through these hills. Homes burned to the ground, fields laid waste, villages razed, churches demolished, and all they'd worked for destroyed. How many died of cold and hunger along this route? How many of the once thriving farmers and shopkeepers survived to reach the cities of Europe, only to live as lean filthy degraded beggars? The ones who made it were lucky. But Lord! They must have been pissed."

"HIMMELREICH," Emily read the sign at a village entrance they had come upon.

Means 'Kingdom of Heaven,'" Jeff translated. "According to what I read in the guidebook, it was named by the railroad engineers after they had finally completed the line through the valley."

Late in the afternoon, they drove right past the sign Jeff had been looking for. He spun the Volkswagen around and headed back to the gravel road. They drove about five kilometers over a snow-dusted pasture to the picturesque village. At first they were disappointed because the steeple they'd seen from a distance topped a modern church, not the ancient building he'd read about. There were a few houses, a small town hall with a post office inside, and one bed-and-breakfast inn.

"Shall we look it over?" Jeff asked.

"We've got to sleep somewhere," Emily answered.

"*Sprechen sie Englisch?*" Jeff tried his best German with the woman standing behind the pastry counter.

"A little."

"We're looking for an old Lutheran church where we believe my ancestors might have come from, but the one across the road looks too modern."

The *Frau* walked over to the window and pointed toward a grove of trees. "It iss mor den one thousant jahr olt. Vas Catolic, den it vas Luteran, four er five hundret jahr go. No many peoples know or care of it. Sometimes ve habe . . . uh . . . have bus of tourists. You welcome go in. Der key ist on der vall insidt post."

They thanked her and walked down to the town hall to get the key.

In the dim light of dusk, the shrine seemed afloat on the shadows. A round stucco room attached to the older-looking brick section must've been an afterthought. Sitting on top of the high-pitched roof, the bell tower was capped with a conical cover resembling a witch's hat. On the peak was a weather vane.

"To ward off evil spirits," Emily said.

"Careful Em. Don't stumble over that rock. Whoops! There's another one. I think we're in a graveyard, but I don't see any names. It's too dark to see anything. Guess we'll have to wait till morning."

———————

Settled in an upstairs suite of the inn, Jeff turned the television to a quiz program while Emily leafed through the brochures. She found one about the church and handed it to her husband who translated as he read: "Even though this is a small village, a short distance from the noise of modern times, it nevertheless has a big story. It was settled early, then came the *Iro-Schottischen*, Irish-Scotch, monks who brought the Gospel into the country . . . ."

Emily lay down on one of the trundle beds while Jeff finished reading the rest of the history to himself. He learned that like many other small communities, this one had been shielded from the outside world by vast stretches of impenetrable forests until the eighth and ninth centuries when outsiders came in to Christianize and destroy pagan worship and bind the church in allegiance to the Holy Roman Empire.

During this era, a farmer donated his land to a monastery whose brothers built the church. When the Protestant Reformation swept Germany in the early 1500s, a preacher introduced Martin Luther's teachings. Literally overnight, the small community of believers transformed from Catholics to Lutherans.

"How did you know where to find this place?" Emily asked, peeking her head out from under the down comforter.

"I just did." Jeff turned out the light and went to bed.

"What makes you so certain this is the right town? Did you live here in another time?" she asked, only half-joking.

"Not that I recall," he played along. "You know I believe in an afterlife, although not necessarily the kind where the soul comes back to the earth in another body. But Em, I know this is it. I can feel it in my blood."

"Perhaps the monks who brought the Gospel here to this area also brought the worship of Satan."

"Good grief! Can't you get your mind off that stuff? This is supposed to be a heavenly vacation, and it's rapidly going to hell."

Ignoring his attempt at levity, she kept talking. "Jeff, *do* you believe there's a Devil—give me a straight answer this time. Please don't patronize me with a history lesson."

"As I've told you before, I really don't see how you can have God without the Devil."

"Well, to tell you the truth, I'm not even sure I know who God is anymore. Wish I could still believe he was the same kind old man I prayed to as a child," she said before drifting off to sleep.

At daybreak, Jeff turned the metal-forged key, which looked like an old jail key, and pushed open the thick heavy wooden door which had been cut in an arc and attached over the opening with massive hinges. Boldly, he took a step back through history. The mini-cathedral stood as a witness to time: to Roman soldiers, Catholic priests, robber barons, religious wars, uncounted civil uprisings, two world wars, and now a divided Germany.

"Amazing . . . simply amazing," he whispered reverently, as if stumbling upon the Holy Grail. Each huge stone in the floor was placed and expertly fitted to the next. The seats were hand-hewn—benches really, fourteen rows on each side of a center aisle—a board wide; enough to sit on with no back. A roughly cut 4-by-6 ran along the top to keep a person from falling backwards.

With the energy of a ten-year-old exploring an old deserted house, Jeff climbed up the creaking steps to the loft. Resting on a pew, he looked down into the sanctuary, trying to absorb it all: the feelings, the furnishings . . . the spirit of the place.

The baptismal font had been carved from granite into the shape of a large chalice. The raised pulpit would have allowed the preacher to look those sitting on the front row of the balcony right in the eye. On the main floor, the congregants would have been looking up all the time. This arrangement kept the proper authoritarian perspective in front of the congregation. People below—church above. The implicit message: Clergy were nearer to God than illiterate peasants could ever hope to be.

Angels floated in heavenly mosaics on the windows. A panorama of Christianity unfolded around the walls. In one picture, Jesus with a pierced side was tied to a cross—no nails: a St. Anthony's, not the traditional Latin cross. A soldier armed with a spear stood beside him. Several wooden crosses and crucifixes decorated the sacred edifice. They were crude, but surprising in their detail. On one Jesus-figure, both arms had been hacked off and the cross on which he hung had been cracked in the middle.

"Damn! God! Wonder how long ago it was desecrated? Is this where it all began? Where all the rage came from—in little villages just like this? People were fed up with both the Roman leaders and the Pope and acted out by desecrating the symbols of Christianity, perverting the mass, destroying sacred rituals, rebelling against the God who didn't stop the long-continuing destruction of their homes, their old beliefs, their ways—rebelling against the God who didn't save them."

I sound like Emily, he thought. As if I've walked into some terrible knowledge and can't see a way out. And that's not the reason I'm here.

Looking down into the church proper, the tone of his prayer changed drastically:

Dear God. Here my ancestors were baptized and confirmed, bound in holy wedlock, and in the end, laid to rest in the ground outside these walls. So much to see. So much to absorb at one time. I'll do what Em says, "Be still and let it speak to you." I'll simply sit here, close my eyes, and listen.

After several minutes, perhaps an hour, Jeff walked back down the stairs to the chancel. For the first time he noticed a door to the right. Opening it, he entered a room which was about a dozen feet square. A sturdy table in the center held accouterments for worship: silver chalices, candelabra, hymn books, and offering plates.

On the wall to his left was a plaque—a roster of Lutheran ministers who'd served the church after it split away from Catholicism.

There it was. Third on the list:

Johanne Kleinreich—1530-1545

The bristly auburn hairs on his arms stood straight up.

In the Black Forest, it was already the first day of spring. In Chestnut Ridge, South Carolina, it was the last day of one man's life.

Chapter 8

T rying to deaden truth,

Fred Crabtree sat at the bar drinking. Three beers didn't do it; weren't strong enough to make him not see the old man standing by the juke-box chewing on a cigar. Impulsively Fred picked up a napkin, grabbed a ball-point pen lying on top of the cash register, and scratched in seeth-ing letters:

> I bet you thought I'd never remember who you are and what you done to me. What you done can't be forgiven and I will never forget it again. If I ever find out your takin dirty pictures of another kid I will see you hang. If all your friends in high places keep on coverin up for you I will kill you myself.

The young man paid his tab, handed the bartender a dollar bill and, on the way out of the joint, slapped the threat into the old man's hand.

Placing the napkin under the light, the old man read it, then stag-gered back to his table. Downing another shot of whisky with one hand, with the other he reached into his coat pocket for a lighter; first relight-ing his cigar, then using it to ignite the flimsy paper from the cheap side of life. He dropped the note into an ashtray and watched the words char to obscurity.

Oughtn'ta make threats, boy, he thought to himself. A promise is a promise.

By the time the sun came up, J. D. Reid Jr., whose newest job descrip-tion called for keeping Olde Towne Cemetery neat and clean, had al-ready changed the oil, sharpened the blades, and gassed up the city's

14-HP wide-cut lawn tractor. He was cheerful as always, but today happier than usual because this would be the first mow of the year. Adjusting the seat to accommodate his long legs, he climbed on the mower, turned the ignition key, and took off toward the oldest section of the graveyard making a joyful noise: "My soul's been anchored in de Lord . . ."

Coming up on the Rheinhart plot, he thought he saw something hanging from the limb of the huge live oak and quit singing. "Another one of my visions," he said to himself, blinking his eyes, looking at the ground to make sure he was mowing straight. "Or maybe an early-mornin' haint." Since the accident, he'd often seen haints wandering around town, although it had been almost a year now and he tried not to think about it much.

He nearly died, they'd said. But even worse, he'd seen a friend, Arnold, and a cousin, Ezra, burned—buried alive. Couldn't save them. Lead man on the pothole crew and he couldn't help them at all.

The three men had been working on the shoulder of the bypass when a transfer truck jackknifed in the middle of the highway, its tail end knocking over a tack wagon filled with steaming hot liquid asphalt—hot tar—dumping it all over the three men. The sticky stuff was burning like hell fire, melting off the top layers of their skin and they couldn't wipe it off.

The last things J. D. heard were the helpless moans of Arnold and Ezra—

Next thing he knew, he was heading through a long tunnel toward a bright light; then he was in the hospital looking up at another bright light with a bunch of people standing around his bed—his wife and mother, even his white friend, Jefferson Klein—all looking very worried before breaking into wide smiles when he asked, "Wat ch'all doin' here?"

"Thank you Jesus . . . thank you Jesus." His wife and mother lifted their hands and voices toward heaven.

J. D. had been lucky. Arnold and Ezra had died on the way to the hospital. His own pain was terrible, mostly from the poison fumes that burned his windpipe and lungs leaving a fiery ache in his chest that never went away. After several weeks had passed, the city put him back to work mowing grass. He missed his old job. For a man who couldn't read or write, who couldn't even talk plain most of the time, he'd done pretty well to make it to boss man of the city's pothole crew.

Maybe mowing grass wasn't so bad after all. He thanked God everyday that he was alive to work and support his family, and that he was still able to sing tenor in the Happy Holler Gospel Choir.

Man, how he missed Arnold and Ezra. Sometimes when he was sitting on the front porch of his house, out of the corner of his eye he'd catch Ezra wandering up and down the street. One time when he was working downtown, he'd actually seen big Arnold standing on the street corner with the homeless people listening to China Doll preach.

Closer to the tree, J. D. glanced up just before running into a body dangling upside down from a tree limb.

Was it real? Or was it his mind playing tricks again? Stored somewhere in the confusion in his head was a story about another lynching; a story he had heard many times growing up on the Campbell plantation.

Deciding that it was a real person, a real dead person, he slid down off the machine and went hurdling tombstones across the vast graveyard. He ran through the gate and panted his way down Church Street, finally reaching the Justice Center. Rushing up the steps three at a time, through the doors and into the hallway, he was hollering over the pain in his chest, "Where's Mr. Tom? I needs to talk to Mr. Tom. Quick."

Chief Paxton walked out of his office. "What the hell's goin' on?"

Immediately upon meeting the 'law,' J. D. changed to calm, composed, speaking perfectly plain. "There's been another hangin', sir."

"What do ya mean another?" Paxton pointed his right index finger at the messenger. "Boy, ya better keep ya big mouth shut. That was a long time ago. And if you start talkin' about it, next thing ya know that woman of yours is gonna become a widow-woman."

"But Mr. Tom, ya gotta get down there."

"What's the hurry, boy? If a man's dead, he's dead, and there ain't a damn thing we can do about it."

Driving through the cemetery gates with a detective by his side, Tom Paxton felt a rush of adrenaline like he used to get after scoring a touchdown for the high school football team. It had been a long time since he remembered a white man getting murdered in Chestnut Ridge. As a sophomore in high school, he'd heard kids at the pool talking about the accident, which he knew—because his daddy had told him so—that it wasn't really an accident at all.

Any murder in this town was bound to generate a lot of excitement and guess who'd be quarterbacking the whole game? He parked the cruiser just outside the old Rheinhart family plot.

"Well, I'll be, it's the Crabtree boy," the detective said, even before they got out of the car. Sporting a long pigtail reaching almost to the ground, the body with some type of object stuffed in its mouth was easy to identify. Except for sneakers and socks on his feet, he was completely naked.

"Sure is," Paxton said, getting out of the car, immediately noticing a stab wound over the heart and a vacant spot in the genital area. "The boy had it comin' to him with everything and everybody he was messed up in."

"Would you look over there?" The detective pointed to a weather-worn concrete box covering an above-ground coffin. "It's his—" He turned around and keeled over, expelling his morning's eggs and grits all over the pitted stone lamb in the corner.

Paxton pulled a handkerchief out of his pocket and handed it to his brawny subordinate, momentarily turned wimp. "Wipe off your face, man. Looks like a mob killin" to me. Hope they stabbed him first. I can't stand the thoughts of anybody havin' to live through what they did to him. Maybe they were gay bashers. I remember hearin' in a police-academy lecture that the penis-thing is quite common in homosexual killings. Never seen one myself, though."

"Could be a drug deal gone bad," the detective responded, apparently having regained his machismo.

Tommy walked over to the car to get a knife from the homicide kit. Back at the tree he told his partner, "When you get right down to it pal, unless there's any prints on his body, or we can find the knife—and that's not likely because this looks like a professional job—all we got is some evidence that proves nothing except that he suffered some kind of awful . . . probably some sort of retribution for disloyalty to somebody."

Chief Paxton reached up and cut the rope wondering whether he had released the boy *from* or *to* hell.

———————

Danny Evans had been monitoring the police scanner on her office desk when she heard a body had been found. Big news! After picking up a camera and spiral notebook, she walked, almost ran, down to the cemetery to find that the entrance gate had been cordoned off with yellow tape. A city cop was standing sentry.

"What happened?" Danny asked.

"Miss, I can't say, except as you probably heard, there's been a lynching. The police chief said he'd be holding a press conference at noon on the steps of the Justice Center."

As Danny was about to leave, a hearse pulled up. When the cop turned around to unlock the gate, the reporter flashed a press ID and hopped in beside the driver.

"Pleased to meet you Miss Evans. I'm Dave Keller with Keller Funeral Home."

"Do you know who it was?" Danny asked.

"Yes, but I can't tell you."

"Mornin' Danny." Paxton winked at the reporter as she stepped out of the hearse.

"Mornin' Chief." Danny looked at the body bag already stuffed and zipped shut. "Can I take some pictures?"

"It's a free country."

The reporter spent a few minutes photographing the crime scene, including two pieces of rope still hanging from the death limb and the grave markers inside the wrought-iron fence. Pointing to a bloody glob on the concrete box, she asked. "What's that?"

"If you don't know, I ain't gonna tell you," Tom grinned.

"It's a guy thing," explained Dave Keller, apparently trying to be funny. No one laughed, so he asked, "Are you gonna call for an autopsy, Chief?"

"Why should I? It's pretty evident to me what happened."

"Poor boy's got no family as I know of," the undertaker said. "We buried his grandmother a few years ago, so I'm probably stuck. If nobody calls to claim his body in a few days, I'll put it in the incinerator and toss his bloody ashes in the dump."

"I thought it was standard procedure to conduct an autopsy in a murder case," Danny was saying to Dave as he and Paxton's man loaded the body bag into the hearse.

"Ma'am, I'm just doing what I'm told and that's to pick up the remains, and I'll be a suck-egged mule before I take another loss for some white trash nobody else cared about either."

Chief Paxton patted his buxom, twenty-something secretary on her bottom. "First get me a cup of coffee, and then I want ya to get Dr. Emily Klein's number."

"Yes sir." The woman opened a telephone directory. "Here it is. I'll dial it for you." Before anyone answered, she gave the phone to her boss and walked over to the break room to get coffee.

Emily's voice drawled on the recording: "I'll be out of the office until Monday, March 27. If this is an emergency please call ....." Weird, he thought. When I saw her last week, she didn't tell me she was going anywhere.

He looked up her home number and dialed it. There was no answer.

"Get Gladys Lentz ... Mrs. Jacob Lentz ... she lives on Main Street ... on the line," Paxton ordered his secretary when she came back with the coffee. She made the call, transferring it to the chief when the party answered.

"Good morning, Miz Lentz. This is Thomas Paxton," he greeted the lady like she would have expected a southern gentleman to do. "How are you?"

"I'm just fine, thank you."

"That's good. The reason I called is, I'm lookin' for Emily and there's no answer at her office or her house."

"Is something wrong? Are the children all right?"

"No ma'am ... I mean yes ma'am, everything's okay. But I do need to talk to her about one of her clients, a Fred Crabtree. He's been murdered and—"

"Emily and her husband are in Europe. They should be getting in on Sunday night."

"Okay then. And how have you been doin'?" It was the second time he had feigned interest in the condition of a woman he could care less about.

"Very well, thank you. I count my blessings every day. Don't know if you've heard or not, but I'll be breaking up housekeeping in a few weeks and moving into Whispering Pines."

Not really giving a damn about how the old woman was doing or where she was going, he poured a pack of sugar into the now lukewarm coffee, trying to think of a way to end the conversation.

"And how's your daddy getting along?" the old biddy asked. "I heard he had a stroke."

"Just as mean as ever," he affected a laugh. "They have him in physical therapy now, and as you know, he's a tough ol' geezer. Sorry Miz Lentz, somebody's on the other line," he lied. "Would you do me a favor? As soon as Emily gets home, how 'bout you have her give me a call? Okay?"

———————————

Sitting at the breakfast room table in the house she and Jake had built during the Depression, Gladys, comfortable in a rose-colored duster with a Peter Pan collar, lifted the phone off the wall and dialed Phil's office. He was out so she left a message on his answering machine. "We need to talk . . . soon. The Paxton boy called. They found a body hanging in the cemetery and think Emily might know something."

Not consciously planning what she was about to do next, Gladys hung up the phone and walked over to the dining room. What a mess, she thought. The table and floor were covered with a lifetime of dishes and doodads, many of which she would have no room for in her new apartment.

She opened the top drawer of the buffet and retrieved a newspaper clipping, long protected between two small pieces of cardboard. Taking it across the foyer to her formal living room, she sat down on the claret-colored Victorian sofa, now covered with a white sheet, and read the article one more time:

> Jacob Lentz, owner of Lentz Abattoir, was fishing from the old railroad trestle that crosses the Roundtree River with his brothers-in-law Dave Keller and Philip Owens and friends Earl Elliott, Casey Paxton, and Cleat Klein. At about 9:45 on the morning of June 4, Mr. Lentz suddenly fell into the lake. He was struggling toward the swimmers' area and was within fifty feet of the opposite bank when the city lifeguard noticed him and jumped in the water. By the time he reached Mr. Lentz, the man was unconscious. Several swimmers formed a human chain to the shore and hauled the large man in. For more than an hour, the lifeguard applied the new arm lift, back pressure method of artificial respiration, chanting "out comes the bad air, in goes the good."
>
> A few minutes after the accident, an ambulance bearing oxygen arrived. Attendants and volunteers kept the oxygen mouthpiece over the victim's face and took turns applying pressure. At 10:45, the oxygen in the tank ran out shortly before Dr. Bill Wilhelm, county coroner, came to the lake side and declared Mr. Lentz dead by accidental drowning.

Jacob Lentz is survived by his wife, the former Gladys Keller, and two children, Emily (13) and Jimmy (18).

Funeral arrangements are incomplete.

Gladys carefully placed the clipping back into the drawer. I never understood why he drowned, she thought. He was such an excellent swimmer.

She walked across the room and opened the Steinway. The long-time widow sat down at the piano and began to play their song: "Dear One, The World is Waiting for the Sunrise," a hit when she and Jake were teenagers, revived in the late forties by Les Paul and Mary Ford. As her long graceful fingers glided effortlessly across the keyboard, big tears—not more than a dozen—drizzled down her face, smudging her rouge-red cheeks.

At noon, standing behind a podium on the old courthouse lawn, Chief Paxton talked directly to J. D. and his wife Evie who were sitting on the couch in front of the television in their modest brick ranch-style house in Happy Holler. "Shortly after seven this mornin', a city employee discovered a body, who we've identified as one Fred Crabtree, hangin' upside down from a tree in Olde Towne Cemetery. A few hours later, an anonymous call came in at the police department from a man claimin' he'd seen the victim leavin' the new *Mona Lisa Bar and Grill* about two in the morning with two African-American males in some fancy dark green car with a New York license plate. This call and what we know about Mr. Crabtree's criminal record, as well as the scant evidence found at the scene, lead us to assume that this murder was the result of a drug deal gone bad. We will keep you informed of further developments."

The camera panned the crowd as it dispersed.

"Look, why der's old Wilbur Lee and Otis." Evie pointed at two men with their backs turned who were walking down the street toward the old ice house. "And over der's China Doll."

"Glory be," J. D. grinned. "Der go Jefferson's pappy widen' by on his motor bike."

"I skeerd, Mr. Reid." Evie never called her husband by his given name.

"Donchu worry none woman. I jus' *found* de body. The law knows I had nothin' to do wit' it."

"Dat's not what I mean. 'Member durin' de riots way back yonder? Won't be long for dey be comin' down here in de holler lookin' for—"

"I sez, donchu worry. I always be wit' chu." The forty-eight-year-old man looked out the window at his yard. New grass planted the previous fall seemed a foot high; a white dogwood was in full bloom; the pine tree outside their bedroom window was dying at the top and leaning toward the house.

One day, I'll bring it down and dig us up a little goldfish pond in its place, he thought in clear English.

When the regular Thursday night poker game in the bank's fallout shelter which had been constructed during the Cold War was over and those who were not part of the top echelon had left, the leader spoke: "To tell you the truth my brothers, it's time to call in your favors. As y'all read in *The Gazette* this evening, the chief said the body had been a mental patient. And we all know who his shrink was." One by one, the patriarch looked each of his comrades in the eye and in a deep slow raspy voice gave the ultimatum: "The bitch could ruin us all. We've got to find out what she knows."

Chapter 9

Without leaving any clues except the shards of glass on their bed, they had been raped. In their own house. Their safest place. The jet-lagged travelers, having arrived home late Sunday evening, had left their luggage in the car and kicked off their shoes in the foyer, heading straight to the bedroom.

"It's freezing in here," Emily said.

"I do feel a little draft." Jeff switched on the lamp. "My God! The skylight's been knocked out. Somehow they bypassed the alarm. Had to be professionals."

Bureau drawers had been scavenged and left wide open. Bras and panties and socks and shirts were strung all over the place.

"Yep. Looks like we had company. Wonder what they were looking for? What they got?" Emily was speaking calmly.

"Careful, Em, watch where you—"

"Ouch!" She hobbled out to the landing, sat down on the top step, and leaned over to take off her sock. After plucking the sliver of glass out of her toe, she stood up again and stepped over to the front window, trying to avoid seeing her reflection in the pane as she looked down at the yard. "Don't see signs of anybody. Do you think we should call the police?"

"Naw, it's too late and they couldn't do anything tonight anyway. Let me go take a look downstairs and then we might as well go to bed."

A note was taped to the mailbox lid: "Emily. Please call me as soon as you get back in town. Tom."

Walking into the building and looking around, she felt as if she'd been raped again. Inside her private office, the tape had been yanked from the answering machine, the computer monitor was glowing, and the file cabinet had been pried open, its contents strewed all over the floor.

First thing she did was call her husband. "How dare anyone come in here and tear things up? I feel so . . . so violated." Her automatic shock of numbness from the night before had tripped over to gut-felt rage.

"What did they get?"

"I don't know yet . . . I'm just too upset to try to figure it out."

"I'll be right over. You should go ahead and call the police."

She hung up and dialed the Justice Center. "Tom Paxton, please."

"May I ask whose calling?" The voice was sweet, syrupy.

"Tell him it's Emily Klein . . . *Doctor* Emily Klein."

Tom came on the line. "Oh, dahlin, I thought you'd never get back." As casually as if he'd been announcing a community watch meeting, he said, "I don't know if you've heard or not, but Fred Crabtree was murdered while you were gone . . ."

She struggled to listen; to take in what he was saying.

Before she had a chance to tell him her office had been ransacked, he said, "I'll be right over. We need to talk."

Jeff and Tom showed up at the same time and Emily met them on the porch. Everybody talked at once.

Jeff about the house; he didn't know about the murder.

Emily about the office.

Paxton about the murder: "Was the most gruesome sight I've ever seen. The old boy's pecker had been neatly chopped off and—"

"Don't you talk like that around my wife," Jeff yelled.

"Oh, Jefferson. She's a big girl now," the chief snickered. "Hears grosser stuff than that everyday, I'm sure."

"Now, come on fellows. Don't act so juvenile."

Tom frowned at her. "Show me your file on Crabtree . . . if it's still here in all this mess."

"Can't do that. Anything I have on him is confidential."

"But he's dead. What difference does it make?" Paxton bent over to pick through the records scattered across the floor.

"You can't do that," Emily practically screamed.

"No, you can't do that," echoed Jeff, clenching his fists as if preparing for a playground fight.

Emily lowered her voice. "All my client records are confidential and you have no right to touch them."

"Dr. Klein, I want to see Mr. Crabtree's records and if you don't let me . . . I've gotta go now . . . but I'll be back with a subpoena this afternoon."

"Won't matter," Emily told Jeff as Tom stomped out of the office acting like a spoiled child who didn't get his way. "They're sketchy generic notes. My detailed notes are on the floppies in the safe, and unless a particular client signs a release, I'll guard them all the way to the Supreme Court, or jail, if I have to. In my opinion, knowing that whatever one 'dumps' in the therapy office will always be confidential, even after you die, is what makes therapy work."

"Serves him right," Jeff said. "The shitass is gonna be back with a subpoena for nothing." He helped her straighten up a little then called his secretary to tell her he wouldn't be back till Tuesday morning. Emily canceled her appointments for the day and followed him home.

Walking together through the family room, Emily noticed that the cover on the rolltop desk was not completely closed. "I thought I locked it before we left for Germany. I'd hidden a tape in the back, intending to take it in with me this morning to put in the safe, but in all the excitement of last night, I forgot to."

She rolled the top back and scrambled through the bank statements in the back corner, sighing with relief upon seeing that Fred's last words were still there. Without explaining a thing to Jeff, she went running upstairs and put on a bathing suit.

Back down at the pool, she swam hard and fast, forty or fifty laps, till her body said: no more.

To cool down, she climbed out of the pool and sat with her legs in the water. Her heart begged to cry, but a program was running in her mind—

Don't cry.
Don't feel.
Don't ever get too close to anyone.

Stiff as a marble angel hovering at the gate of some unknown world, Emily stood outside the Rheinhart family plot. Anyone would've expected her to break down at the crime site, but she didn't. Almost every client she'd seen during the previous month had wanted, had needed, to talk about the murder, but her own thoughts and feelings about this matter had been negligible. The therapist had been forced—by professionalism—to listen to their fears and their questions without divulging how devastated, how guilty, how responsible she felt.

Rumor in town was that the case had already been closed. Nobody in authority seemed to want to know what happened. But two things Emily was sure of:

Fred Crabtree had told.

Fred Crabtree had died.

Casey . . . Casey . . . Casey. The name banged inside her head like a hammer on a gong.

Still, she couldn't cry.

Forcing a deep breath, the distraught woman approached the waist-high door hanging precariously on a single hinge. One pull on the handle and it fell to the ground, smashing her toes.

She couldn't feel the pain.

Kicking the door aside, Emily stepped through the opening and looked around, seeing things she'd missed earlier when standing by her client during his abreaction of the ancestor-worship ritual—or whatever it was. Pieces were missing from the rusty wrought-iron fence. Whether built to keep things in or out, it was useless now, except as a support for creeping Carolina jasmine. A live oak, its lower branches trimmed carefully away, loomed over the graves, each with a weather-beaten stone of a different size, shape, and message. One was a cross. Another held a sculptured olive branch. In the corner, a pitted-stone lamb guarded a baby's tomb.

The place where her client had remembered being pornographed triggered a wave of chills. Taking time to recover from the primitive emotional reaction, Emily closed her eyes.

Afraid to look.

Afraid she'd see his mutilated body hanging from that tree.

Or his blood.

Fred Crabtree was gone. He would never call her again.

Emily closed her eyes and tried to pray but no words came.

Why should she pray to a God who had once allowed a child, and then the adult he became, to suffer so?

Opening her eyes; quickly closing them again. Her mind protected, showing her a spirited child singing in the daylight, leaping over scatter rugs of wild yellow crocuses, splashing through clear streams, and chasing butterflies.

Chapter 10

I t was not a dream:

I am a baby crawling around on the floor — shiny hardwood floor, slick — in the room at the end of the hall; in the blue bedroom in the house on Main Street. Three beds: Mommy's, Daddy's, and my cherry-wood crib. I smell roses. But it's cold outside and no flowers are blooming. Mommy is asleep in her bed. Daddy picks me up and carries me to his bed. I am flopping upside down on his fat belly.

Emily threw the one-legged rag doll down on the guest bed and rushed to the bathroom. When the revulsion passed, she went to her own bed where Jeff was sleeping.

At 12:18 on the dot, she awoke as she had many times before. A clear refined woman's voice said: "It happened at this time."

It was a dream:

Masked men slash my tires. I take the car to the Goodyear store. Call Jeff to pick me up, but he's not at home, not at work. I get on the public bus and sit on the back seat.

"No," the driver says." You cannot sit there. That is for the coloreds."

I move to the front. The bus nears my old house on Main Street but I don't pull the bell rope. Somewhere along the route, everybody except me gets off. I ride to the end of the line. The bus stops. The driver opens the door. I get up and walk through the door, down the steps. A heavily tarnished silver disk is lying at the side of the road. I squat down on it and begin to slide back toward town. Spinning fast . . . faster . . . faster until it breaks down into pieces of excrement. I get up and run —

The alarm sounded. Jeff shut it off and rolled over to give his wife a 'good morning' hug. "Did you sleep okay?" he asked.

"Sorta. I dreamed a lot."

"Nightmares again?"

"Not really. One was rather interesting. Wanna hear?"

"Sure."

She'd described the first part.

"So you were left sitting flat on your butt in a pile of shit," Jeff teased.

"That's one way to look at it. But there's more. Up ahead were two roads: one to a lush green valley; the other was narrow and rocky going straight up a mountain. Either I had to decide to go to the peaceful valley, knowing I'd never get home, or I had to struggle up the mountain and cross to the other side to reach my goal."

"Which road did you take?"

"I'm not sure. When the alarm went off, I was walking around a mountain . . . around and around a mountain."

"Emily dear. What's the matter? You look pale. Have you been sick?" Wearing a casual house dress overlaid with a crisply starched cotton apron, Gladys Lentz was standing in the hallway outside her new apartment.

"No Mama, not sick but—"

"That's good. Come on in and have a seat. When you called and said you were coming over, I mixed up a batch of Tea-Time Tassies. They're almost done. When you were a little tot, you liked them better than anything I made."

They sat down on stools at the bar which separated the kitchen from the living area.

"I'm not sick, Mama, but I'm really upset because—"

"How do you like my new love seat? There was no way I could keep that big old sofa and my piano both. Not enough room. And why are you so upset?" Again, Gladys didn't give her daughter a chance to answer. "Honey, I've been so worried about you lately. Wish you'd quit working so hard. Those crazy people . . . they're tearing you to pieces. If you keep going as you are, you're gonna go crazy, too. And then what would I do? You know me, I just wish you'd get back in the church—"

"Will you please listen to me? Last night—" Emily's breathing was becoming shallow; her vocal chords tightening, making it even more difficult to speak. "Last night I had this memory of someone molesting me . . . don't even think I was old enough to talk . . . it had to be Daddy. Who else would I have been around like that?"

"How in heaven's name could you bring back something that happened when you were a baby?" Gladys got down from the stool and walked over to the built-in oven. She removed the tin of tiny pecan tarts and placed it on a cooling rack on the counter.

"Well I did . . . at least I think I did," Emily said.

The mother turned around, glaring at, scolding the daughter. "You must've been dreaming. Jake Lentz, my precious Jake, was a very good man, a Christian man, God rest his soul. When you were sick, he was the one who mostly took care of you; worried an awful lot about you; was always taking you to doctors."

"Why? Why did I need to see doctors?"

"I don't exactly remember."

"It wasn't a dream. Mama, I was wide awake. Listen to me. I just need you to listen. I was holding the Raggedy Ann doll Uncle Dave gave me for Christmas one year . . . you remember, the one with the missing leg that Jimmy cut off."

"I'm sure he didn't mean to."

"No, that's not true. He threatened . . . I've never told you this, but when I was only seven, he took me to his room and threw me down on the bed . . . Mama, he was five years older . . . and he—" This time Emily was interrupted not by her mother's voice, rather by a picture in her mind: A mommy standing in the hall looking in. Something was wrong. No good mother would've stood by letting anybody hurt her daughter. But the memory of Jimmy was clear. Always had been. "—he told me: 'if you tell, you die.' And I believed him because I never told . . . not until just now."

"Why are you suddenly coming up with all this stuff?" Gladys had turned her back toward Emily and was scooping out the tarts with a fork and—carefully, so they wouldn't crumble—placing them on a crystal plate. "Did I tell you? I got a postcard from him the other day. He gave me his address, let me know he's okay, and asked to borrow a few hundred dollars."

"That's wonderful. I wish him well, but please Mama, I need you to listen to *me*."

"Then tell me." She faced her daughter again. "I'm right here."

Consciously relaxing her jaw muscles, Emily tried again. "Last night, I was upstairs in the big rocker holding the doll. All of a sudden, I had this strong sense of being little and crawling around in your bedroom and—"

"How do you know it was my bedroom?" The interruption sounded almost accusatory, but if it had been, the accuser was now satisfied to look down at the flowers patterned in her apron and smooth their non-existent wrinkles.

"Because my crib was next to your bed, it was like I could see you there . . . and he picked me up and carried me to his bed, so I had to be little. You were in yours . . . asleep. As I was saying, I felt like I was in that room again, and Daddy was flopping me up and down on his big belly like a—" The words rag doll stuck in her throat.

Gladys casually set two gold-rimmed cups and saucers out for coffee. "He didn't have intercourse, did he?"

Emily was unexpectedly stunned; it was the first time in her life she could recall her mother ever uttering a sexually explicit word in her presence.

"Cream?" Gladys offered, pleasantly.

"No thank you." The daughter's southern-bred manners were automatic. "Are you suggesting that molesting a baby is acceptable if it doesn't include penetration?"

"That's not what I said, but I do hope you can forgive him for what he did . . . if he did anything. Certainly hope I didn't spend all those years trying to teach you God's ways and His glory of forgiveness for nothing . . . if you don't forgive, you're just letting the Devil in, you know. Doesn't pay to hold a grudge, Honey."

"He's dead, Mama. Surely I can feel anyway I want to about the dead." Shame was turning to betrayal. Betrayal to anger. "And if, as you say, he didn't do anything, what's there to forgive?"

"Let me fix you some lunch." Gladys didn't seem to understand that heartfelt questions, any questions, deserve answers. "When you were upset as a child, food always seemed to calm you." She pushed the cup across the counter, then walked over to the refrigerator.

Emily accepted the coffee, unaware of anything but her mother's bland expression. She wasn't hungry, but that was hardly the point: she wasn't a child now and wasn't going to allow herself to be stuffed with food so there would be no room for feelings.

Her mother was busy setting out a loaf of home-baked bread and freshly made chicken salad. "Please don't say anything about this to anybody else, especially your brother. He couldn't handle it."

"Oh, like I'm really going to hear from him, right? Who can't handle it, him or you?"

Gladys set out silverware and two plates and climbed back up on the stool. Nervously making little balls of the sourdough bread, she rambled on. "Don't see how he could've hurt you . . . I never let you out of my sight . . . if he did anything, I didn't know it. One thing's for sure, as God is my witness, I never hurt you. But he could have, I think . . . not sexual . . . it's just sometimes he'd use a belt to—"

"I don't recall any whippings by Daddy."

Yet, she did remember her mother welting her legs with a long thin hickory stick, assuming that in those days when 'spare the rod and spoil the child' had been preached from the pulpit, everybody routinely got switched. Suddenly, the grown woman who rarely cried heard the burst of a loud sob escape the effort of her control.

"Get hold of yourself," Gladys said sternly, seeming to recover her own senses. "I've never seen you in such bad shape."

Forty-seven-year-old Emily yearned to be held and comforted, to hear her mother say she was sorry it happened. She wanted to crawl into her mother's lap on that big rocking chair and hear her say once more, as she used to, "Now, now, little one . . . sleep. It was only a dream, my precious, just a dream . . . everything will be all right in the morning."

Instead, the woman looked at her daughter as if seeing through a veil and after a moment said quickly, "What you need to do is forget the past, Honey. Get on with your life. You should try and do what I do. Just turn everything over to the Lord."

"Turn it over to the Lord? We must be talking about different gods. The God I know expects me to do something on my own and I'm try-ing." Emily stood up, bristling almost, raring to turn everything over to her mother and run away as fast as she could. "I should get back to work."

"Wait just a minute, dearie."

Emily waited obediently as her mother boxed up the Tea-Time Tas-sies and gave them to her to take home. As the daughter was going out the door, love offering in hand, the mother said, "Thanks for stopping by."

Before Emily reached the elevator at the end of the hall, she heard piano music seeping through the walls of apartment #303 at the Whis-pering Pines Living Center. A familiar tune it was, but she couldn't re-member the words . . . something about the sunrise.

Gladys Keller Lentz had mastered the art of denial every bit as much as a weather forecaster who can stand in front of a camera saying the sun is shining when the viewer can see rain drops pelting behind him on the windowpane. If the woman had been such a good mother, how come it was Sue Weaver who baked her cookies? Listened to her read and helped with her homework? Made her frilly dresses for birthday parties and tutus for dance recitals? If Jake had been such a good father, how come it was Dick Weaver who had magically pulled pennies out of her ear, played mumbletypeg, taught her to ride a bike and pumped up her basketball and her self-confidence?

Although Emily had left the apartment, ridden down the elevator, and walked across the busy lobby to the parking lot, started her car and driven herself across town, she'd remembered nothing of the short trip until she found herself under the corridor of willow oaks drooping over the west section of Main Street.

She parked in front of the white frame house where she'd spent her happy growing-up years. Another family lived there now. Perhaps another little girl roller-skated with her mother up and down that long wide hall, or squatted at the end of the driveway to 'cook' mud pies for all her imaginary friends.

That night, Emily dreamed she was pressing a red mole on her left breast and a long black snake slithered out. Predictably awaking at 12:18, panting in terror, the internal message was clear:

There is something dark and evil inside of me.

The Weavers. They would remember her childhood; her mother; her daddy. She'd called them on Saturday morning, asking if she could stop by for a visit in the afternoon.

"Do come," Dick had answered. "We always enjoy talking with you."

What shall I say . . . ask? Emily was thinking when the door opened.

Reaching to give their 'adopted' child a hug, Sue was saying, "So glad you came. Dick's back in the den." Emily followed Sue through the house. "Dick, look who's here." He stood up about to shake hands but instead turned the greeting into her second big hug of the day.

For twenty or thirty minutes, they sat around talking about the children, the weather, local politics, gardening and lots of other things common to both generations.

"It's really ironic you came by today," Sue said. "We've been going through some old pictures and picked out a bunch we thought you might want. Why don't you and Dick look through them while I go stir up a few mint juleps?"

"Sounds great, but go easy on the whiskey." Emily winked at Dick. "Y'all know I've never been much of a drinker. Do you remember when you used to let me taste yours? Mama would've killed you if she'd known you let a drop of alcohol pass my pristine lips."

Sue smiled. "Your parents were probably too wrapped up in their own lives to have noticed."

"That's not the way Mama remembers it," Emily said, still reeling with disappointment from the previous day's visit to Whispering Pines. "One reason I came is to see if y'all could help me remember some things about my daddy. Strangely, I have only a few memories of him and they're not all that great."

"As far as I know, he was a good man," Dick said. "Very generous. Always helping out people who were down on their luck. A big contributor and money raiser for the March of Dimes, as I remember. Too bad he didn't live to see polio eradicated." He opened a white shirt box and started flipping through the photos. "Look! Here's one of you sitting on top of the ice cream freezer. Wasn't she a cute little thing, Sue? Always smiling or giggling when she was around us."

"Emily, I don't know what your memories might be," Sue said, "but we have wonderful memories of our little 'Emma Wee Wentz' and often reminisce about the little incidences that happened. Like the way you used to love to show us how you could write backwards, about as fast as forwards, and read it without any trouble at all."

"You really were a smart kid," Dick added. "Except maybe when you were never able to figure out how I pulled a penny out of your ear."

They were all still laughing when Sue stood up, saying, "I'll go fix the drinks while y'all keep looking through the box."

Dick picked out a few pictures, telling little anecdotes about each one till he came to one showing several men holding up fish on strings. "Just look at this, Sweetie. It's probably the last one I took with your daddy in it. As I remember, he and a few of his buddies had just come back from a deep-sea fishing trip and wanted me to get a picture of their catch." He pointed to a young-looking Jake Lentz. "Your daddy's holding the biggest one. Looks like it might be a king mackerel. There may be a few others in there of him and your mother and there are lots of you." He placed all the pictures into the box and put the lid back on. "They're all yours."

"Thanks a lot. I'm sure Carol and Matt will love to see them. My folks never took any snapshots. For that matter, I don't even remember a camera in the house. The only pictures I have of me are from school and those that my friends and their parents took. Now Jeff, his daddy made oodles of them."

"Yeah. I recall that Cleat used to have a darkroom in the basement of his apartment. Quite a craftsman, your father-in-law . . . when he wasn't drinking too much."

Sue came through the door with the drinks and a tray of cookies and cheese straws and set them on the table. Emily picked up a chilled glass and took a sip. "Very refreshing, Sue, thank you."

"Do you happen to remember any of the circumstances of your daddy's drowning?" Dick looked at Emily.

"Not really. I don't know anything except what I've read in an old news clipping. And that it happened on my thirteenth birthday, the morning I got back from camp that year.

Dick glanced at his wife, as if asking approval for what he was about to say.

Sue was shaking her head. "She should know."

"Well, Honey," Dick began, "there were rumors around town for a long time that it wasn't an accident. Your daddy'd been fishing from the old railroad trestle with Cleat, your uncle Dave, ol' Earl Elliott, and a bunch of other guys. You know the crowd. From from what I've heard, they all ran around together from the time they were boys. All except for Phil Owens who didn't come to town till during the war. They kinda picked up where their daddies had left off, like a next-generation born to run things . . . and born knowing it, most of them."

He stopped talking long enough to gulp the mint julep—not exactly the southern way.

"Well, as it turned out, nobody claimed to have seen him fall across the railing. They said he was just there one minute and then he was gone. A lifeguard dived in and pulled him out but he was already unconscious, I guess, and they never could revive him."

"What do you mean by rumors. "Did people think he killed himself? Or . . . you're not talking about foul play, are you?"

"As far as I know there was never an autopsy or any further investigation." Rather adroitly, Dick had tiptoed over her question. "Like I say, you know the crowd he ran with. At least since you've been grown, you know what I mean. They were pretty much every one of them a pillar holding up some corner of this town's economy, or its future, some way. Nobody was going to ask them any awkward questions, no matter what they might've been thinking privately. And they didn't. Ask any questions, I mean. Not even old Casey himself. Tommy was just a kid then, like you and Jeff. Looking back though," he grinned, "seems to me he'd already decided he was gonna take over his daddy's job, sooner or later. He was a rough kid—"

"That's for sure," Sue interjected. "We really got worried when you started going out with that boy."

"Yeah, the chap was rougher than a lot of folks knew, I always thought. Maybe they didn't wanna know then—but I'll bet they've noticed, now that he's Chief Thomas Paxton."

Emily had not expected to come here to talk about Tom Paxton so she changed the subject back to herself. "Well, regardless of what happened, however he died, it threw me into premature adulthood. With Daddy gone and Jimmy in the service, it seemed like Mama chose me for her confidant and best friend."

"She was always mature for her age, wasn't she Dick?"

"Yes you were, Emily. You know, we never saw you cry or even get angry. You were so . . . so polite. I guess that's the word."

"And brought so much joy to our lives," Sue added.

For another hour or two they sat around sipping drinks as Emily listened to the Weavers retell many of the little incidences that had happened.

Trying to remember something, anything, about the man, Emily stood alone on the railroad trestle looking down into the deep waters of Roundtree River where Jacob Lentz had splashed feet first into eternity.

"Yes, Daddy, it's just what I wanted. I'll treasure it always. I'm glad you remembered my birthday early. You won't forget me while I'm away at camp, will you, Daddy?"

"Forget my little baby. Why, I don't rightly think so. Daddy's little girl, turnin' thirteen . . . can you imagine that? Where's the time gone? You were always such a pretty thing in your fussy dresses and them socks with the lace on 'em and them white shiny shoes with the bows on top . . . always such a good little girl . . . Daddy loves ya . . . hear me now? And Mama'll get you to the bus on time."

That year, she'd had some kind of religious experience during junior-high week at Camp Chrismont. On the last full day, the day before her birthday, campers had been instructed to find a special rock to carry in a candlelight procession to the top of the mountain to be used in building an outdoor altar. Upon placing the rock on the pile, each camper was supposed to make a personal vow to God.

Emily remembered praying: *Dear God. I promise I will always be good to little children.* Immediately, a warm peaceful feeling had come over the teenager. A connection with the cosmos, perhaps. Pastor Miller would've called it the Holy Spirit.

When she'd come home on Saturday morning, Uncle Dave and Uncle Phil were waiting in the church parking lot with grim expressions on their faces.

"Emily darling, there's been a terrible accident." Uncle Phil tried to put his arms around her but she pushed him away. "Your daddy fell over the railroad trestle and . . . and drowned."

The rest of the day had been a blur.

At the viewing of the body on Sunday afternoon, the funeral home had been packed with lots of sympathizers. Dressed for the role in a black silk dress with a matching pillbox hat and spiked, open-toed black leather heels, Gladys stood by the open casket relishing the accolades bestowed upon her newly-late husband.

Men and women, some of whom Emily had never remembered seeing before, would look at her, tell her not to cry and say things like:

Your daddy was a good man.

It was God's will.

He's in a better place now.

Daddy's little girl had wanted to believe what they said but for some reason she was positive Jacob Lentz had gone straight to hell.

As the memory was floating away, Emily heard the lonesome, drawn-out moan of a train's engine somewhere off in the distance. And smelled coal smoke.

Night train . . . night train . . . coming around the bend.

Impossible! Steam engines went out in the '50s, didn't they?

Reaching into the pocket of her warmups, she put her fingers on the last present her father ever gave her. She took it out and carefully examined the heavily tarnished 1887 silver dollar. Printed above the lady's head were the letters: *E Pluribus Unum.*

At the moment, Emily Lentz Klein, Ph.D., her mind dampened by the early Sunday morning fog, couldn't even remember what the Latin words meant.

Chapter 11

Emily no longer had a choice.

If she wanted to remain a therapist, if she ever hoped for peace again in her own soul, she'd have to go where she didn't want to go—even as her clients so often found they had to—into the past . . . deeper and farther than she herself had ever plunged. She made an appointment for Friday afternoon, June 9, 1989, to see Dr. Julie Jacobson, a Charleston psychologist and medical school professor, an internationally-known expert in clinical hypnosis, and a published author about her experiences as a child of Holocaust victims.

"May I have your permission to tape the session?" Julie asked as Emily handed her the paperwork she had completed in the waiting room.

"By all means. Is it okay if I lie on the couch looking the other way? I think Freud would like that."

"Of course, whatever makes you most comfortable," Julie laughed, pushing the record button.

From somewhere outside herself, Emily listened intently to the two voices in the room:

It's been a long time. My records show you were last here in the late seventies as the therapy requirement in graduate school. Weren't you in one of my hypnosis classes, too?

Yes, and I must say that has proved to be the most valuable class I took. My very first client was MPD, and if I hadn't understood some of the principles of hypnosis, I don't know exactly how I would've worked with him. That's probably one reason I feel like I'm coming apart now. He was killed almost three months ago.

An accident?

No, it was a gruesome murder, and I'd rather not talk about it today. I know I should be feeling sad and angry and all that—

How *do* you feel?

Nothing really. Right now, just numb. But I realize that's self-protective. If I could only cry about it. But if you remember from the other time I was here . . . crying . . . I've never been much of a crier. Wish I could. Occasionally, I'll cry at sad movies. Or when I get really angry. But I didn't come here just to talk about the murder.

So how do you think I can help you?

Well, until recently, I thought everything was going fine. Then my husband and I began having some problems. I think it has to do with my work . . . he doesn't think I'm spending enough time with him . . . and to put it frankly, our sex life has about gone kaput . . . but that's not all the problem.

What else is there?

To tell the truth, I've been wondering if I might have been sexually abused as a child.

Sexually abused? I don't remember our talking about that when you were here before.

I didn't have those feelings then. But now sometimes when I'm in bed with my husband, I can hardly stand for him to touch me, and sometimes I sorta blank out when we're making love. And I wonder if that's why I've gained so much weight . . . so I won't be attractive and he'll stay away.

There could be many reasons for sexual problems. Is everything all right physically?

As far as I know, but it's been several years since I've seen a doctor. Except for my weight which goes up and down, I'm pretty healthy. I get a lot of exercise, mostly swimming. But lately I've been real hyper. Not even the self-hypnosis you taught me, which I'm pretty good at, seems to help calm me down. It's like I'm . . . I'm . . . revved. Sorta like the feeling I get when I look in the rearview mirror and see a cop with his blue light flashing—except it won't go away. Sometimes I don't sleep but three or four hours at night. And sometimes it gets so . . . so unbearable . . . I wonder if the only relief would be a complete meltdown of my senses . . . to get to the core.

Are you menopausal?

Not that I know of. I had a hysterectomy when I was only thirty-two . . . they left the ovaries . . . no, I don't think it's that . . . at least I've not had any hot flashes.

Emily, I really believe you should get an examination to rule out any physical causes for your symptoms.

I know. I know.

Does anybody in your family have a history of manic-depressive illness?

Not that I know of. You don't think I have that, do you? . . . My father could've been . . . that couldn't be it. I never get depressed. Most of the time I handle things pretty well.

Is you mother still living?

Yes, and she's doing fine; recently moved into a retirement center and appears to be adjusting well. The inside of her suite looks like a picture out of *Southern Living*. I doubt if her life-style will change very much.

Have you told her about the problems you're having?

I tried to, but I suppose she's just not ready to listen.

Your children?

They're doing great. Just great. Someone asked me the other day what I thought the most important accomplishment in my life was, and this may sound self-serving, but I told her it was my children. They never gave us one bit of trouble, and now they're both responsible, independent adults.

Other than the murder, which I imagine has been quite traumatic for you, is there anything going on with your clients that could be triggering your symptoms? Is it possible you could be experiencing secondary posttraumatic stress?

Anything's possible. But I've worked with lots of traumatized clients for ten years now . . . why would my reaction just now be showing up? What I really want to do is explore this sexual abuse idea . . . anything that would help me get my marriage back on track. Now don't get me wrong . . . we have a good marriage . . . the best-friends type . . . only want to make it better.

Have you considered marriage therapy?

Yes I have, and I'm certain my husband would go if I insisted, but he thinks we can work things out on our own . . . and I do too, really, if I could just get myself settled back down. What I was really wondering was if you could perhaps, through hypnosis, help me find out if anything really bad happened when I was little. I was wondering . . . could you help me redissociate?

Redissociate. That's an interesting term. Never heard it used before. Are you telling me you want to dissociate again?

That's correct. If the symptoms I'm having result from forgotten trauma, I'm bound to have various ego states who are holding those memories. If I could access them —

But Emily, that would be risky. It'd take a lot of courage to deliberately evoke buried memories, especially since you're coping quite well. You're a professional person. Successful.

The way I see it, I can't expect my clients to do what I'm unwilling or afraid to do, and I believe that using clinical hypnosis, which as you taught me can open the window to the unconscious, might help me open up any locked-away memories and feelings.

I suppose that's possible, since we know that the hypnotic state appears to be a type of controlled dissociation.

True, and I'm beginning to wonder if someone used it on me to try to make me comply with their wishes.

Tell me about your dreams.

Interesting you should ask. Just the other night, I dreamed I saw several children rushing to get an elevator before it closed. And they all made it except one little girl who remained standing outside frantically pushing the 'up' button as the elevator was going down.

What do you think it meant?

How can I be sure? But one interpretation is that the children were ego states; the elevator—

Looks as if you may have already found some of the dissociated aspects of yourself.

More like they've found me. As I was about to say, the elevator may symbolize the route to my unconscious where the dissociated parts, if I have any, stored the memories so they wouldn't interfere with my life as an adult. Those parts hid away, and now they're trying to get my attention.

Voilà! Looks as if they did it. You've been all stirred up for some reason.

I won't go crazy if I let those hidden parts resurface, will I?

I don't allow my clients to go crazy.

That sounds pretty confident . . . don't think I could say that to any of my own clients. Speaking of memories, one night several weeks ago, I did experience what I believe was a memory that had been repressed or dissociated—a memory of my father using me for fellatio. For months, I'd been waking up at 12:18 . . . well, one night when I woke up and looked at the clock, I heard a voice saying, "It happened at this time."

That must have been your unconscious speaking.

I certainly hope it was my unconscious and I'm not crazy and there aren't any ghosts in my bed . . . what do you think it meant?

What do you think it meant?

Okay, I forgot. You therapist. Me patient. To answer your question, my gut feeling is that my daddy molested me when I was twelve to eighteen months old. That toddler had no words to describe the feelings of being touched, rubbed, licked. Or it could mean that he molested me at 12:18 every night. Or both.

I think you're angry with your mother.

Where in the world is that coming from?

Well, you certainly have every reason to be angry, and it seems reasonable to assume that you're holding her responsible for what your father may have done to you.

Served me up on a silver platter, she did.

What did you just say? I couldn't hear.

I said, I don't feel any anger toward her. If anything, I should be angry with him. My mother said she didn't know. I guess she couldn't have helped what he did.

Emily, about memory, I'm sure I don't have to remind you of the research that shows that some memories are true, some false, and some are partly true and partly false.

I realize that. In fact, I have a very vivid memory of diving head first into the bathtub and going for a swim when I was three or four, which couldn't have happened. But what I'm talking about now is a different presentation of what I believe are memories—or at least clues to what happened to me when I was little.

Tell me about them.

There's not enough time to talk about them all, but lately I've been seeing things just before I go to sleep at night . . . hands with long slender double-jointed fingers coming toward me . . . a shadow of a man standing over me, and sometimes I wake up coughing and gagging. One night, I saw a vivid image of a baby's tiny fist on what seemed to be a foot-long penis. Where else would such a picture have come from, if it were not a memory? Do you believe those were things that happened to me before I could talk?

I can't answer that for you—we really don't know much about pre-verbal memory.

I understand. It'll be up to me to decide what's true for me.

That's right. And as I'm sure you know, memories are not necessarily exact depictions of things that happened at an earlier time, and they can be distorted by things that happened between an original event and the time in which the memory is recalled. There may be parts of experiences that don't even make it to long-term memory—and even if they do, a person has a tendency to fill in gaps so that a logical narrative can be created.

I know that some images, like the one I had the other night, are only symbolic. With my eyes closed, I saw a man's buttocks on one side; a woman's breast on the other. Down in the left-hand corner was a screw . . . just a screw all there by itself.

(Laughter) Your unconscious appears to have a sense of humor.

And there's another thing I remember. Throughout my early childhood, when I'd lie down at night and couldn't go to sleep, I'd do some deliberate imagination, 'going into my story,' I called it. A lot of times I'd be on a metal table and a doctor and his wife—I thought she was his wife . . . could've been a nurse—tortured me. And you know what, I enjoyed it sometimes. The feeling . . . it was a lot like the revved I told you about earlier.

Interesting.

But you didn't answer the question. (Laughter)

Remember. Me therapist; you patient. All kidding aside, we both know you're going to have to find your own answers to your questions.

Sorry, Julie. I didn't mean to get smart again. But this being on the other side is rather uncomfortable. Reminds me of my recurrent dream where I'm swimming toward some illusive island and think I might drown before I get there . . . if indeed there is a place to go.

Where would you like to go right now?

If you tell, you die.

What?

I was just thinking about . . . to be honest, I was hoping we could get right on with things. Something tells me that I'm not supposed to be remembering what happened, that bad stuff will happen if I do. But I know where that comes from. A client—the one who was murdered—remembered and told me something that might help identify one of his perps, and two weeks later they found his—my very first client's—mutilated body hanging upside down in the town cemetery. I'm not worried about being killed, because I don't even know what it is I'm not supposed to tell . . . and now I'm just rambling, or free associating . . . and what I really want from you is to help me discover what it is I don't know. It's as if my mind has been programmed to 'not know' and by golly I want to know . . . I've *got* to know, and that's why I'm here. That's why I came back to the expert.

Are you ready to go into trance?

Oh yes. Thanks for hearing, for understanding what I really want out of this; for not making me go through all that therapy-talk first; for trusting your client to know what she needs.

Well, close your eyes then . . . now take a deep breath. Relax and allow yourself to release the tension that has built up. Release the tension and relax the muscles . . . allowing those muscles to feel more comfortable . . . more in tune . . . and as you take a real—ly deep breath, allow yourself to think of a place where you feel safe and comfortable. . . . If you've found that place, nod your head.

Julie, it's not working. I can't seem to relax. Can't think of a safe place. My clients are always able to visualize safe places in hypnosis and I can't see a darn thing.

That's okay. You can still go inside. As you take another real—ly deep breath, allow your mind to become receptive to new ideas, new directions, and new learning. And as you continue this journey inward, opening up memory files like those in a computer, allow yourself to take stock of what your current goals are in seeking to redissociate. The early learning you received, this learning can always be changed; this learning can be given up if it is no longer necessary to continue to follow its rules and dictates. Any form of learning can be changed. The fruits of learning are flexible. They can be stored temporarily. They can be tossed temporarily . . . And now it's time to give up old, antiquated learning that no longer has any particular relevance in your situation. So you can be restored, so you can move toward new goals, so you can be free, so you can be yourself . . . And what's happening right now, Emily? . . . What are you aware of inside? . . . What thoughts are coming in?

I have an image of a bank vault, the kind holding safety deposit boxes. The door is open to the vault and I have stepped through the thick walls. Looking around I see hundreds of drawers, little ones on top, big ones on the bottom. The vault represents my unconscious. The boxes keep my memories of negative things in a safe place until I'm ready to open them and look at them. They hold my feelings, sensations, behaviors, and thoughts. Many boxes have been opened, the contents examined, and put away again so they don't interfere with my present life. Some boxes stay open all the time; they hold a lot of good memories. Many boxes have never been opened. I'm curious. I've an insatiable need to open more boxes. I don't know how many more. To open a safety deposit box, two keys are needed. With your support, I can begin to open the boxes.

That's really a powerful image. Now I want you to take another deep breath and hold that right arm and hand up: lift it and focus your attention. Lift it in the air. And you see, your ability to take action to lift that arm matches your ability to choose what lines of learning you want to maintain and what lines of learning you want to give up.

I hear what you're saying. Things are different from when I was a little child.

Of course. Now you're a professional person, and you're free to choose to learn new things and to clear your mind of things that are too repetitive, that block you, that wake you in the night. You can begin to toss out those things the way you might clean out that bank vault or delete the documents on a computer. The important thing is that you can choose; you can pick and choose the new, and you can toss the old if you like. You can restructure things because, although there may be a little girl inside who was treated like a toy, there are also other parts who are grown up and mature, who can make decisions to choose new goals, even if those goals involve making your life more pleasurable, more enjoyable.

And more comfortable.

And in a way this is a new type of learning for you. One that is Emily-oriented. So Emily can get the things she wants and be the person she wants to be, whoever that is. And that's perfectly all right . . . take a deep breath now and imagine what it feels like to be liberated, what that would feel like, what that would be like, how it would be experienced. Perhaps it would be a sense of feeling free, of not having to be a certain way, of not having to hide feelings, or deny feelings, but to be Emily in the full spectrum of her experience. To be free to be happy. To be free to be sad. To be free to be angry. To be free to be and experience whatever it is she is experiencing. It's all right to set new goals and to make decisions you want to make because they enrich and enhance your self-image, and not because they're designed to please another person. And so this is a deliberate time when you can pick and choose and sort; when you can make choices; when you can decide what to keep and what to toss; when you can choose to take on new learning. Now, take a deep breath and allow yourself that experience. Tell me, Emily, what you are aware of . . . now . . . in your right hand.

It's in a tight fist.

Open that hand. Open it. Open the fist. Open it. Move it. Become aware that it is a tool for you to use, and you can choose how you want to use it. As you continue to open up the memory files, you can choose what you want to keep, and what you want to throw away or delete. This is something you can be thinking about. Now take another deep breath . . . count backwards from five to one . . . and you can open your eyes to the here and now.

Julie took the tape out of the recorder, labeled it, and handed it to her client whose eyes had become fixed on the recessed light overhead. Holding it like it was the other key to the vault, Emily sat up and read the label: "Old Learning vs. New Learning,"

Emily Lentz Klein was not a robot whose behaviors were controlled by handlers, but a human being with a free will. Learning, not programming, was a more palatable way to describe her early conditioning, whatever it may have been. To help her client, Julie didn't have to know about sophisticated programming techniques. The gifted psychologist seemed to know all about human behavior, learning principles, and the unconscious.

"I trust you can help me with some new learning. Although it's a two-hour drive, I'd like to start coming down on a weekly basis for a while at least. Could you see me on Friday afternoons? My family has a beach cottage not too far north of here, so if I wanted to spend the night, I could."

Julie opened her appointment book. "Want to start next week? That'll be June 16. What about three o'clock?"

"That's good. I'm beginning to understand that before tossing out those memories, which are no longer useful, I need to look at them and try to figure out what's happening in my present life that's pulling them out of the closet." Raising her right arm once more, the client ended the session, "And I think I just might've figured out how to use this hand."

Chapter 12

Kneeling at the communion rail
was discomforting. Emily's hands, reaching to accept the bread, were sweaty and cold. "Take, eat . . . this is the body of . . . take, drink . . . this is the blood of . . ."

When the pastor put the chalice to her lips, she obediently followed his command.

Dear God, she prayed silently before leaving the circle, *what is happening in my life? I feel like I've become the observer of a drama whose characters all look like me, and talk and sound like me, but don't always act like me. Playing different parts. How can I go on like this?*

Hurriedly, walking down the aisle—almost running, as if a spigot on her adrenaline line had been locked wide open leaving her in high gear without a way back to neutral—she became mindful of the chatter in her head.

Psychologist heal thyself.

But first you must see the wounds.

And feel.

Back in her seat, in First Lutheran Church where she had been baptized, confirmed, and married, Dr. Emily Lentz Klein—good wife, mother and daughter, successful psychologist—bowed her head and began a spiritual journey the unenlightened would have called mental illness.

Chapter 13

A long time to live with one woman, Jeff was thinking to himself on the Fourth of July as they rode through the lowlands. He didn't like Emily's little sports car; she wouldn't ride in his rickety pickup, so they'd compromised with a Volvo to use for traveling.

It was the week of their twenty-eighth wedding anniversary and he'd chosen the scenic route to the coast. The Campbell family had vacationed on the island since the early nineteenth century. When Carol and Matt were little, Jeff had introduced them to the joys of his own childhood: shrimping and crabbing in the creek, building sand castles, frolicking in the surf, fishing, sailing. Now, his major decision each day was whether to spend it in a hammock reading or to sit on the deck in deliberate solitude watching the waves roll in. On hot summer days, Emily liked to swim out past the breakers, lie on her back, and just let her worries float away on the tide.

He glanced into the rearview mirror. "Wish that juvenile jackass would get off my rear end. Think I'll slam on breaks and let him run all over me. See if he likes a lawsuit as much as he likes his little game of hot-pursuit!"

"I'm pretty sure the Klan did it." In characteristic non sequitur, Emily ignored Jeff's road rage for the displaced anger it was.

"Did what?"

"Killed Fred Crabtree. Or had it done."

"Good Lord! So this is about that boy. It's supposed to be a romantic vacation—a whole week's celebration, just you and me—and you still got dead Fred in your head."

"Great poetry," she said without smiling. "And no, Mr. Klein, for your information, it's not about Fred. It's about me."

The whole world doesn't revolve around you, he wanted to say, but held back, concerned that she was more emotionally fragile than he'd ever seen her, and he certainly didn't want to do anything to make her literally go off the deep end.

"Jeff, was your daddy in the Klan?"

"How am I supposed to know?"

"I believe mine was."

"What makes you think so?"

"Because last night, as I was drifting off to sleep, I had one of those, what they call hypnagogic hallucinations . . . it's as if I were there and it was happening all over again . . . I was sitting in the car—it was the red Oldsmobile so it must have been 1949 or after—sitting with my mother. She was on the passenger's side and I was in the back seat and we were parked on a lane in Olde Towne, looking toward the Rheinhart plot where they found Fred. I could see people marching off in a distance and they were all wearing what looked like white sheets and those conical hats with cloth over their faces . . . you know with holes cut out for the eyes like you see in the movies, like that old silent one, what was it? *Birth of a Nation*—"

"Maybe you were remembering a movie."

"But it didn't seem like one. And if it wasn't, why in heaven's name was I there? And why were Mama and I waiting in the car?"

"Even if your daddy was in the Klan, it wasn't your fault."

Seemingly satisfied with his response, Emily was quiet for a long time as they passed through picturesque small communities full of history and pride trying to hang on to life, trying to change with the times as fast as they could. Towns dying in their own speed traps—each with its one cop—waiting to get a share of someone's vacation money. Most had a water tower, an old movie theater, a small textile mill, and a church on every corner.

Having become almost extinct with the development of synthetic fibers, cotton fields were back. Wild flowers bloomed along the roadside and poison ivy crawled up pasture fences. Shacks holding TV antennas were being replaced by mobile homes with huge satellite dishes. Yards were decorated with kudzu vines, Confederate flags, and old Chevrolets balanced on concrete blocks.

"It was Casey Paxton."

"What?" She'd forced him to switch gears in his thinking. "What about Casey Paxton?"

"Well, I guess since Fred's no longer around, I can tell you what he said the last time I saw him. In fact, I brought the tape along. It's in my briefcase and I'll play it for you right now if you want me to."

That's just what I need to hear on the way to paradise—a dead man from hell, he thought, but was too sensitive to say.

His wife put the tape in the slot on the dashboard and played it all the way to the last incriminating line:

. . . the last thing I ever recall Mr. Casey tellin' me was if I ever ran when I wuz supposed to perform or if I ever told anybody what my job wuz, he said there'd be the devil to pay; and the payment would be my life—me. And he said to me if I ever 'member what they done to me, I'll have to kill myself. And that I oughta keep the knife with me always in case I had to die.

"It's evidence, Jeff. Fred told and he was killed. Do you think Casey had it done?"

"Who knows. What you have there proves absolutely nothing. What are you going to do with it? Take it to your old pal Tom."

"Oh, shut up."

He did.

She didn't.

"But Jeff, perhaps it *was* the cult that did it."

"What cult?"

"A satanic cult maybe. That's what Fred thought it was."

"Who knows if Fred's abusers were really worshiping Satan? They might've just been making dirty movies." Jeff signaled and pulled into the parking lot at the old Swamp Fox General Store in Hamptonville. "I wish that man had never walked through your office door and into our lives." He slipped on his sandals. They both got out of the car and headed toward the run-down building constructed out of recycled barn wood. It looked about the same as it did in the fifties.

Dressed in standard beach attire—Bermuda shorts and T-shirts with sunglasses now resting on the tops of their heads—they looked like any other middle-aged couple making their traditional rest stop on the way to a week's worth of rest and relaxation.

Walking in over the squeaky wooden floor sprinkled with peanut hulls, a comfortable smile spread over Jeff's profile as they strolled past a dusty case of knives, an old-fashioned carousel of nails, and a cage of crickets revered by fishermen in the lowlands as the best bait for the bream in local ponds.

Except for the signs in the back (from *Men* and *Women* and *Colored* to 'Men', 'Women' — and 'Private'), not much had changed since the times their families before them had made the pilgrimage to the beach in the '40s and '50s. It made him feel good, that sense of continuity.

At least they let blacks come inside, Jeff thought, opening the door to the rest room. A lot of places had not.

Coming back out, he glanced at the old porcelain water fountain in the corner; rusted beyond use, a relic of discrimination in its own right. In the eyes of memory, he could read the unconscionable sign hanging above it: *Whites Only.*

After stretching a little, they picked up a few packs of cheese crackers and Jeff reached into an old cooler which opened from the top, nostalgically lifting two green-glassed, bottled, soft drinks. "When I used to come here as a kid, you could buy a six-ounce one for a nickel; a dime if you took the bottle with you," he said to a customer standing behind him in line. He paid with a five-dollar bill.

"See ya next time," the young clerk's voice followed them out the door.

"Salt marshes, ocean spray, sand, and oysters, here we come!" Jeff proclaimed, buckling his seat belt. A few miles down the road he brushed his hand across Emily's breast.

"Stop it." She slapped his hand, pushing it away.

"Just checking to see if you're buckled up . . . you used to enjoy that."

"But, I can't stand it right now. When you put your hands on me it's like they're . . . dead."

"My hands?"

"No silly, my boobs."

Neither so much as smiled and in silence they continued the trek, passing acres and acres of tobacco roasting under the midsummer sun. Empty tar-paper shacks stared at the road like small monuments of defeat, while crumbling road-side produce stands overflowed with homegrown peaches, watermelons, Silver-Queen corn, and juicy Big Boy tomatoes.

"Gonna find her . . . Ba Bump! Gonna find her . . . Ba Bump! Been search-in . . . Ba Bump!" Singing along with an oldies' radio station, Jeff tapped his fingers on the steering wheel attempting to lighten things up a bit.

"Remember the first time we ever went to the beach together?" Emily asked above the final chords, reaching over to turn the volume knob down. "We were juniors in high school."

"I believe I do. That was the night I told you I loved you and you tucked into your shell faster than a turtle ducking a sea gull's beak."

"I've never understood exactly why I acted like I did," she said, thinking about that night after the prom.

They'd joined a caravan of cars to Windy Hill, now North Myrtle Beach. In those days, the beach, a wilderness away from today's high-rise hotels and condos, had more sand dunes and fewer cottages and plenty of secluded places for teenagers to do what teenagers do.

No wonder she hadn't taken up smoking or drinking after that night when she'd sat around a bonfire following the gang, trying to inhale tobacco smoke, coughing, gagging. A few sips of beer had put her in a quick stupor and she hated it, that sudden feeling of being out of control.

Jeff must've been pretty high because he offered to carry her on his shoulders. She remembered thinking she was so fat she might break his back, although she'd weighed only 115 pounds. Later they huddled on a blanket at the water's edge to wait for morning and were rewarded with the most beautiful sunrise she'd ever seen.

"I love you," he whispered in her ear, waiting for her to return the declaration. For some strange reason, Emily was petrified; couldn't say a word. Springing to her feet, she kicked off her flip-flops and ran down the beach and onto the pier, not stopping till she reached the end. Looking into the ominous water below, she felt the urge to jump. Smelled death. Thought she saw eyes.

"What happened?" Jeff came from behind, putting his arms around her waist.

"I don't know." She squirmed away. "But I feel like throwing up."

"I can understand why," he had said, kicking a rank fish's head off the pier.

Before crossing the Intracoastal Waterway, they stopped at the *Bridgewater Fish Market* for fresh shrimp and oysters. After leaving with the day's catch in the cooler, they had to wait on the drawbridge for about ten minutes to allow a yacht to pass under. A florist truck pulled in line behind them. When the bridge was back in place, the truck followed them over the sandy road, the last mile to the cottage.

"For Mr. and Mrs. Klein," the driver announced almost formally, placing the vase on the front step, unabashedly extending the palm of his hand to Jeff. "Thank you sir," he smiled, looking down at the picture of Andrew Jackson on the bill just placed in his hand.

As the truck was pulling away, Jeff picked up the card, tentatively giving it to his wife, then unlocking the door. With Emily following, he carried the vase inside and placed it on the entrance table.

"It's from Mother." She began to count the roses: "One, two, three, four . . . twenty-seven, twenty-eight. One for each year. Isn't that cute?"

"What does she have to say?"

"It says, 'Sorry I won't be able to be down there to celebrate with you, but I'll be praying for you. May you have many more years together.'" Wadding up the note like it was used facial tissue, she carried it into the kitchen and tossed it into the trash compactor.

"Why are you so angry?" Jeff was standing behind her. "Is it because she's back there with her sweetie-pie Phil. I saw in the paper that he's Grand Marshal for the parade this year."

"Will you lay off that crap? They're nothing more than good friends." Emily sneezed. "Get those stinkin' flowers out of here, please. Mama knows I'm allergic to roses. I wish she'd just give her money to the poor."

Jeff obliged, taking the vase outside and setting it on the lower deck.

Back inside, he chided, "You should be ashamed, my dear bride. You know her heart's in the right place." He walked over and patted his wife on her bottom. "How about a skinny dip before supper? It's almost dark and I didn't see a soul on the beach."

"And afterwards, we'll be all smooth and wet, and we can hide behind a dune and make passionate, romance-novel, bodice-ripping love, right?"

"I'll second that," he drawled, pleasantly surprised at her apparently recovered ardor.

Get it over, she thought. He was above her, moaning in pleasure. She tried to focus on the stars speckling the sky and the waves pounding at the shore. Relax, breathe deeply, don't panic, you won't suffocate, her mind suggested before going blank. For how long, she couldn't tell. When she next saw him, he was standing, reaching out with strong supportive hands, drawing her up from the sand. And without saying anything, he pulled her close to his body, held her tightly, kissed her passionately.

A firecracker exploded somewhere down the beach.

"Man that was powerful," he laughed softly.

They dressed silently then walked back to the cottage holding hands, stopping on the patio to light the makeshift grill Cleat had rigged from four concrete blocks and a piece of sheet metal.

While Jeff went inside to devein the shrimp and do whatever he had to do with the oysters, she went upstairs to take a shower. Not noticing that the steaming water was turning her skin red, she heard the voice again:

Thirteen.

Puzzled, she tried to think of something else: the upcoming wedding . . . would she still be able to squeeze into the size twelve mother-of-the-bride dress she'd bought in Atlanta? . . . Should her mother and Cleat sit next to each other? . . . What about Phil?

When Emily went back downstairs, Jeff was dumping the oysters, which had been steaming in a burlap sack, onto the picnic table. "Be careful, Honey," she warned. "Don't let that blade slip. It could lay your hand wide open."

Shucking oysters on the island had always been a ceremonial feast for the Campbells and their guests. Standing in a circle around a table, each person awaited his or her turn to receive the morsel, open the calcareous shell, look for the mythical pearl, remove the body, dip it into one of the red hot sauces carefully prepared to test the stamina of the consumer, and partake of the delicacy. Emily had always hated the family ritual. Right that minute, her stomach was churning like custard in an old-timey ice cream bucket at the thought of those salty, slippery, slimy, almost raw globs of grey matter sliding down her throat.

"Don't you worry about me. I'm always careful," Jeff assured. "One thing my daddy taught me was how to use a knife. Sure you don't want to try an oyster tonight?"

"No thanks. But I'll take some shrimp when they're ready. Do you want me to bring the fixins out here so we can eat in the moonlight?"

"Great idea. The wind's blowing just enough to keep the mosquitos away."

Everything was going fine—they were laughing and talking about their twenty-eight years of wedded bliss—until Jeff looked at his watch. "It's almost eleven and I need to call Dad to see if—"

"Dammit Jeff! It's our anniversary." She had tried to keep her mouth shut, but exasperation pushed it open. "Sorry about the cussing, but I just remembered what that half-drunk bastard—sorry again—what your daddy called me last summer when he was here . . . when he insisted on taking pictures of me lying on the beach in a bathing suit."

"What did he call you?"

"A beached whale. He had no right to make fun of me like that."

"I'm sorry, Em. Why didn't you tell me?"

"Ah, that's okay. I know you can't control him," she replied with a semblance of resignation, "but it's worse when he's been drinking, which is most of the time. Why do you think I feel so disgusted when I'm around him?" Before giving her husband a chance to respond, she answered her own question with another vicious attack: "Because I just can't understand why you always stand there and let him slap us both in the face with his attitude and don't call him on it."

"Now calm down, Em. You're getting loud again . . . . I'll tell you why. Because Grandmother taught me to back up and take water. To do what you can to keep a conflict down. I'm sure my daddy didn't mean anything by what he said."

"Would you please quit defending him?"

"Would you please quit picking on him all the time? I'm certainly not a psychologist, but I wonder if your anger at him should really go to your own daddy . . . now that you know what he did to you."

"Maybe so, but it's hard to hate a dead man. And I don't know for sure that he did anything."

They looked at each other for what seemed a long time. Neither seeing nor knowing how it might end.

Don't tell him about the voice. Not now. Was it her own or an unthought-thought?

"I'm going to bed now," she said, dispassionately.

"Yes. You need some sleep."

"Yes. I need some sleep," she repeated, as if bland repetition were a benediction of some sort.

Under the covers, loud thoughts twirled around in her mind in cadence with the ceiling fan: *Yes, need to sleep . . . Gladys' daughter is tired now. And nobody wants to hear about it, including Gladys. Sleep. None of this is happening, don't you know. There are no evil people in the world who torture little children and animals.*

After a while, she gave up her quest for sleep and went downstairs where Jeff was washing dishes. "Honey, I think I'll go down to the water. Wanna go with me?" she asked.

"You bet."

A few minutes later, they were standing at the end of the pier watching sparks from a pregnant moon glittering across the waves like flashbulbs popping in a darkened arena. In solitude, their thoughts meshed: remembering their different versions of the story of "The Night They Fell in Love."

"What are you thinking, my little princess?"

"About the time you carried me on your shoulders."

"Me too."

They stood wrapped gently around each other for a long time.

"Want me to carry you now?"

"Sure . . . if you think you can lift a beached whale."

Chapter 14

Aghast at the idea of having to give his daughter away, the father of the bride paced back and forth through the church library. "But that's what daddies are supposed to do," Carol had said, having planned a simple traditional wedding. To avoid inviting everybody they knew, she'd chosen to be married in the historical Lutheran church on the edge of town with a seating capacity of less than one hundred fifty. No regular worship services had been held at Mt. Hermon since 1985, the last being a celebration of its 150th anniversary.

A lot of Chestnut Ridgers had been brought up in the Mt. Hermon community, once considered way out in the country. The chapel out there had special meaning to both sides of the family. Gladys had been the preacher's daughter. She and Jake, Luella and Cleat, in their turns, had all been in Luther League together.

Many times, but only when Emily and her mother weren't around, Cleat had told how a bunch of good ol' boys would make moonshine whiskey in a still that was down by the branch below the back cemetery gate. What they didn't drink on the spot, they'd haul up in a mule-wagon to hide in the dirt room in the basement of the church.

Who in the world would have known an operation like this—certainly not one for the Lord—was taking place on church grounds? Jake and his father, of course. Preacher Keller, the father of Gladys, would have known. Jeff suspected his Grandfather Klein had also been one of the partners.

Looking for something to take his mind off the gentle anguish of losing his daughter to another man, Jeff picked up one of the anniversary booklets. By force of habit, he skipped directly to the history section, to the only interest he'd ever really had: the larger Past was what captivated him. He so often wished Emily could see it as he did: that the larger perspective was all that mattered; that you'd never get that perspective working only with peoples' hideously tormented (as she never ceased to tell him) individual pasts. That's where she was wrong, he thought, beginning to focus gratefully on the picture of the building and the distraction of words on a page.

Migration from the Black Forest to Carolina was a result of tragic events in Europe's history. During the religious wars of 1618-48 (a series of wars that started as a conflict between Protestants and Catholics in Europe which, in the end, reduced the population of Germany by half), armies lived off the land, taking livestock and burning homes, forcing people out. After the major conflict was over, bands of terrorists still roamed the countryside, robbing and murdering those peasants who had somehow managed to survive the scourge by the Imperial troops of the Holy Roman Empire.

Our forebears had already endured the horrors of starvation, disease and persecution. In the 1670s, they recovered just in time to be attacked by the French king and subjected to the greed and cruelty of French troops. Homes were burned again and peasant families, once more, pushed out into the snow. When the War of the Spanish Succession came to the Rhineland area, history repeated itself and the lands and the people who clung to them were re-devastated.

Facing exile, they followed the Rhine to the Netherlands where there were vexing delays at toll points on the river, then often waited as long as a month or more for a ship to take them across the English Channel to England where the British government, who didn't want them either, sent them on to the new colonies in America. Many of the ancestors of church members here at Mt. Hermon came over as a group on the ship, *Patience*, in 1748.

It took from six months to a year to complete the trip from the homeland of the Black Forest area to Pennsylvania. And a dangerous passage it was, in boats not much larger than today's deep-sea fishing vessels. That kind of voyage must have tested their last reserves of courage and strength. Crossing the ocean took from six to twelve weeks. Greedy captains failed to provide adequate food; storms threatened to capsize ships. There were many passengers who did not survive to reach their new home. Those who made it to the grand New World were often indentured—placed under contract as virtual slaves—to pay back the inflated expenses of their passage.

Jeff stopped reading for a moment and gazed out the window at the old tombstones, thinking about how disappointed he'd been with his daddy's reaction when he'd come home from the Black Forest, excitedly sharing the joy of having found the church of their German ancestors. "What's the big deal?" Cleat had asked. "It ain't whatcha come from that's important in this ol' world, it's whatcha do with whatcha got."

Feeling sad, but not sure if it was because of the imminent wedding or the impossibility of ever 'doing his father proud,' Jeff looked back at the booklet.

When permanently freed of their contracts, there was little good land left in Pennsylvania. In the late 1700s, they began to migrate down toward Carolina, where the countryside with its mountains and valleys and waterways reminded them of the beauty of old homes lost. One of the first things they did when they arrived in these environs was to establish Mt. Hermon, a German Reform church. They called one Preacher Keller, a direct ancestor of the Reverend Keller who was at Mt. Hermon in the early 1900s, from the homeland.

According to still existing old records written in German in the 1830s, a few men in the community had been disgruntled with what was then happening in the church. They signed a protest against "nightly activities taking place in the community." The translation reads further: "As members of this body of Christ, we are duly concerned about the frolics taking place on holy grounds. They are unchristian and demonic. As Christian parents, we pledge that, on our plantations, as far as it lies in our power, we will admonish our children against them and will not allow frolics of any nature."

On an August evening in 1835, one George Klein and one Frederick Rheinhart called a meeting to organize what, in fact, became Mt. Hermon Lutheran Church. The first building was a crude log structure painted red. Now, at that time, people believed in evil spirits. Someone apparently associated red with the Evil Spirit and burned down the structure to get rid of Satan. They built another which was destroyed when General Sherman marched though this area during the Civil War.

After the war, they rebuilt it for the third time. A note in the church register of those years described it as "a substantial frame 30' by 50', an elegant and commodious church. The congregation has from the beginning had preaching twice a month and—

"Come on, Dad." Matt had come into the room. "They're ready for the procession to begin."

"I'm on my way." But being a man who never could leave history unfinished, he stole a quick glance at the final words:

—while it has many members, there are those whose spiritual life is not what it should be."

And laughed softly to himself over them. Twas ever thus, he thought wryly, replacing the booklet neatly in its stack. "Where's your mother?"

"Dad, for chrissake, Mom's already seated. Everybody's waiting on you."

"I'm coming, son, I'm coming. Have I ever let you guys down?"

"You haven't forgotten your lines have you? That sounds like a cover story to me . . . a class-A diversionary-tactic," Matt groaned in mock hysteria.

For a split second, Jeff realized that before long he'd be losing his son as well. Some pretty young thing with beautiful eyes and beautiful manners and all the rare qualities with which Emily had taken his own heart would . . .

He put his arm around his son's strong shoulders and said confidently, "Lead-on Horatio!—before I run from the task ahead." They walked out of the library together like two men; not one man and a boy, anymore.

"Who gives this woman to be married to this man?"

Standing in the sanctuary with his daughter on his arm, the father-of-the-bride answered, "H-her m-m-mother and I." Then turning away as Brad stepped forward to take Carol's hand, to take his place, Jefferson Winslow Campbell Klein went to sit beside Emily Lentz Klein, his own childhood sweetheart, his rock of ages.

Emily wondered if anyone else had noticed Jeff's stuttering. Usually he only stuttered around Cleat. Well, it didn't matter today. Fathers are famous for being nervous at weddings. And mothers. When the congregation stood to sing "O Perfect Love," she opened her mouth, but nothing came out.

Before her stood the young couple, waiting to pledge a lifetime of love and loyalty and commitment; behind sat Gladys and Cleat and Grandmother Campbell as if wedging Jeff and Emily between the past and future. Gladys wore beige lace; Cleat, a business suit; Grandmother, a pink linen suit with a broad-brimmed straw hat and white gloves.

The sins of the fathers are visited upon the children to the third and fourth generations. Emily was hearing one of those verses stored in the noisy Bible her mother had implanted in her mind from such an early age. Go away, she thought, and the next thing she heard was the minister announcing: "Ladies and Gentlemen. I present to you, Mr. and Mrs. Bradley Amato."

After the picture-taking was over, Emily tugged on Jeff's sleeve, whispering, "Before we leave for the reception, I need to go to the rest room. Be right back."

At the foot of the basement steps she saw the room in her flashback where she had been forced to parade naked in a circle of people dressed in robes. Frosted windows were on the east side. At the far end, a miniature altar held a small gold cross.

Emily stood stock-still, rooted to the intangible spot between Then and Now—feeling at once stoic and dreadfully accelerated—realizing that before this moment, she'd remembered only in fragments: the windows and table, a penetrating cross, faceless antagonists, hands.

Perhaps a child ego state stood side by side with her now, as the adult, the professional therapist, tried to see through both lenses of time—to reconstruct in the analytical mind of her adulthood, the 'service.' Behavior, affect, sensation, and knowledge were coming together in an *in vivo* abreaction: a momentary reliving of an event, including in some measure, a visceral impact (the physical aspect often called "body-memory") allowing her to reassociate most of the experience which had been outside her awareness for more than forty years.

As a toddler, having hardly any physical or verbal vocabulary at all, she had parceled out the early experience, including all its 'religious-framework,' allowing her to go on consciously learning and accepting, without disturbance, her mother's Christian teachings.

One part of her brain saw what happened; another relayed the physical shock of the moment to her body; another kept her from recognizing any face which might have been known to her; another had learned, over time, to enjoy the erotic throbbing which nature had meant to save as an overwhelming joy for her someday.

'Emma Wee Wentz,' as she'd called herself at three, had been sexually assaulted in a house of God: the church of Jeff's childhood; the church of his father before him, and the church of their ancestors before that.

And her own father's church.

And her mother's.

Unto the third and fourth generations.

Chapter 15

D o not exploit a client.

The therapist sat at her desk, rummaging through a shirt-box full of old black and white photographs, contemplating a deliberate violation of her own moral code, not to mention a clause in the American Psychological Association's "Ethical Principles."

But if she didn't do it, she'd be giving up the only clear opportunity she could see to squelch the rumors emanating from her own unconscious. Like muddy water spurting from the concrete fountain in the old Confederate cemetery, rationalizations came into her mind: First, the woman is dying and called for me to come to her house to see her. Perhaps she wants me to know the truth. Second, she's not really a client. Just someone dropped into my office by the U.S. Government. Third, she's not really a friend either.

Friend. The word seemed strangely out of place, so separately had their lives evolved. On the other hand, from the first day Linda Lou Lackey had re-entered her life a little over a year earlier, Emily had discerned an unexplainable connection.

"Do you 'member me?"

"Of course, I do."

Hidden under a weary surface of wrinkles was the face of the little girl who had sat right in front of Emily in the sixth grade. In the summer of 1988, Disability Determination Services had referred her to see if, in addition to lung cancer, diabetes, high blood pressure, and rheumatoid arthritis, she had a mental condition. Well, who wouldn't with all she had gone through?

"I wuz a Lackey—Linda Lou Lackey—but now I just go by Lou." Emily was reaching out to shake the nicotine-stained hand, as if three decades or more had not happened at all since they'd last seen each other. The frail-looking woman bypassed the gesture, substituting a firm hug, then pulled away, making eye contact. "Well, I 'member you real good."

"What do you remember?"

Minus a few front teeth, Lou grinned, "You used ta tell me not ta worry . . . that everything would be just fine."

The psychologist had no idea what the woman was talking about; no recollection of ever befriending the scrawny little girl who'd lived over on mill-hill in a shabby company house, often coming to school wearing dresses made from discarded feed sacks with tiny blue flowers printed all over them. It was hard to forget how Miss Amanda Jarrett had mercilessly picked on Linda Lou because she couldn't seem to do her work. That child must've held the record for holding geography books at arm's length: five minutes for every spelling word missed, and if an elbow bent, even slightly, the old witch would rap it with a wooden paddle.

Back in the testing room, for a half-hour or so, they had talked about the town, the times, a few scattered school-days memories. Life had not been kind to Linda Lou. Born her grandfather's daughter with her mother's syphilis and never learning to read or write much, she'd quit school in the eighth grade to marry a man in his twenties. Shortly after their fourth child was born, her husband was killed in a sawmill accident and she had gone to work, first in the cotton mill, then at Syn-Tec.

"Why are you unable to work now?" Emily was expecting Lou to say it was because of physical problems.

"My nerves is shot an' I jus' can't keep up."

"How long have you had nerve problems?" The psychologist wished the question hadn't sounded quite so inane.

But Lou seemed not to have noticed and gratefully accepted a soft drink, appearing to be giving the question due consideration. "All my life, I guess. My mama, she's in a nursin' home now, told me last time I wuz out there, she had ta put me somewheres at nine or ten . . . 'cause of nerves."

"Was it a hospital?"

"All's I 'member wuz, they taken me ta some kind of army hut, one of those big round metal things, to get me better . . . an' when it got dark they put me in a little white cabin-like thing to sleep . . . there wuz other kids out there with beds in a row . . . not too far away from home though. At daytime, they took me back ta the hut where I 'member bein' strapped down. There wuz doctors an' nurses standin' all 'round. Hollerin' at me." Linda Lou had indeed become nervous talking about the experience, patting first her arms, then her forehead with her fingertips. "Put little things on me that stung. Left marks—ya wanna see 'em?"

"I don't need—" but Emily was too late. Lou was pulling up her blouse showing a few distinct red blots beneath the bra line.

"Electroshock," Emily said, not sure whether aloud or in her head, wondering what made her think such a thing.

"What?"

"Nothing . . . nothing to worry about. Go on, now—I didn't mean to interrupt you."

"Well, my daughter, she tried to find out where it wuz at ta get my records, but ain't nobody seem ta 'member such a place that was at a hospital 'round here anywheres."

As Lou was describing those childhood experiences, Emily began to feel nauseous. "I'll be right back," she said.

Returning from the rest room, the psychologist began the testing protocol that the Department of Social Security required.

Upon completion, Emily's formal report stated that the claimant, a slow learner, displayed symptoms consistent with generalized anxiety disorder and that, in her current condition, she would be unable to tolerate the stresses associated with day-to-day work activities.

When Lou found out that she had qualified for disability, she had called to thank Emily for helping get the checks started and asked if she could stop by once in a while just to talk. Feeling sorry for the unfortunate woman and perhaps a little guilty for living on the other side of life, Emily had said that would be quite all right.

The bond between the two women had been cemented one day, six months later, when Lou wandered into the office, spilling bits of a fractured childhood all over the waiting room floor.

"Help me. Please someone help me. I'm dying."

"Excuse me." The therapist interrupted a session with a client and walked out to the waiting room where Linda Lou Lackey, appearing as cold as the icy chill of that early January morning, was shaking all over. As Emily reached for her hand, Lou fell forward, flinging her arms around the shoulders of her childhood friend. "Help me. I'm dizzy . . . feel drunk . . . I'm freezing . . . so scared."

"Take a deep breath," Emily supported, helping Lou lie down on the couch.

"Stop it!"

"Stop what?"

Not answering, Lou's eyes glazed over.

Emily went back into the therapy room where the ten o'clock client was reaching for his jacket. "I'm sorry—"

"Don't you worry about it, Dr. Klein. Whoever's out there needs you more than me right now. I'll see you next week." The fifty-year-old bank executive from two counties away was in therapy, supposedly dealing with grief over his wife's recent death; more accurately, dealing with guilt for having had an affair with a young teller, even as his wife was dying of breast cancer. He left through the back door.

When Emily returned to the waiting room, Lou, with her eyes now closed, was talking, shuddering: "There's a big light above my head . . . so cold, my butt's on cold metal . . . men wearing dresses. Oh my God! There's a saw at the end. Please don't . . . I'll be good. Stop it! Stop it!"

Emily knelt by her side. "Lou, it's me . . . Emily Klein . . . Emily Lentz. I'm right here by your side."

The woman's voice changed to an awful composure. "There's a rag around my head . . .my eyes . . . can't see where I'm at . . . cold . . . so cold. Make me drink somethin' . . . Koolaid . . . no, not Koolaid. Salty. Nasty. Blood. Oh my God! They make me drink blood. Somebody yanks off the rag. Somebody in a Halloween suit."

"What else do you see?"

"Animals hangin' all over. Bloody . . . people dressed up like animals . . . the smell—it's awful." Gagging, coughing, Lou opened her eyes.

"What happened, Lou?"

"He came down over me." Lou stuck her right hand between her legs. "Hurt me bad down there. Then a bunch of 'em took turns." Lifting her hand, she made a fist and began to beat on a throw pillow, squealing, "Dirty, smelly . . . bastards."

"Did you see any faces?"

Lou was quiet for a long time before responding. "One. When he wuz done doin' it, he took off his head." As if surprised by her own answer, she explained: "A funny lookin' head with horns stickin' out . . . and he wuz laughin' . . . he looked down at me laughin' . . . like I wuz some kind of baby doll or somethin'. "

Crossing her arms over her chest as if trying to get warm, Lou began to explain what she had just remembered. "My papaw, he taken me out in the country ta some kind of a buildin' . . . very cold. And he carried me down some steps, tore off the rag. A bunch of guys wuz waitin' at the bottom . . . it wuz bright . . . a real bright light. The walls wuz bright white, you know the way sun's on snow—that's it—those walls wuz made of little snow-blocks . . . a man . . . I 'member he wuz wearing white shoes under that black dress thing . . . or it coulda been a white dress . . . let me think . . . no, it was a white robe, you know like the preacher wears over a black . . . maybe it was a skirt . . . anyhow he puts money in Papaw's hand. The Bull! That's what I heard somebody call him. He was a white man. I know that for sure but his hands were black. Must've been wearing gloves like he didn't want ta get his filthy hands dirty. Anyhow, he lifts me up on the table . . ."

Lou stopped talking aloud, apparently continuing the memory in her head. Without comment, Emily waited a long time, giving the woman a chance to do whatever she needed to do.

"When it wuz all over," Lou was talking again, "they put the rag back on my eyes. This other guy, he picked me up and taken me back upstairs. Next thing I know, I wuz wakin' up in my own bed at the house."

"Lou, what you've just seen in your mind and felt in your body may have happened, but if it did, it was a long time ago. You're a big person now and they can't hurt you anymore," Emily said in her detached, therapist's voice.

But something inside her head shouted: **Lou's memories. God, make them false!**

Clearly back in the present, Lou sat up. "Did I ever tell ya where I wuz born and raised? It's the very same house I live in now. Me and my husband, we bought it back yonder when the mill wuz sold out and they went and got out of the house business."

"No, I don't think you ever told me that," Emily answered, desperately needing to drift into the woman's blatant denial.

After Lou had left that day, a stunned psychologist went into the therapy room, lay back in the recliner and escaped to self-hypnosis, giving her unconscious a chance to repress the message blindly delivered that day by Linda Lou Lackey. To bury it as deeply as she could in the convolutions of her brain.

"There it is!" The psychologist shouted to herself when she got to the very bottom of the box of pictures that the Weavers had given her.

Every cell in Emily's body flooded with adrenaline.

A thousand times revved!

Painfully, revved!

Like waking up in the midst of a nightmare.

The answer to her most terrifying question—uncontrovertible evidence—lay at her fingertips. In that unobtrusive picture of a half dozen men back from their deep-sea fishing trip.

––––––––––––

Shivering under a tattered patchwork quilt in the sparsely furnished bedroom of the little house where she'd lived her entire life, Linda Lou Lackey grabbed the glossy photo from Emily's hand, placing it a few inches from her eyes. "Where'd ya get this?" she asked, looking at her visitor as if she'd just flown straight in from hell, probably forgetting about the desperate call she'd made the day before: her request to see Emily one last time.

Pointing to the third man on the left holding up a king mackerel as long as his arm, Lou shrieked, "Where did you get that? He's the meanest man I ever did see . . . the goddammed Bull!"

As quickly as thunder follows lightning, Emily's delusion of a safe and happy childhood split from **Before** to **After**.

Lou's eyes rolled upward; the lids closing as she fell back flat on the bed. Corpse-like, the woman left Emily in silence, all alone with thoughts racing around in her head like old cars in a demolition derby:

Never should have shown her the picture.

She's going to die and it's my fault.

I'm a murderer.

She's got to be mistaken . . . he was a good man . . . that's what Mama said. And Dick Weaver, too.

Somewhere in the frigid hot room, a clock was ticking: *Can't be . . . can't be . . . can't be.*

If there is a higher power in the universe, and some invisible force directly intervenes in the lives of individuals, and if there is a purpose to everything that happens under the sun—in God's name, what does all this mean?

Emily wanted to run home. Straight to the strong arms of her soul mate. But first she had to take care of the woman who, like a dead character in a horror-movie coffin, was rising up again.

Stiffly balanced, Lou opened her eyes, asking softly, "Who is he?"

Surely the woman must have noticed the terror convulsing through Emily's body, rumbling like a developing earthquake near the fault line, but asked again, this time loudly, adamantly, "Who is he?"

"He was . . . my . . . my daddy."

With both hands, Emily covered her face, trying to hide her deep sense of immorality.

The odor of tobacco steamed though the spaces between Emily's fingers and she felt Lou's cold, rough hands on hers.

"So help me God. I didn't know. I'm so sorry." Lou pulled Emily's hands apart and spoke to her eyes. "Don't ya worry now. Everything's going to be just fine."

The wounded had become the healer.

Emily wanted to believe the words the dying woman had given back. But an unknown something was curling through her insides, crushing to pieces the person she'd thought she was.

Feeling as if she were running in slow motion, Emily heard herself wailing, "It was Daddy! Daddy! My daddy was a monster!"

Jeff saw his wife coming down the walk. Dropping his rod and reel on the pier, he rushed toward her. "What in the hell are you talking about?"

They met on the gangway. Standing at the rail, their ragged reflections rippled in the shallow water below as she described the encounter with Linda Lou Lackey, trying not to omit any details.

After almost forever, Jeff spoke. "The woman could've been wrong. Out of her mind. It's been so long ago . . . perhaps the face she remembered was only similar somehow to your daddy's face."

"For God's sake, Jeff. You don't understand, do you?" Emily asked, feeling that his reaction was too calm, too minimizing.

Wrenching her hands loose from the railing, Emily began slashing the air in front of her dry-eyed face, as if to remove the sight. "It was Daddy! My daddy!" Anguish surged up from the pit of her stomach until the wails finally changed to whimpers like those of a child who can't find her mother.

When Emily came back to herself, she pleaded, "Let's pack up and go to the coast for a few days. I've gotta sort all this out in my mind."

"But Hon, don't you remember? I promised Dad I'd fly him up to Slicky Rock tomorrow to pick apples. Tell you what, if that hurricane tearing up the islands bypasses us, I'll take you next weekend."

"Well, I'll be damned. You son of a . . . as usual, you'd rather go with your old man than me?"

She didn't wait for his response; didn't expect a truthful answer. Jeff would never admit that he was continually seeking recognition as a good son. If she brought this up, he'd only throw it back in her face like a shot of cheap whisky. And he'd have reason to. Because, wasn't she forever trying to be a good daughter to her mother?

You should've never told her about your memory.

"Shut up."

"But I didn't say anything," Jeff said.

The dam on her reservoir of resentment burst wide open and she couldn't close the floodgates fast enough. "Then you go to hell and I'll go to the beach by myself."

"If you'll just wait till I get back, I swear I'll go with you."

"Forget it," she spit.

"Go on and go then. You're gonna do what you want to do any-way." Jeff made his classic reply to their now endless differences of opinion. He headed toward the house, leaving her alone in the darkness spreading over Lentz Mill Pond, immersed in the maelstrom swirling through her mind.

Bull! Bull! Bull!

She tried to think of something else. Of ships at sea and of old soldiers turning their vessels for home; praying, as they surely must have, to make landfall before an enraged Neptune carried them all away in the dark.

Thirteen.

The voice again.

How's that possible? —is Neptune laughing? Somewhere in the dark there may be thirteen of them watching for my searchlight; depending on me. Maybe I am crazy and my ship . . . the Good Ship Fam-i-lee won't make landfall either.

Who do crazy people pray to when their ship is sinking?

Perhaps Jeff hadn't as yet understood the impact Lou's revelation would have on their lives. In the same way the Hubble Space Telescope probing through the sea of space and finding life on one of those far-away planets would change the history of the universe, what she'd just learned about her father would surely require her to revise everything she knew, or thought she knew, about her childhood.

Now she was being forced by that evidence to begin the process of realizing that in some measure—a measure she couldn't yet fathom—the life she thought she knew better than anyone alive, all the days of Emily Lentz Klein from the morning of her birth through today's setting sun, had somehow been a lie.

But how much of it?

Were there people who knew the truth?

And if so, had they been watching her all these years, laughing behind her back? Or watching for some other purpose? Waiting to see if, or when, the fabric of her identity might tear?

She'd heard too many horror stories, witnessed too much honest anguish over the years from the ordinary human beings who'd come through her office door seeking help, to believe that wasn't possible. Anything was possible regarding humanity: people were murdered everyday; tortured to death in third-world prisons; starved or worked to death in re-education camps; maimed by police in first-world jails, burned in ovens; blown up by bombs as they walked down the sidewalk carrying their babies in their arms; or snuffed out in pornographic films.

Anything was possible when dealing with the human race.

Even this.

Without waking her husband, Emily got out of bed at three o'clock in the morning, dressed, threw a few things in an overnight bag, and left for the beach. Two and a half hours later, she was sitting on the draw-bridge with very little remembrance of the trip. Highway hypnosis, she and her colleagues would've called it. Clean-cut dissociation, she admitted to herself. Normal.

All day long she meandered aimlessly up and down the beach as her brain analyzed the data it had been inundated with the previous day.

What am I supposed to do with such dreadful knowledge? Publish it in the local paper? Go on television? Tell someone's mother? Keep my mouth shut? That I can do. It's part of my training.

Near the inlet, she stooped, frantically digging in the sand. For what, she didn't know.

————————

Not wanting to die, the woman felt compelled to kill herself. Rocking. Faster and faster. Staring blankly across the golden dunes, across the black water to the edge of nothingness. She got up from the cane-back rocking chair on the top deck of the beach cottage. As though being controlled by some experimenter pushing a remote button, she went down the steps, across the boardwalk to the beach and up onto the lighted pier. Like a wooden soldier, she marched to the end, paused for a moment, glanced at the "No Diving" sign in the corner, kicked off her flip-flops, climbed up on the rail, surveyed the undefined horizon— and jumped.

Her feet hit the shell-paved bottom, giving her the sensation of having jumped on a pin cushion. Instinctively, a strong swimmer's kick went into action. Using her arms, with support from her buoyant fat cells, she crawled up the heavy salty water until she reached air. After a few minutes of treading on the ocean's restless face, she spotted a flicker on the old lighthouse at the north end of the island. I can make it, she thought, just before a breaker sent her gyrating under water, trapping her in an undertow.

No you can't. You have to die.

The masculine voice was deep and low.

If you remember you die.

If you tell you die.

Images tumbled around the sudsy water like clothes in an old front-loading washing machine: naked women dancing backwards around a fire; a scowling face with protruding cheek bones, bushy eyebrows in a puff of smoke and fire—Neptune? The Wizard of Oz? No, she recognized the face. It was Mr. Earl, the druggist, with red eyes beckoning: "Come to me . . . you are mine," he said, jamming a needle into her tiny arm. "Sleep . . . sleep . . ."

Now I lay me down to sleep,

I pray the Lord my soul to keep.

Ifishudi . . .

The adult surfaced again, bringing up two choices: to kill herself by programming or to reach the 'ship of safety.'

"No child . . . it's not there anymore . . . you must be your own ship now . . . Go back, beloved. Take my hand." The feminine voice was clear and polished and strong.

Something touched Emily's palm, beyond the icy tow and drag of the water. Raising her head suddenly from the waves, the swimmer looked back—only in that moment realizing how far she was from land. In one motion her body turned toward shore as her voice screamed, "No . . . no . . . no," into the nothingness of Neptune's churning, whirring, spinning, empty face. Fully conscious now, she was gasping and choking and flailing, tasting the salt of terror in her mouth like a live thing. She felt her arms begin to cut the swells in slow, deliberate, controlled rhythms, gathering strength for the journey home.

Everything will be just fine.

Next thing she knew, her sticky wet motionless body was lying supine on the gritty sand—

Alone on the beach. Alive.

Overhead, a sea gull cried plaintively. For several seconds, maybe minutes, she observed its plight. Ostracized from its flock. Flying into the wind. Making no forward progress. Standing still. Not moving forward. But not falling down either.

Emily stood up and slowly walked back to the cottage. After taking a hot shower and dressing in a purple knit shorts outfit, she ate a poppy seed muffin, drank a glass of grapefruit juice, and took a long nap—a day-long nap.

The wake-up call came at 6:00 PM.

"What's happening, Em?"

"Nothing much." Failing to mention the suicide attempt, doubting if she ever would, doubting if that's what it really was. Why would a strong swimmer have tried to kill herself by drowning? If it hadn't been so terrifying, it would've been funny.

"Are you keeping up with the storm track?" Jeff asked.

"No, I haven't even had the TV on."

"Well, they're saying Hugo's already devastated the Virgin Islands and will hit Puerto Rico tomorrow."

"Jeff—"

"It looks as though it's heading straight toward Charleston. So you better pack up and come on home. I've called our handyman down there to go by and board up things tomorrow morning. Gotta go now," he said, as if the approaching storm was the only reason he'd called.

And she said, "Okay then. I'll leave in the morning. See you sometime tomorrow afternoon," just as if the approaching storm was the only thing that mattered.

"I love you," he said.

She clicked the receiver in place, having nothing more to say about nothing.

———

At dusk, Emily walked barefoot over the long shadows on the beach, hoping to find a very special tiny shell. *Look, Mama! Sandime!* Carol, or was it Matt? called out in her memory. Every one in the family had always gotten excited when someone found a fragile baby sand dollar that had washed ashore.

She paused to stand in the rippling surf. As the outgoing sand buried her feet, she listened to her thoughts:

Until I began working with survivors of what appeared to be organized groups of pedophiles, my inner and outer states of being remained as divided as land and sea.

Now I realize that even though the land, or outer me, is basically solid; the sea, or inner me, is full of mysteries and sunken memories.

Ego states, swimming within that sea, are beginning to surface in the forms of images, voices, thoughts, odors, body sensations, and dreams. Are they memories? Or merely my imagination.

With the recent revelation by Linda Lou, my sea has become turbulent. To find peace in my soul, I will have to know what happened to me as a child. Not unlike the way the FAA investigates planes which have crashed into the ocean, I will be required to conduct my own search. Looking for a black box where the answers are hidden. Neatly subdividing the area to be searched into grids, taking material from each section, examining the data, trying to solve the crime when I don't even know if there was a crime . . . not sure whether my daddy was a criminal or not . . . all circumstantial evidence.

I must go deep. When I know what horrors are there, I can bring them to the surface one by one—face them, one piece at a time, learn from them—and then allow the wreckage to float away until it's banished forever in the briny waves.

Riding in with the tide, a large, nearly-perfect conch shell—rare for that part of the beach—docked at her feet. Glancing at her watch, Emily noted that it was 7:37. She picked up the shell and placed it over her ear, listening to the whispers of the sea.

As the moon—big, round, and orange—began to slip up through an envelope of black clouds, she prayed—

Dear God . . . please let morning come quickly.

KNOWING

Chapter 16

"All we can do now is watch and wait," the governor was saying. "But first I've got to get off this stupid highway and get home," Emily talked back to the voice coming across the airwaves.

Since leaving the island five hours earlier, she'd been in bumper-to-bumper traffic with natives and tourists, running for shelter. The wind jostled her car, the setting sun was beginning to cast a pumpkin-colored dome over the Midlands, and she still had twenty miles to go.

"Chances of the storm of the century hitting the Carolina coast are steadily increasing," a forecaster warned through the static. "Hugo's center is moving toward the northwest at twelve miles per hour. The military has brought aircraft inland and sent ships to sea to ride it out."

Before going home, she stopped by her office to pick up the mail and check the answering machine. There was only one message: "Hello. My name is Larry Lackey. Lou's son. It's early Thursday morning, and I called to tell you that my mother died peacefully in her own bed about 7:30 last night—7:37 to be exact. It was the cancer that finally got her. She was such a fighter though, until the very last. Dr. Klein, I just wanted you to know that Mama thought the world of you."

Near midnight on September 21, 1989, the autumnal equinox—a day when light and dark are approximately equal all over the earth—a monster storm, packing 135 miles per hour winds and pushing a fifteen-foot wave surge, hit Charleston, then unexpectedly swept inland.

Through the night, Jeff stood at the bedroom window watching longleaf pines dropping like pickup sticks. When the gracious chestnut oak near the pond crashed to the ground, his wife curled under the down comforter and went into a deep sleep as if willing herself to a windless place of safety.

Emily Lentz Klein, the interminable insomniac, slept through Hugo.

Early in the morning, Jeff drove out to the plantation, zigzagging through fallen limbs and power lines strung all over the road. Neither the original house nor his grandmother's more modern Winslow Manor had been damaged.

Grandmother Campbell was in the parlor trying to calm her companion who was hysterical because she couldn't get in touch with her son. Jeff sat down beside Nina Belle, placing his hand on her knee. "I am sure J. D.'s fine, Miz Reed. Phone lines are down all over the place. But I'll stop by on my way home to make sure he's okay."

Jeff burst through the hole in the little brick house in Happy Holler. Too late. Impaled by the splintered limb of a pine tree, J. D., clad in jockey shorts, had met his final moment with eyes open, looking toward his reward. Wearing a bright colored housecoat, Evie was sitting quietly at her husband's side, her hand over his, as though trying to hold him for just a little longer.

Two weeks earlier, the men had been down at the river when J. D. casually remarked, "Bro, I got a feelin' dis be de las' we be fishin' togeter." About that time, Jeff hooked a twenty-two pound catfish and, in the excitement of the moment, never followed up on the comment.

And now his first true friend was gone.

In reality, the Klein/Reid friendship had never been allowed to mature. The two boys, grown to men, had never known how to discuss why their relationship had been infected. Racism in Chestnut Ridge, no different from other parts of the country, was analogous to a disease nobody talked about, or even gave a second thought about. The Blacks who had coped successfully in the days before the civil-rights movement had, of necessity, developed pretense to an art. Their survival had depended on being able to disguise their true feelings and thoughts: smiling when they were angry; laughing when they were sad; and dancing when they wanted to commit murder.

Emily would've called J. D. dissociative, his real-self hidden by stereotype, prejudice, and ignorance. But if he were, was it only in a societal sense and not very personal? Or if it were only a further consequence of physical self-preservation, then where did those thoughts and feelings hide? In what kind of closet? For how long?

The man couldn't read very well and if there had been special education in their day, teachers might have called him mentally handicapped. But he wasn't; he knew too much. At least till the fifth grade, he did. Before then he'd said he could read and write and had even won the third grade spelling bee. One summer morning, all that had changed when Nina Belle had found her son sitting on the front steps of their house with cuts and bruises all over his face and his mouth swollen shut. She'd told everybody, including J. D., that he must have cracked his head on a rock. Which her son readily believed and which belief he'd carried into adulthood.

When J. D. had started talking again, the words were not always pronounced clearly or correctly except when he was angry or singing. "When he be mad, he can talk real plain," Evie had reported more than once.

Jeff bent over and closed the man's eyes. Placing his hand on Evie's shoulder, he consoled, "I'm so sorry. I'll do anything I can to help you get through this."

"It be God's will. I know it. Mr. Reid's in a better place now."

Evie wept.

Tearfully, Jeff unfolded the patchwork quilt at the foot of the bed and tenderly, reverently, spread it across the body.

The house could be restored; the memories recalled. But Jeff would never go fishing with his friend again.

———

Hugo had been unforgiving. No respecter of class or color. In Black Bottom, dozens of mobile homes had been leveled to the ground. Many lavish residences in Chestnut Ridge's historical district—known for their size and ostentatious asymmetry—had sustained major structural damage. At the coast, home owners were not allowed on the barrier islands to assess the damage.

On Friday afternoon, the Kleins flew down to the shore in their biplane. From high above, they could see a new channel splitting the island in half. Salt marshes meandering the west side of the island looked like giant jigsaw puzzle pieces. Shrubs and sea grasses were already turning brown from the effects of ocean spray. Swooping low, they scanned a paradise bombed by nature: a refrigerator here, a stove there; doors, windows, and furniture scattered across the dunes; boats piled up on each other like stacks of cordwood.

No way could the couple have prepared for the feelings that came over them when they spotted their cottage, blown clear of its pilings, barely standing in the middle of a road piled with sand as high as the mailboxes along its edge. A side wall was detached, leaving the structure appearing as if it had been a giant doll house ravaged by a little girl in the throes of a temper tantrum.

Looking through binoculars, Emily pointed to the kitchen where all the cabinet doors had been blown away, leaving a lone box of Morton's table salt sitting on the top shelf.

"When it rains, it pours," she said, too softly for Jeff to hear.

Cricket Cassidy was bored. No electricity. No hot water at the shop. All by herself on Friday afternoon, usually her busiest time of the week. Danny was out drumming up personal interest stories about Hugo for Sunday's edition, provided they could get the presses running in time. Their landlord had taken off to the mountains with his dog earlier in the week, asking her to take care of the cat.

She figured this would be a good time to take a look in the basement; to find out why the old man stays down there so much. Sometimes they'd even heard him rummaging around in the middle of the night. When they'd signed the lease, Mr. Klein had made it clear that even though their apartment had an access door, they had no business going down there. He'd padlocked the door from the basement side. Of course, that had made Cricket and Danny even more eager to snoop around.

Carrying a small flashlight in her back pocket, she unlocked the door and went into the other apartment, almost stepping on Puffy Poo who was lying in wait just beyond the threshold. The feeble cat stood up and brushed against Cricket's legs. How could such a grumpy old codger have such an affectionate cat? she wondered.

After setting out fresh food and water and cleaning out the litter box, she walked down the hallway and opened the basement door. You shouldn't be doing this, her conscience was saying, but a part of her, excited as a cat burglar—she chuckled at the thought—was egging her on.

With Puffy Poo leading the way, Cricket slowly descended the steps, waving the flashlight around like a detective in a mystery movie.

What a mess! But a neat mess. Everything seemed to have its place. Whiskey bottles filled a big bin in the corner. Stacks of musty magazines lined the side wall. A dark, wormy-pine captain's chair and table were positioned below a single light bulb in the middle of the concrete floor. Under the high point of the steps stood a gun safe just like her daddy's.

A brown cigar box hanging over the top edge caught her eye. Standing on tiptoes, she reached up, knocking it to the floor. The lid flew open, strewing the contents all over the place.

Feeling like that cat burglar caught in the act, still holding the flashlight in one hand, she quickly picked up the box and sat down in the captain's chair to examine the find: five yellowed envelopes bordered with quarter-inch slashes of red, white, and blue. The name, Private Cleatus Adolphus Klein, followed by an APO address was typed on the front. There was no return address.

Trusting that the batteries in her flashlight would hold out, Cricket opened and read each letter, all typed by some girl named Katherine on patriotic stationery that matched the envelopes.

Cleat, my love, my dearest darling,
I do not know how to tell you this, but remember the last time we were together? Well, I must have counted the days all wrong because I have missed having the pip this month and I have been sick a lot in the morning. What are we going to do? My father will kill me if he finds out I am carrying your child and I do not know how my mother will react . . ..
I will always love you,
Katherine

Cleat, my love,
I cannot believe you reacted the way you did to my last letter. I tore it up knowing that you could not possibly mean all those terrible things you said. I am sure you are the father of this baby because I have never been with another man. That is, if you are a man and plan to take as much responsibility for this bad luck as I do. . ..
Love always,
Katherine

Dear Cleat,
I am sorry I talked so hateful to you in the last letter but you don't know what it is like being here all alone with our terrible secret. Now that you told me you will be leaving for Germany after basic training, I do not know what I will do. . ..
Love,
Katherine

Dear Cleat,

Our secret is out. Mother caught me vomiting this morning and I told her the truth. Needless to say, she was very upset and called you some very bad names. She went right to Daddy. Well, I do not think you had better come to our house when you get home next week. My daddy said he would have Bill Wilhelm, who is almost a doctor now, take care of it.

My daddy called our baby an IT! And worst of all, he has no compunction about having it murdered or risking my life in so doing and Mother, who had calmed down a bit, said, "We will do no such thing. We will send her to Atlanta to stay with my sister until it is born and then she can give it up for adoption and nobody in this town will ever know how much our daughter has disappointed us; how much she has disgraced the Campbell family name."

Cleat, I am eighteen years old and my parents are still trying to make decisions for me.

Sincerely,

Katherine

Cleat,

Since you will be home soon, I decided to write and let you know my plans whether you want to be part of them or not. I have decided to keep our baby, even if it means I lose the love and support of my parents. Since you have not replied to any but my first letter, I now believe that I have already lost your love and support.

If you should decide to do what society considers honorable and marry me, I will be agreeable to that for the baby's sake. We will have to elope and trust that my parents will forgive us and accept you and our child into the Campbell family.

Katherine

Sadly, Cricket folded the letters, placed them into the proper envelopes, and neatly stacked them in the cigar box. As she was stretching to place the box back on top of the gun safe with one hand, still holding the flashlight in the other, she noticed a faded label, written in a backhand that was barely legible: "Letters from KC—1942."

"Come on, Puffy." The cat followed her up the steps. "Wonder what ever happened to poor Katherine?" She knew what had happened to Cleat. He had become a bitter old drunk. Though she despised her landlord, she did understand him a little because he was a lot like her old man who'd lived out a miserable life way back up in the 'Georgie' mountains.

"Too bad about what happen to J. D. Jr., ain't it?" The older man swatted a mosquito off his cheek. "Hear'd dey gonna bury him quick since der's no aircondition. In de morning at sunrise, I hear'd."

"Dat's a strange time to funeralize a man, but if dat's what his woman wants, dat's all right by me." The younger man relit his pipe, taking a long draw.

"Looks like World War I all over again," said the older.

"Indeed it do," agreed the younger.

On Saturday morning after the storm, Wilbur Lee Jackson and Otis Washington sat swinging their legs off the plank platform, watching the citizens of Chestnut Ridge darting around like lunatics scrambling for ice, water, flashlights, batteries, and candles. At their backs a placard flapping in the breeze advertised, "ICE HOUSE — Arts, Antiques, Garden Accessories."

Most people considered Wilbur Lee an antique in his own right. Come October first, he'd be ninety-eight, but his mind was as clear as the blocks of frozen water he'd once pulled from the galvanized cans in the ice-making tank. There was a time, using the cable overhead to run the crane, he could harvest as many as a dozen at a time. He'd slide the ice cakes out into the storage room and cover them with sawdust to keep them from melting too fast.

For almost a century, Wilbur Lee had been a silent observer of the town and its people. As a chap, he'd gone with his father into every house in town to help carry ice blocks to their kitchens. After he had come home from World War I, he made the deliveries himself until everyone had replaced their old ice boxes with refrigerators.

Sometimes during the Depression, Mr. Jake would send him up to the mountains to bring back a load of moonshine whiskey. When he'd get back, his boss man would always stuff a couple bills in his pocket and give him a few pint jars full of the brew. Wilbur had often told the fellows he hung around with, "Man, it wuz good stuff." To tell the truth, he never really drank much. Mostly kept it around in case of snake bites.

Mr. Jake used to sit on the platform doling out ice chips to the children, colored and white, who stopped by the plant to cool off on hot summer days. Until that terrible accident down at the train trestle, he'd kept it running to make ice for his meat business, or for fisherman to take to the coast or families in town to churn homemade ice cream. By the time the man died, automatic ice-making machines had popped up everywhere and the widow-woman Lentz closed down the plant.

In the '60s, Miss Gladys had rented the place to a couple of guys who poured the ice tank with cement—so it wouldn't be dangerous to fall into—and refinished the old plank floors. They filled the building with artwork and shelves holding dusty old books, tarnished silver platters, pewter vases, and other old-timey pieces.

Held up by steel rafters, the inside of the brick building had survived Hugo's fury. Outside, terra cotta pots filled with fall flowers, molded birdbaths, and wooden picnic tables had been broken up and scattered around the place.

It was cleanup time. All over town, National Guardsman—sent in to prevent looting, to clear roads, cut trees, and deliver generators—were setting up tents and supply wagons.

"Never seen anything like it," said Wilbur Lee. "Ya know it's awful bad when de Friday night high school football game gets called off."

"Me neither," said Otis, who was in his eighties "Praise God, we's still livin', and looks like dis ol' place made it through de storm all right. Sometimes I wonders if we wuz better off without 'lectricity and runnin' water. Den we wouldn't miss it so much when de Lord take it away."

They watched Miss Emily get out of her car and walk into her office in the house where Mr. Jake's mother had lived during her brief marriage.

"Yessir Otis, if I didn't know better, I'd be thinkin' dat young lady over der be de ghost o' Miss Hannah. Somethin' 'bout dose eyes—not lookin' down on nobody, dat fine lady."

Wilbur Lee had loved Hannah Rheinhart with his whole heart, even as a child. His family had sharecropped for her daddy. After coming home in the afternoons from the one-room school in town, she'd take him down by the pond and show him what she'd learned. The young girl taught him to read in the days when Negroes weren't even allowed to go to school. It was a romantic love on his part. If he'd been white, he'd have courted her and asked her to marry him, even though she was several years older than he.

But that couldn't be.

Closing his eyes, Wilbur Lee went back to that lovely, terrible spring day when Miss Hannah had married into the Lentz family. He'd helped his mother do the decorating for the wedding, carrying in the ferns and roses and setting them where the bride-to-be directed.

After the ceremony, Miss Hannah had asked him to drive the carriage down to the station. Loading the couple's bags on train #36—he'd never forget the number of that train—he stood with tears blurring his vision, watching it roll off toward Washington, carrying the beautiful woman with big brown eyes and long soft curls away to her honeymoon.

It would've been better than heaven to have been able to hold her in his arms.

Leaving one eye in the past, he opened the other and gazed toward Olde Towne Cemetery.

They said the church had been full of flowers for her funeral: lilies, roses, and gardenias. Miss Hannah had taught him about the delicate gardenia: "Don't touch it or it'll turn brown and die."

Less than a year after her wedding day, she'd been touched by the evil: they called it scarlet fever. But she was a brave woman and had stayed alive, some said by pure determination, until her baby was born. Mr. Peter Lentz, Hannah's husband, had named the boy Jacob.

"What is it dat Miss Emily does anyways?" The sound of Otis' voice brought Wilbur Lee's train of thought back to the platform.

"Uh. . . . she's a psycho somethin'. One of doz head doctors. Dey tells me she helps people wit problems. Too bad she couldn't of done somethin' about her ol' man. But if you ax me, Mr. Jake wuz good in his own way . . .when he weren't drunk. 'Member when I work for him at de meat house . . . fifty cents a hour he give me and a little extra when I clean up dat basement. Ain't got no idee what all dey done down der. Dey did play poker right much. But I never seen such a mess sometimes after Saturday nights."

"What kind of mess?"

"Things like likker bottles and cigarette butts. Once't or twice der wuz even blood all over dem dirty white walls. Where dat came from only de good Lord know."

Over at Miss Emily's office, a woman was riding up the ramp in a motorized wheelchair. "Why dat be de Rucker girl. Wonder why she be seein' Miss Emily?" Otis asked. "Ain't nuttin wrong with her. She may be crippled, but she shore ain't crazy."

Everyone in the black community felt that little Maggie Rucker had done them proud. In spite of the polio, she'd made something of herself.

"Now guts, she's got a plenty of," Wilbur Lee added. "Takin' on dat ol' doctor wit' all his money and all."

———————

"They've gotta stop! They've gotta stop! God help me! They've gotta stop!" screamed the hysterical woman who had just rolled into the waiting room.

"Who has to stop? What has to stop?" Emily asked, sensing an immediate bond with the woman slumped down in her wheelchair, crying, gasping for breath, whimpering.

"The snakes. I saw the snakes and—"

"Everything's okay. There're no snakes in my office." Emily had come into town on Saturday morning to see if her building had been damaged, and Maggie Rucker had showed up without an appointment.

"I'm so glad you're here, Dr. Klein. I would've called first, but all the phone lines in town are dead. Can you see me today?"

"Sure. Give me a few minutes. I was just mopping up some water around the back door. But first let me get some forms for you to sign."

The therapist got a medical/social history for Maggie to complete, then finished her housekeeping chore.

"You can come on back now."

At the sound of Emily's voice, Maggie managed a weak smile and handed over the papers.

When both women were settled in the therapy room, Maggie began the conversation. "I'm so sorry. I was acting like a child. It's not really the snakes . . . I'll probably always be scared of them. It's the seizures that have to stop. Yesterday afternoon, I was wheeling around the park down by the river and my puppy started barking. I looked up and on the tree limb above, there were two black snakes. Probably harmless, probably trying to get away from the rising waters left by Hugo. For whatever reason, my body begin to shake all over. I couldn't stop it and blacked out for a few seconds, maybe as long as a minute."

"Is this the first time something like that's happened?"

"No. They started after—" Maggie anxiously fiddled with her shoulder-length pageboy and changed the subject. "You may have heard about my charges against Dr. Wilhelm?"

Emily nodded affirmatively.

"Well, right after filing the charges I began having these . . . these blank spells and if they don't get under control soon I might lose my driver's license. Then what would I do?"

The therapist wondered how this attractive woman drove at all, but obviously that was not what she'd come to discuss. "You must be under a tremendous amount of pressure."

"You can say that again. I've gotten threatening phone calls. Even found a dead chicken on my porch one morning. But that's to be expected if you defame one of the icons of the community."

"Have you always remembered what he did?"

"How could we forget?"

Noticing, but not saying anything about Maggie's use of first person plural, Emily looked down at the medical history. "Let's see. You were born in 1949. That makes you—"

"Forty."

"Why did you keep quiet for so long about Dr. Bill . . . Dr. Wilhelm?"

"At the time, I felt degraded, ashamed, and powerless to do anything. Wouldn't you, if you'd been raped by your doctor? In those days, white doctors were gods . . . come to think of it, there weren't any black doctors around here. Anyway, no one in the '60s would've taken seriously the complaint of a poor African-American teenager about a . . . maybe it wasn't exactly rape, but it felt like it. Then again maybe it was. He told me he had to do a pelvic exam. Why that was needed for a college physical beats me. So when my feet were in the stirrups, he stuck his rubber-gloved finger into my vagina and manipulated me to what, I now realize, was orgasm." The client paused, waiting for the therapist's reaction.

Emily was silent so Maggie continued. "Well, after I put my clothes back on, he sat calmly at his desk and wrote out a prescription in big letters. Thank heavens, I stuck that in my diary, which is in my safety deposit box right now, and if this mess ever goes to court—that probably won't happen since he's in the town's good ol' boy club—it's good evidence."

Well, what did it say? Emily wanted to scream.

But her client went back to the presenting problem. "The neurologist called my spells pseudoseizures, whatever that means."

"Can you describe them a little more?"

"Yes. They begin with a funny feeling . . . sorta spinning-like. My body begins to shake and I go out. Coming back, I'm usually numb all over. The doctor said they were probably caused by stress, but I believe it's more than that. I suppose there *was* a lot of stress with my going public about Dr. Wilhelm. From the very beginning, the district attorney refused to prosecute and told me that to protect my reputation in the community I'd better keep quiet, because it's just my word against the doctor's, and no one would believe me. That ticked me off, so I reported him to the Medical Board. Later I called that new reporter at the paper. Danny Evans is her name. She's not a native so wasn't bent on protecting anybody, I suppose. It's a wonder they printed it, me being who I am . . . whoever that is . . . and since the article came out . . . can't believe it's been eight or nine months now, I've been accused of all sorts of things. And Dr. Klein, I must say that I'm getting pretty tired of being called a 'low down nigger' behind my back."

Emily couldn't think of a single reflective comment.

"On the positive side, two other women—white women—came to my office and asked how to file similar complaints."

"And?"

"Of course, I told them I'd help in any way possible. They also filed complaints with the board. From what I've heard, the old devil, rather than having to defend himself, surrendered his license. Suppose that's about the best we could expect."

"That's good."

"Yeah. At least he won't be able to hurt another patient."

"Have you always been unable to walk?"

"Oh, no. I caught polio when I was five years old. Supposedly, I was in and out of the Shriners' Children's Hospital several times." Maggie paused as if waiting for a Polaroid shot to develop. "Even now I can still see a frightened little girl looking out the window, waving at her mama who was crying. There was a quarantine at the time and the nurses wouldn't even let the woman come up to hold her own little girl." Eyes filling with tears, Maggie looked down at her small light-colored hands, now resting in her lap. "I can almost hear the swishing of iron lungs in the ward . . . and when they turned one off, you knew another friend was gone."

"Were you ever in one . . . an iron lung?"

"Not that I remember. Around the fifth or sixth grade they operated on my back and I was put in a body cast, Mama said, for about three years. Sometimes they'd put me on a table and spin me around and around where I seemed to float out of my body . . . like looking down at a cocoon with its little curly head sticking out the top." Maggie closed her eyes. Her lids fluttered, suggesting she may have spontaneously slipped into a hypnotic trance and was viewing the moving pictures in her mind.

It was a few minutes before the client spoke again. "When they wrapped that thing around me, I was just a little girl; when they took me out, I had budding breasts and pubic hair . . . I was almost a young woman. But I must've gotten well, or maybe Mama just never allowed me to be sick again . . . or to be a child, for that matter." Opening her eyes, Maggie looked down at her hands again, as if she might have said something too personal.

"So you did get back to walking?" Emily asked, giving the other woman room to recover.

"Yes, I did. But right after I made the accusation against the good doctor, my legs became real weak again. It was . . . well, it was quite a shock. However, the neurologist doesn't think it's postpolio syndrome; doesn't think that's what's causing the seizures either but she's not sure what is. Thinks it might be psychological and suggested I call you because you've helped a lot of her patients. You know, I thought I could handle it myself until yesterday afternoon when I reacted as I did to those snakes."

"If you decide to work with me in therapy, we'll certainly try to figure out what may be triggering the seizures. Are you having any other problems?"

"Well lately, we just haven't been able to sleep. You know, weird dreams, I suppose from all the stress."

"What have you dreamed?"

"Marvelous stuff," Maggie laughed. "Plumb full of demons hovering over us like cartoon-vultures. And flashing lights. And kids screaming like we all used to in scary movies in the days when Blacks had to sit in the balcony." Her voice grew somber and she said rather flatly, "Sometimes we wake up feeling completely paralyzed."

"That must be terrible," Emily empathized. "It's possible your nightmares represent archetypical images. Have you ever heard of the psychiatrist Carl Jung?"

"The name sounds familiar, but right off the top of my head I couldn't tell you a thing about him."

"He was an early student of Freud," Emily explained, "but later developed some theories of his own in a rather different vein. He came to believe that certain universal images and ideas are a part of what he called the 'collective unconscious'; ideas common to people all over the world, and thus expressed in their arts, myths, religions, and fairy tales."

"Well that would be lovely. Just lovely." Maggie sounded almost as if she felt she were being patronized. "I hope that's what it is, but I have to tell you, a lot of them seem so real, we wake up sweating."

"In addition to PTSD from what Dr. Wilhelm did, you could be suffering a delayed stress reaction as a result of the medical procedures you endured as a child. They must've been quite agonizing."

"I don't ever remember hurting," Maggie said, looking surprised at the directness of her own answer. "How could that be?"

"Perhaps you were able to imagine you weren't hurting." Because of her medical history, Emily had every reason to suspect that the woman had developed dissociative defenses.

"Never thought about it that way." Maggie looked at her watch. "I should be going. My aunt's expecting me for lunch. Don't know what we'll have since the power's still off. Probably pork and beans and a can of sardines . . . not exactly soul food," she grinned. "Already I feel much better, just talking with you. But there're some other things we'd like to discuss. Could I make another appointment, please?"

"Sure, let me go get my book."

Emily came back into the room. "What about next Wednesday at one?"

"That's good. We'll see you then." Maggie rolled over to the door, braking for a moment, then turning her head around to look at her new therapist. "There's one more thing I meant to tell you."

"What's that?"

"Well, it's just that when I wrote to the Shriners' hospital for my records, they couldn't find any."

Sitting alone on the back pew at the Holy Ghost House of Worship, Jeff let his grief take over as he watched the stream of guests flow by, paying their last respects to the deceased. He was the only white person in the church. Mrs. Campbell would've come, but she was in the hospital, having fallen and broken her hip trying to pick up limbs on Saturday afternoon.

The only illumination was the pure early sunshine streaming through the open windows. In the church, a simple frame structure with the outside vestibule sheltered by the roof, two aisles separated the pine pews into three sections. A narrow seating area, where slaves once sat when it was a white church, edged the top of the sanctuary. Down front, the center of a low platform was enclosed by a rail marking the chancel and the sections for the choir. A large central pulpit loomed over the communion table.

The casket was surrounded by flowers wilting in the unrelenting heat and humidity. They were mostly sprays of dyed carnations arranged in designs: crosses, open Bibles, hearts, and a fish. The pall bearers had rolled the body into the church a half hour before the service was to begin. Plenty of time for good-byes.

Jeff walked down front to take his place in line behind Wilbur Lee and Otis. When it was his turn, he looked down to see a smile of natural happiness preserved on the face, its wrinkles etched deep by a lifetime of struggles. The man was lying with his huge hands crossed over his chest, dressed in a white polyester suit—peaceful, pure and clean for the Lord. A boutonniere on the lapel had been sprayed yellow to match his tie.

J. D. Reid Jr. was dressed to meet his maker. He looked fine.

As Jeff walked back to his seat, a woman in a center pew began to sing, "Soona will be done-a with de troubles of de world . . ." More a wail, as if she'd taken the dead man's feelings to release for him. Other mourners joined in, singing the old spiritual first sung by their ancestors during slavery.

"In my Father's house are many mansions . . ." A deep resonant voice drew Jeff from his meditation. The church's pastor was leading six men dressed in elaborate liturgical garb down the aisle. J. D. would've been very proud. In his culture, the number of preachers at the funeral was directly proportional to how dedicated the deceased had been to the Lord.

Next came the family. First was Evie, supported by her oldest son. She was wearing a black dress. A veil on her hat hid her tears. The son's wife and the other three children and their spouses followed in birth order.

Jeff felt a touch on his shoulder. It was Nina Belle, mother of the deceased. She grabbed his hand and pulled him into the procession: the highest honor her family could bestow. He entered the reserved section, even before the aunts and uncles and cousins who were lined up according to how close they had been to the man whose life was being celebrated.

The relatives waited in the pew while Evie went up for her last viewing of the remains. Standing over her husband, she caressed the memories of a life well lived. At one point, appearing to weaken with the burdens of the world, she fell gracefully to her knees. Two undertakers clutched her arms, bringing the widow back to her feet.

Slowly she reached out and touched her life-mate's stone-cold face, then leaned over to impart one final kiss. Bracing herself on a handle of the casket, she shook her head, weeping quietly. After what was judged a reasonable time, the men gave her a nudge and ushered her back to her seat.

Now it was Nina Belle's turn. And Jeff's. They walked forward together and stood side by side at the casket. "I should be in that box . . . it's unfair he went before me," Nina Belle whispered.

"He was my friend." They were the only words Jeff could speak before leading the grieving mother back to her seat.

As the funeral director was closing the casket, a pale-skinned woman with white hair and pink eyes that never stopped moving, dressed in brogans and a wool coat, came down the aisle pounding a tambourine. It was China Doll, the town's most famous nut. Before she 'got religion,' or 'went crazy,' or whatever the case might have been, she'd been known in Black Bottom as the 'whore of the holler.' By all accounts, she'd been a sweet child until she became a teenager and got herself pregnant every year or so. Nobody ever talked much about what happened to the babies.

Each day she made her rounds, and in the past few years she'd even ventured uptown to preach in front of the courthouse. Sometimes, she'd stand there, pointing her finger at passersby and those sitting on the wooden benches, and tell everybody if they didn't get away from the Satan who lived right here in Chestnut Ridge, they were going straight to hell. When she'd speak in tongues, she scared the little children. But mostly when she came around, people, even the homeless bench-warmers, would scatter and move somewhere else.

China Doll walked up and looked in the casket, announcing loud enough for all to hear, "This one's for you." She went over and sat down at the piano and began playing, then singing along in an angelic voice, improvising with shouts and extra-long-held notes, "There will be peace in the valle-ee . . ."

This surprise by the woman, who obviously had a gripe with a Satan who was very real to her, threw the audience first into a mild state of shock, then ecstasy, as they joined in her oddly-heartfelt rendition of the old hymn.

When China Doll had done her number, she shuffled down the aisle and straight out the door, never looking back.

Nina Belle had once told Jeff that during a family's bereavement, all feelings of private derision are put on hold out of respect for the deceased. J. D.'s friends and family had honored this tradition by respecting, at least for the moment, even China Doll, the outcast of outcasts.

"We will follow the program," said the pastor, regaining control of his service. After the church secretary had read the obituary, the other ministers participated in the review of a life well lived: praying, making special remarks and giving condolences to the family; acknowledging flowers and other gifts; reading notes from those unable to attend; offering the Prayer of Comfort; and concluding with the eulogy.

As the family recessed out of the church, all of J. D.'s friends and assorted relatives, rhythmically tapping their feet on the floor, joined in singing the chorus of his favorite Negro spiritual, a legacy to his faith in a better life ahead:

Ain't no danger, danger, danger,
Danger in de water.
Ain't no danger in de water.
Git on bo-o-o-ard, git on board.

Hugo had been an equalizer. Amid the symphony of chain saws, the townspeople had pulled together: Black and White; rich and poor; young and old.

On Friday afternoon, a week after the storm had maimed the town and its citizens, Jeff and Emily had stopped by the hospital to visit his grandmother. Later, they went out to check on things at the plantation. As they were sitting on the veranda drinking iced tea, Henry Kiser came up the driveway in a logging truck. The former German POW got out and walked over to talk with the Kleins.

"Have a seat, Henry," Emily said. "Like something to drink?"

"Just what I need, Miz Klein. I can't take this kind of work like I used to."

She poured him a glass of tea.

"How're things going?" Jeff asked.

"Fine. Everything's under control. The crew's trying to salvage as many of the pine trees as possible on that thousand acre patch that Hugo tramped over. You know, working out like this reminds me of the days when I first got over here. Did I ever tell you and your wife about the time when—"

It would probably be a story the Kleins had heard many times before, but they were polite enough to listen again.

"—we stacked those logs on the trucks to look like they were full, when actually we'd left a hollow hole in the middle. But for eighty cents a day, what did they expect?"

"Eighty cents a day?" Emily asked.

"Yes ma'am. The farmers paid the government three-fifty a day for each prisoner. And we got eighty cents to use at the commissary. I still feel a little guilty about it though—playing tricks on Mr. and Mrs. Campbell that way because everybody sure did like your grandparents, Jefferson. They didn't treat us like prisoners at all."

"Well Henry, from what I've heard, due to the short labor supply caused by the war, that kind of cheap labor was a boon for the community . . . and my grandparents, too. Papa Campbell used to tell me stories about the POW's. I remember him saying that y'all were merely human beings obeying orders from the German government and that he couldn't fault you for that."

"Yeah, most of the soldiers I came over with were assigned to the timber industry." Henry took a big gulp of tea. "Work in timber wasn't easy. Cutting and loading the logs on trucks was dangerous. The production quota was high and not easy to meet. The weather was dreadful and the heat was unbearable. And the bugs. I could stand the flies, but I never got used to the mosquitos. As I just said, I was lucky to work for your folks. They were fair and honest and always provided plenty of food and water when we were working."

"I'd never heard about the POW camp," Emily interjected, "until recently when Jeff mentioned that his daddy was a guard out there when he got sent home from the war. Nobody ever taught us in U.S. history that our country kept war prisoners, did they Jeff?" Not giving him a chance to answer, she kept talking. "Wonder if they got the same treatment American POW's got in Germany?"

"Don't know about the others, but as for me, I think getting captured by the Allies in France was the best thing that ever happened to me. When I first heard Hitler had replaced the Christian cross with the swastika, I knew he was at war with us Christians as well as the Jews and you better believe I wasn't proud to be a German in those years."

"How old were you when you were captured?" Emily asked.

"I was barely eighteen when I was called upon to defend the fatherland. And only nineteen when they shipped me over here."

"That must've been awfully scary."

"Not really, Miz Klein. When I first saw the neat white buildings set among the tall pine trees, I knew God would help me get through whatever I had to. Folks, to be honest, I didn't mind life outside the prison as much as I did inside. There were a few fanatical Nazis in our camp who tried to rule the other, usually younger, prisoners. They set up an inner discipline committee and doled out various punishments to the fellows they thought were fraternizing with the enemy. One of my comrades lost his finger in what they said was a sawmill accident, but we all knew it wasn't an accident. Some of the Nazi-types had held his hand under the saw blade because he was seen talking to one of the black women who served our food."

"How terrible." Emily poured a little more tea into Henry's glass. "Chopping off fingers. That must be a universal punishment in barbaric societies. I've heard that Satanists do it."

"And the Mafia," Jeff added.

"I don't know anything about Satanists or the Mafia but to finish the story, there was a two-week period when I didn't have to go to the plantation. Looking back, I believe I was a subject of sorts for some type of drug testing program. Rumor was, our captors—that's y'all," Henry smiled, "were trying to find a truth drug . . . could've been marijuana they gave us to smoke. As I remember, I was taken to the infirmary for several days in a row. They'd stuff a cigarette in my mouth and make me smoke it, which wasn't too bad because it made me feel great . . . high. And then they'd have two men in civilian clothes ask me a bunch of questions. None of us minded it at all. Any way you look at it, smoking dope was much better than going out to work in the forests, and I didn't know any secrets to tell anyway." Henry took a last swig of tea and slung the remaining ice over the porch rail. "I gotta run now."

"Keep up the good work," Jeff said, as Henry walked down the steps. Then he asked Emily, "Wanna walk with me down through the woods? I'm almost afraid to, but I really need to see how much damage we have to deal with."

"You bet. I could use the exercise."

Hand in hand, they headed toward the cabin down by the river that formed the southern boundary of the plantation. Walking over the scattered debris on the logging road, Jeff noticed where Hugo had scribbled graffiti all over earth's fine artwork: a still life—purple asters, goldenrod, milkweed fringed by scarlet-leaved staghorn sumac—decorated the pasture; deer and turkey tracks formed abstracts in the sand.

"Look at that!" Emily exclaimed, as they came to a clearing just above the river bank. The cabin had blown down, it's logs entangled in uprooted, dying honeysuckle vines.

"The old cot still stands," Jeff said, kicking at the soggy canvas with his hiking boots. "Wonder how many times we've made love here?"

"Good Lord! The world has come apart around us, and that's all you have on your mind?"

"Well, this was our little shrine. Remember the first time we kissed?"

Their hideaway had always been special. Little more than a shelter to get out of the rain, it was too rustic for the hunters, and the muddy, shallow water didn't even attract fishermen. As children, they'd explored these grounds together when Gladys had come to play bridge with his grandmother and her friends.

"I remember," Emily smiled. "We were in the sixth grade. But when I got to the seventh, mother forbade me to go to the woods with you anymore. 'Didn't look good,' she'd said."

"You never told me that."

"I never quit coming down here with you either, did I?"

At the ever-flowing spring, Jeff filled an old tin dipper he'd found hanging on a tree limb. "To the love of my life," he proclaimed, offering his princess a drink. They shared the icy-clear, uncontaminated water; then, like old times, lay side by side on the river bank watching the clouds float gracefully through the sky.

"How could a loving God allow such a horrible thing to happen to J. D?" Emily asked, then answered the question herself. "Perhaps it was God's way of getting him out of his suffering."

"I don't know Em. Before the accident, he didn't seem to have any major problems; even seemed to be coping fairly well with his chronic pain. You know, from something he said when we went fishing together the last time, I'm beginning to wonder if he sorta suspected he wouldn't live too much longer.

"A premonition?"

"Who knows? His death was so—killed by a tree."

"It wasn't the tree's fault. Hugo pushed the tree over . . . so I guess he was killed by an act of God. Right, Jeff?"

"For heaven's sake, accidents happen."

"I was just kidding," she said.

He tugged at his wife's elbow, pulling her closer. "I always wanted to tell him the truth about the night he lost his speech."

"What truth—what do you mean?"

Jeff took a deep breath. "Okay, if you really want to know. One night . . . I was about nine or ten and Dad had let me take J. D. coon hunting with us down on the other side of Black Bottom. It was about midnight, when we saw Sheriff Paxton and some other white men come through the woods chasing a young black man who'd been run out of the bus station when they found him peeing in the men's room. I remember my daddy telling us to get in the back of the truck and stay out of the way. Dad took off running, too. Well, they chased him until he fell over trying to cross the creek down there. I saw it all. They dragged the poor man, screaming and kicking . . . they dragged him over to a tree, and Casey pulled off his belt—"

"How terrible! J. D.'s falling on a rock, like his mother said he probably did, would've been easier to accept."

"Will you let me finish?" He gave her that wilted would-you-please-quit-interrupting-me-look. "As I was trying to say, Casey Paxton came over and told us to get out of the truck . . . and the sheriff grabbed J.D. by the neck. He didn't touch me, but I suppose that's because Dad was there and he knew my dad would make sure I didn't talk. Anyway, Casey grabbed J. D. and took him to the front of the truck and slammed his head against the hood, over and over, putting the fear of the devil in that poor little boy, saying something like: 'Boy, if ya tell anybody, even ya mama, I'll cut your tongue out and you'll never say another—'"

"How long have you known it wasn't a dream?" Emily interrupted, this time compassionately.

"I knew all along. I'd always tried hard to forget, but it kept coming out at night . . . I was with a group of men who murdered a black man for sport."

"You were only a kid, a child really. You couldn't have stopped what adults were doing."

"But Em, there were other kids there, besides me and J. D. . . . and one of them was your ol' buddy, Tommy—I forgot to tell you he was with Casey when they first came through the woods. Tommy Paxton. He was as bad as me."

She placed her arm across his chest. "None of you, Jeff, not one of you kids was responsible for what a bunch of grown men chose to do."

"But you don't understand. Can't you see? My daddy was part of it. How could he have been involved in murder?"

"I don't know." Like a mother soothing a betrayed child, she wiped the sweat from his forehead. "I just don't know."

"Hold me," he said softly, not daring to move lest she reject him— maybe forever.

Somewhere in the woods they heard another tree fall, toppling in the oversaturated soil, pulling its root system out of the ground to leave a deep depression in the earth.

Chapter 17

"**W**e have to go in there."

"Excu-use me!" Jeff said. "What would we do in there?"

"Diagnostic repairs."

"You'd do diagnostic repairs?"

"No silly. I was reading that sign behind the counter." On the last day of September, they were at the Auto Care Center waiting for her car to be inspected.

"So Em, what's on your mind?"

She looked across the street at the *Mona Lisa Bar and Grill*. "Something tells me I gotta go down into that basement."

Inside the door, a smirking Mona Lisa, life-sized in pasteboard, lured them to the bar. A waitress wearing a long dark straight-hair wig flitted around. She had no eyebrows.

"I like that costume she's got on," Jeff said. "Shows a little more cleavage than the real lady . . . but I'd have to say the skirt's a little short."

Emily tried not to look.

"Two house beers," Jeff ordered when they were seated, seeming to know his almost teetotaling wife was about to need a tranquilizer.

Twirling around on the stool, Emily was not sure if she were winding up or winding down. Coming to a stop, she studied a print of the masterpiece taped to the mirror behind the bar. For a moment she lost herself in its classic da Vinci landscape: roads leading to nowhere, bridges to nothing, crags evaporating into the mists. Coming back to the real world, if you could call this joint real, she motioned for the manager to come over.

With feigned, slurred speech, she took a sip of beer. "I used to play here when I was a kid." The room had become hazy long before the smidgen of alcohol had any chance to take effect. "Would you believe, one time this place was a slaughterhouse? My daddy ran it . . . killed defenseless cows and pigs . . . cut their guts out."

"Really? So that's what the big table in the basement was for. And the rusted saw on the end." The young man shivered. "It's spooky down there."

"Could we take a look?" Jeff asked.

"Fine with me. Watch out for spiders and snakes," he laughed.

Walking down the steps, Emily felt like a child on a Halloween visit to a haunted house. Dampness and mustiness in the room, along with cobwebs streaming from rafter to rafter, created the ambiance of a dungeon. Camel crickets, the only sign of life, broad-jumped across the floor.

Jeff took out his pocketknife and scraped a section of mildew off the wall. "Would you look at this, Em? These are smaller than regular-sized blocks of concrete. Used to be white."

"Snow blocks," she whispered, but he didn't seem to hear. She walked over to a metal cabinet, about six feet tall, narrow but deep, and read the inscription at the bottom: "'Victory Safe and Lock, Co.' Doesn't look like a safe to me. You could put a little kid in there," she said grimly. In her head she heard banging, clanging, and the muffled cry of a child: *Mommy! Mommy!* She pulled on the door, but it wouldn't budge. "Hon, will you help me open this?"

Jeff picked up a piece of metal from the big table and pried open the heavy door. He stuck his hand in the dark box. "There's something soft crumpled at the bottom. And a hard part. And another." Dragging the objects out to hold in the light, they saw that one was a garment of some kind, fashioned out of a broad-weave muslin; the other, a headpiece made from knitted, black wool trimmed with white around the eyes and mouth. Two slick cow horns protruded out of the top sides. "An old Klan outfit."

"How do you know it's Klan?" Emily asked.

"I don't know. I mean . . . I just know, that's all."

Emily rubbed her hands over the headpiece. "The Bull! Lou's memories *are* true. Can we take it home? . . . and the robe, too. For proof."

"That'd be stealing," he said.

"No, it wouldn't." She'd thrown the switch to neutral, the numb gear in which so much of her adult life had been driven. And with the barest suggestion of a Mona Lisa smile beginning in her eyes, declared, "It's my inheritance."

The Kleins walked up the steps, past the bar, across the dance floor, and out the front door. Nobody, not one soul in the whole place, appeared to notice the grotesque bundle Emily was carrying. It was as if they'd never been there. As if it had never happened.

It was all a dream.

"Get over here quick. Your wife has gone stark-raving mad." Gladys was frantic.

"What's wrong?" Jeff asked.

"She's brought this silly costume thing and is saying it was her daddy's and that he wore it to rape one of her friends. Son, we may have to get her committed somewhere."

"Now Gladys, calm down."

"Don't you understand, Jefferson? The girl's in bad shape. I'm trying to settle her down the best I can. . . maybe I should call Dr. Bill to come and give her a shot."

"Of course. Why don't you call the old pervert?" Emily was yelling in the background. "Just like you used to—is that what you did, Mama?"

"Don't call anybody, Gladys. I'm on my way."

When Jeff arrived at his mother-in-law's apartment, the crisis appeared resolved. Mother and daughter were sitting at the table talking in normal tones. Looking at Emily, he asked, "What happened?"

"I told Mama what my friend remembered about the slaughterhouse and—"

"There's no way my Jake would've done something like that . . . he was a good churchgoing man. Don't you remember darling, he considered you his most prized possession?"

"From what I'm beginning to remember, that's for sure."

"What are you beginning to remember, dear?"

"Mama, I told you back in the summer. Now I'm wondering if something bad also happened to me . . . in a basement. And I've had memories—what I think are memories—of other things . . . I think at Mt. Hermon . . . and in another room . . . a loft or something. There was a stained glass window."

Gladys looked at Jeff. "Don't you see? She's talking out of her head."

"And if I am, it's all your fault Mama. You . . . you should've taken better care of me."

"I have no idea what you're talking about." The mother's face got red and she spoke sternly, as if she were addressing an undisciplined child. "If I had . . . if your daddy had been involved in those kinds of things, I would've known it. I always took care of you. Never let you out of my sight. Took you to church every Sunday. Gave you birthday parties. You had friends over. I bought you nice clothes. Don't you think I'd have known if someone was hurting you?"

"Mama, I know you don't want to hear what I have to say, but please listen. I don't want to believe bad things happened to me. I want to deny the idea as much as you do, but the more I deny, the more I learn."

"But he was so protective of you. Always taking you to doctors."

"You've said that before, and I'll ask you again: what in the hell for?"

"Now Honey, you know I didn't teach you to talk like that. Let's change the subject. Your bringing up all these things . . . to be quite frank, it's the worst thing that ever happened to me." Gladys walked over to the piano and sat down.

"No ma'am. Not yet." Emily followed and closed the lid of the Steinway. She sat down beside her mother and tried to seize control of the conversation. "I need to talk, and I want you to listen. When Jeff and I told you we were getting married, you said 'If you make a hard bed you have to lie in it' . . . well, I didn't make that hard bed when I was a child, but I was certainly forced to lie in it. I'm trying to get out of it now. And all I ask is for you to tell me what you know. Please."

"I would if I could but, as God is my witness, I don't remember anything . . . I just don't remember." Gladys opened the piano, put her hands on the keys, and began to play.

Pressing her hands over her mother's, Emily noticed the long slender double-jointed fingers: hands that had always looked to her like she thought a witch's hands might look. "Mama, do you think you're different from every other human being in the world—from every other human mind in existence? Could it be that things happened that you've blocked out?" Gladys was probably grateful that Emily hadn't given her a chance to answer anything. "What if you had a part of you that Daddy controlled, and that part did things you didn't know, or couldn't remember you did, and—"

"If something like that had happened, I would've known it. And if he did take you to any of those places, it was only a few times."

"What did you just say, Gladys?" Jeff asked, but the old woman ignored him completely.

"Please, Mama, please listen." Pretty please, she felt like begging. "That's all I ask. What if that part of you was created when you were a little girl to handle things that might've been forced on you and—"

"I was never hurt. My childhood was wonderful."

"But you once told me that your grandfather used to kiss you in ways you didn't like and that Aunt Luella had said he fondled her breasts."

"Yes he did, but I used to run from him . . . he never got me . . . I didn't let him get me."

"Okay, then. What if you also learned to run from him in your imagination? What if you developed a personality who lived through it and then forgot it?"

"He didn't mean anything by it. Grandfather Keller was a good man, a preacher . . . a man of God . . . as was my father."

"Well then, why would I recall things that didn't happen?" Emily pleaded for logic from her mother. "Fifteen minutes ago I dared to express my feelings, and you immediately accused me of being in bad shape."

"I haven't accused you of anything, little girl . . . it happened—if it happened at all—it was a long time ago."

"Mama, I'm not in bad shape. And I'm not crazy. Fortunately, I'm not like many of my clients who have life-threatening problems because they endured the kinds of things I'm now beginning to believe also happened to me. You gave me so many good experiences as a child: instilled positive values. You taught me to be honest; to help others; to love God. But you also taught me not to be a whole person: not to feel; not to get close to people; not to remember bad things."

"That's true. I always try to hold onto the good, and in my opinion, sometimes it's better not to feel," Gladys said with no emotion at all.

"How many times have I heard you say that? But Mama, you gotta understand that when I can't feel, I can't love. When I can't let people get close to me, they're unable to love me either, to reach me with their love. When I can't remember things that happened to me—yes, even bad things—I've lost a part of myself. I want to find the part of myself I lost."

"All right, dear. Tell me how I can help you."

Not responding, Emily slid off the bench and walked away from the piano, from her mother.

"There's no way you're ever going to stop that stuff," Gladys blurted.

"What stuff, Mama?"

"Turn around so I can see your face." The child obeyed. "You know what I'm talking about . . . the Devil's always been here . . . always made people do evil things. Out in the country . . . they used to—"

"How do you know that?" Emily's voice had gone as cold as her skin.

With a startled look and a jerk of her upper body, Gladys stammered, "From . . . from what you've told me." She looked away from her daughter and son-in-law, lost somewhere, as if the distance between the piano and the window were a thousand miles of menace and memory.

"Mama, what is it? What do you see . . . right now, what do you see?"

The mother's eyes were vacant, her gaze removed, withdrawn to some other place or time.

There was no mistaking the fact that the person in front of her had spontaneously dropped into a trance. Seizing the moment, Emily began to speak in a slow suggestive voice. "Mama, you've said you want to help me. It's possible you could begin to have dreams that would give some answers to my questions."

"I don't believe in dreams," Gladys said almost formally. Her tone was low, but she wasn't completely gullible.

It was just a dream, my precious. Everything will be better in the morning, Emily seemed to hear the other Gladys talking.

"Mama, will you promise me if you do have dreams or memories about any of this, you'll tell me?"

"Certainly, dear." All at once her mother was back—the smiling mask covering the tracks of her momentary walk away from pure control. "If I have a dream tonight, I'll call you first thing in the morning. You can be sure of that." The mask smiled unctuously and said, "I'm so glad we could have this little talk."

Gladys Keller Lentz put her hands on the keyboard. With the grace, dignity, technique, and emotion of a concert pianist, she crossed into yet another world. This one, apparently more to her liking; more of her own making: a reality all her own, perhaps made a very long time ago.

Emily glanced at Jeff who was picking up the box of evidence that her mother had looked right over. "We should go now."

As they left, the strain of "Dear One, the World is Waiting for the Sunrise" followed them out the door and down the hallway.

"That's the only piece I've ever heard her play without sheet music," Emily said. "She always played it when it was stormy outside . . . Me, I never was very good at piano. 'Can't you feel anything?' my teacher would ask. What was I supposed to feel?" She reached for his hand. "Jeff . . . do you think my mother could be—"

"You should know."

"If I didn't know better, I'd probably be confused. She asked me to forget something that she'd said in the same breath had never happened. Or, 'if anything happened, it was only a few times.' She asked me to forgive Daddy for what she said he didn't do. Said she'd do anything to help me. All I wanted was to be heard. So finally she listened and then said my telling was the worst thing that ever happened to her."

"The woman's not going to change," Jeff said. "Whether she's simply dissociative or . . . well, there's no point in asking her for help. Why don't you just leave her alone? She's an old lady. Part of her must have been a pretty good mother once . . . look how you turned out."

His smile came to rest on her like a delicate handmade lace handkerchief, wrapping her numbness in a soothing balm.

When Emily lay down to sleep that evening, feeling as if she'd been unceremoniously shoved overboard from the deck of the 'Good Ship Family,' she heard a timid voice saying, "I'm so scared."

The little girl in Emily would never hear what she wanted: the truth from her mother. Even if Gladys Lentz remembered it all, she would never admit to any of it.

Sitting up, the adult daughter, ever trying to placate her mother, reached over to the night stand and picked up a pen and paper:

> Dear Mama,
>   Please understand. I didn't mean to upset you; I only thought you might help. As you taught me, I prayed to find out why I was having so many problems, why I couldn't sleep at night, and why I couldn't settle down. And then I began to get answers. Maybe I shouldn't have told you about my memories, but perhaps remembering is helping me heal. I forgive you for not knowing. Please accept my knowing.
>   Emily

Later in the week, Emily received a small package in the mail addressed in her mother's eloquent handwriting. She sat down at the rolltop desk and ripped off the brown wrapping paper. A two-page note was taped to the front of a plain pasteboard box.

> Emily dear,
>   Please accept this little gift as a token of my Christian concern for you and don't feel bad about telling me your memories. I'm so glad you did. Otherwise, I wouldn't have known what was going on. I like honesty, and I appreciate yours. Even tho' we can't agree on this situation, I hope we can forget the past, go on with our lives, and live as God intended us to. If you will just turn everything over to the Lord, I am sure you can find the peace you are looking for. Real peace comes with Forgiving and Forgetting, and plenty of love, which I have an abundance of for both my children, even tho' I don't always express it.
>   I don't understand all of this, but I accept it. There's a purpose in all of it, I'm sure. For me, it has made my faith stronger. It's in the past and there's not a <u>darn</u> thing we can do about it.
>   If I've done anything to hurt you, I am truly sorry and ask your forgiveness. I believe more and more that nothing is impossible when you put your trust in God.
>   Who knows? Perhaps God has allowed these things to happen to make you an even better therapist.
>   Love and Forgiveness,
>   Mother
> P. S. I am praying for your full and complete recovery.

Emily crumpled the paper and tossed it into a wastebasket. Reaching into the box, she pulled out a book bound in blue leather, its title printed in gold.

Glancing at the portrait of the woman sitting on the top of her desk, she implored, "Forgive me, Hannah." Then, with all the force Emily Lentz Klein, good daughter of Gladys and Jacob Lentz, could muster, she slammed the new *Revised Standard Version Bible* against the brick wall.

Chapter 18

There was more to survivors of deliberately inflicted trauma than the experts were teaching. To that, Maggie Rucker was a living testimony. Early in her therapy, it had become apparent that the young professional woman had learned to use her dissociative abilities adaptively, creatively, and in service to humankind. By intuitively knowing how to behave 'Black' in the black world and 'White' in the white world, she'd been able to bridge the gulf between the two races better than anyone Emily had ever known.

In the second session, less than a week after the Hugo snakes had terrified Maggie into a seizure-like reaction, the therapist had routinely spent the hour trying to learn everything she could about her new client.

"Tell me more about yourself."

"Okay then. What do you want to know?"

"Why don't you tell me about your childhood, other than the illness, the polio?" Emily asked, wondering how it must've been growing up black and brilliant in a town where most white folks probably considered Maggie just another little 'pickaninny.'

As if she had been reading Emily's mind, Maggie asked, "You mean, how it was to be light-skinned in a black world and dark-skinned in a white world? Used to be that back in the '60s when 'black is beautiful' was the cry, the darker you were, the better off you were in my community . . . I could pass for white in a lot of places . . . and got a lot of dissing because of it. Doesn't bother me anymore though—my skin color. Most of my people now recognize Blacks come in all shades. And I've learned to accept who I am without apology . . . except sometimes I'm really not sure who I am."

Quickly deciding to pursue that last statement at another time, Emily asked, "Are your parents living?"

"My mother's living, and I don't know about my daddy. She had me at fourteen and never told me who he was." Maggie looked down at her hands. "Anybody would know by looking at me that he was white. The only close relative left is her sister who lives here in town. If anybody knows who he was, it'd be my aunt . . . someday I might ask her. Back to Mama, she is a dear old soul, humble and kind. Never will I forget the day I walked in and saw her on her knees in a white woman's kitchen. Guess that's the first time I knew my place. The next time I felt second class was when she sent me to the Village Diner to pick up fried chicken for supper. Never been there before, and when I walked in the front door, an old white man behind the counter yelled at me, scaring me half to death."

"What did he say?"

"Don't know exactly. Except to go around to the back door."

"That must've been degrading."

"Really tore me up. I went home crying."

"What did your mother say?"

"Something like, 'You shoulda knowed better' . . . as if it were all my fault." Although Maggie couldn't remember her verbal assailant's exact words, those of her mother's had appeared even more hurtful.

The client continued to free associate. "I've always felt different. Not fitting into either my family or my community when I was little. My mama didn't have any education—as soon as I learned to read and to understand money, I took over the business matters . . . even tried to teach her to read but she never caught on—although she was a very hard worker. When I was little, she worked as a maid for the Owens' family."

Emily gasped, quickly turning it into a cough. As far as she knew, there was only one Owens family in town—Uncle Phil and Aunt Luella. About everybody she knew in her childhood had black maids who cooked and cleaned. But the white children had rarely known their last names or anything about their families.

"For a few years, we even lived in the servants' quarters on their place. In essence, we were 'House Negroes,' not much different from the black slaves a century before who worked in the master's house. You'd have to say though, we were a step up from the colored sharecroppers who lived on the spacious plantations outside of town . . . but still not as respected as the poor white trash who could get jobs, if and when they'd work, in the cotton mill. Blacks weren't even good enough to be mill hands in those days, not so long ago." She paused as if needing to know how her listener was reacting.

"Doesn't matter if they're rich or poor, a lot of people have to have somebody to hate," Emily responded. "Go on."

"The man and woman probably thought they were pretty good to us . . . gave us their hand-me-down-clothes . . . let us clean their house, cook their food . . . but there was one place the line was drawn."

"Where was that?"

"We were never allowed to sit at their dinner table and eat with them."

Emily thought about Lossie Mae eating alone at the kitchen table in the house on Main Street. "I'm sorry about the way you were treated."

"No need to be. It wasn't your fault . . . it's just the way things were. But when we lived on the Owens' place, it was better than when we stayed with my grandmother. Granny was real tenderhearted. When I was in the second grade, I use to soil my britches. One day I left school to go over to her house to change clothes. When I got there and she saw what I'd done, she took me out to the pasture and made me take my clothes off and put my hand on the electric fence and . . . that's all I remember." Maggie had told the story without seeming to feel any hostility or any emotion at all.

"That doesn't sound very tenderhearted to me." Emily wondered if the electrical torture could have had something to do with Maggie's current seizure-like activity.

"I should explain. Around black folk, when you call someone tenderhearted . . . I guess you'd say it's a euphemism for . . . for . . . I guess you'd say my grandmother was emotionally disturbed." Maggie's speech became louder and faster. "She was a mean old woman. God was she mean! They say she used to put curses on people. I can't say if she ever put one on me or not. When I was in high school, she called me a whore. No reason to. I was fairly attractive and had lots of boyfriends, but I never went to bed with any of them. Granny didn't like it a bit when I went to the white high school. 'We should stay with our own kind,' she'd said."

"You went to the white school?"

"Yes. When the schools were forced to integrate, I was among the first ten black students invited to attend Chestnut Ridge High School."

"Invited?"

"Neither side wanted any trouble so they apparently decided to start with the best students."

"Surely that was a difficult experience for you."

"You could say so. There were lots of ogles . . . some of the kids even spit on me; there were boys who made catcalls when I walked up the steps . . . never got invited to join any of the school clubs. The teachers were about the same. They were no more ready for a black girl to 'sit for learnin'' than their previously all-white student body was ready to sit next to my black body in their classrooms."

"Did you go to the prom?" Emily had always believed one of the main reasons most Whites didn't want to integrate was because they were afraid their kids would begin to date and marry and have racially-mixed children.

"Are you kidding? I knew my place. No white boy was gonna ask me anyway and there were only a few black males, even by my senior year. The Whites hadn't yet figured out that the black boys could play basketball and football and win state championships for them," she said caustically. "But I did go to the spring dance at my old school . . . my mother had taken me to Columbia to buy a dress. First time I ever went in a store where somebody actually waited on me. It was a princess-style. You remember, with that raised waistline like they had. In the most beautiful baby-blue taffeta. I asked for stockings and the clerk showed me the Red Fox brand with the ugly seams in the back. She apparently assumed because I was a Negro, and that's what most Negroes wore, that's the only kind I'd buy."

"What did you do after you graduated?"

"I was awarded a full academic scholarship to State; majored in political science; then went on to law school at Howard University."

"And you came back home to practice?"

"You sound surprised. To answer your question . . . not for a long time. After passing the bar exam, I went up the road to New York. For southern Blacks, New York City was some sort of mystical place where dreams would come true. I worked for the city a year and a half, but didn't see much real opportunity, so I took some bit parts in off-Broadway musicals and trouped across the country for a few years . . . have you ever heard of the Church of Satan?"

"That's an interesting question." Emily had read about the group founded by Anton Levay, author of *The Satanic Bible*. "What made you ask it?"

"Because when we were performing in San Francisco in the early '70s, a couple of strange-looking men came to my hotel room saying, 'Come with us.' They dragged me to their church for some kind of weird kinky service. I don't remember much about it."

Emily couldn't imagine why Maggie would've been drawn to such a place. Or would've so casually mentioned the experience.

"Why did you come back here at all?"

"Well, because a few years ago my mother had both legs amputated because of diabetes, and I came home to help my aunt take care of her."

Maggie was silent for a long time, as if giving insight a chance to develop, before saying, "There's one more thing." Reaching into the basket on the side of her scooter, she picked up a red diary not much bigger than her hand, dumping its loose contents onto her lap. Unfolding a piece of paper that had been torn off a prescription pad, she held it up for Emily to read. Printed at the top was the name: William B. Wilhelm, M.D. Scribbled below his name, address, and phone number were five words, barely legible enough to read:

IF YOU TELL YOU DIE

"My brain is like one of those machines scrambling numbers for a Bingo game—not knowing which piece is going to fall out. Am I going crazy?" Maggie had asked in a later session.

"You don't seem crazy to me," Emily assured.

"To tell the truth, there's a lot of me I don't know." Maggie looked down and began to run her tiny fingernails up and down on her useless legs. "We want to walk again."

"Pardon me, what did you say? We . . . who?"

"All of us."

"Who are the others?"

"The same that was already," Maggie replied in a deep voice.

Emily had no idea what the answer meant, but thought it sounded profound.

"Could I talk with them?"

"I don't know who 'them' is . . . are."

The last thing Maggie remembered, so she'd later said, was Emily asking if she could turn the camera on.

Extending the session, Emily had played the tape, introducing Maggie to the dissociated parts who'd come out to talk with the therapist: Maggie the Angel, who took her silver-rimmed glasses off and looked around the room; Maggie the Confused, who put the glasses back on and looked at the ceiling,; and little Mag who took the glasses off again.

The child alter looked down at the necklace holding a Tuareg cross and yanked it off. When Maggie, the host personality, came back to awareness, she asked in her usual voice, "What is my cross doing on the table?"

As the picture on the screen turned to static, Maggie spoke with serious astonishment, "Videos don't lie."

And the therapist began the education process, the difficult task of helping her client understand both the positive and negative sides of dissociation.

Finding herself in that drug house in a candle-lit room smoking crack with strangers had been Maggie Rucker's 'great awakening.'

Party Girl had later explained to Emily: "I . . . we're not addicted to drugs. I just thought Maggie needed some fun, needed to get away from all the pressure of being such a hifalutin' respected member of the community."

Maggie, the host personality, had been appalled, incredulous. Two months earlier, she hadn't even known about Party Girl.

Through therapy, she'd come to understand why her life had always seemed intermittent. Now it was possible for her to sense when a new traumatic memory was about to emerge. Together, therapist and client would attempt to plan and pace its emotional release or abreaction, processing it in bits and pieces over a number of sessions to keep it from being overwhelming. This way her activities as an attorney and a musician would not be as likely to be affected.

The snake memory was different. It had all come into Maggie's head as she was sitting in the therapy room with her eyes closed:

The little girl wrapped in wet wool blankets is strapped down on the bed in a hospital room. A doctor wearing a surgical mask comes into the room carrying two boxes. One is black with dials on it. The other is wooden, about the size of a banker's storage box. He sets the black box on the bedside table. He sets the wooden box on the floor.

"Now, now little girl," he whispers. "This won't hurt a bit."

She looks through the thick lenses of the white man's wire-rimmed glasses into his magnified scary green eyes. He carefully removes the blankets and runs his hands over her soft skin, first picking up one arm. Moving it up and down and all around. Then the other. Next, a leg. Moving it up and down and all around. Then the other.

"Beautiful Baby. You are as supple as a lamb on its—"

Suddenly he rips off his mask—

Next thing little Mag knows, she's standing at the side of the bed with both feet in the wooden box. The doctor is saying, "Margaret Rucker. If you ever tell anybody what just happened in this room, I will find you and put your feet into this box of snakes again and they will bite your toes over and over and you will never be able to walk again."

Maggie opened her eyes, rubbing her forehead. "Whew! What an experience. I was there and not there. Even now my feet are stinging."

"Would you like to tell me about it?" Emily asked.

"Of course. It was so real to me, I just about forgot you weren't in there, too." The client went over the memory in detail, then interpreted, "I don't know exactly what he did to hurt me—I can only assume it was sexual—but two things I now know for certain. It couldn't have been snakes in the box. Nobody would've gone to all the trouble to capture a bunch of snakes. Anyhow, those mean guys wouldn't have been able to control snakes, but . . . the black box . . . it had to be electroshock: something very easy to control. But why, Emily? How could a doctor who's pledged to heal—to do no harm—hurt me like that?"

"I don't understand it either," the therapist consoled. "Perhaps someday it will all make sense. Now what was the other thing you know for sure?"

"I will walk again, that's what I wanted to tell you."

"I believe you."

"Thank you, Sister Emily." Feeling as if she might have crossed some boundary, Maggie explained, "In my African-American culture, calling someone sister is the most affectionate, appreciative term you can use."

Chapter 19

"**Y**ou be's careful now,"
Nina Belle said, watching the hunched over mistress of Winslow Manor descend the curved staircase. With a cane in her left hand, Mrs. Campbell let her right hand slide down the bannister. The resident matriarch was dressed for company in a beige linen suit and a blouse printed with the colors of fall, accented with her favorite earrings: tiny shellacked cotton bolls, a gift Jefferson had crafted for her when he was in the Boy Scouts.

"I'm doing fine, thank you. It's so good to be on my feet again. I just thank the good Lord for giving me and my family one more Thanksgiving dinner together." She smiled at her companion, "And that includes you, Miss Nina Belle."

"Well ma'am, dinner's 'most ready. Warmin' in de oven. Now youse just go on out in de front room and wait for de kinfolk."

"That I'll do. My heart's fluttering just a bit, but I'll be all right."

Nina Belle helped her mistress hobble into the parlor and sit down in a Queen Anne's chair upholstered in maroon mohair. "Now ma'am, if you needs anything, just ring."

"Thank you." Mary Katherine Delacroix Campbell glanced at the old-fashioned bell pull, still in use in her houseful of memories. Then, for a moment or two, her eyes fixed on the large-as-life portrait of her deceased husband hanging over the mantle. Clasping the broach over her heart, she talked to his spirit:

Oh dear Winslow, oh how I miss you. As I do our dear Katherine. I loved her so much, and I know you did too. You just didn't always know how to show it. Always stern. Sometimes too harsh with our baby. But Lord, how you cried when your little girl ran off and got married. So did I. But not anything like we both cried when she took her own life. Where did we go wrong, Winslow? If only she'd come to us, we could've helped. We could've saved her from that no-good drunken Klein boy. Everybody in town must've known he was running around with that strumpet of a school teacher. Everybody but Katherine, that is, until she found them together in their own apartment that morning. Poor girl, our beloved daughter. She'd be so proud of Jefferson and his family.

One thing I am sure of, Colonel, I know you were never unfaithful. Always accounting for every minute you were away from the plantation; even shared with me your biggest secret of all, which I shudder to think about in this day and time. But in those days, things were different, weren't they, Sweetheart?

Perhaps someday I'll tell Jefferson. When he's a little older, wiser, more tolerant of the foibles of people. . . . just whom am I kidding? I won't be around long enough for that. And our dear grandson is too idealistic about the way people should be.

From the pie-crust table beside her chair, she picked up a little book that she'd recently found stuck between two larger ones in the glass-enclosed bookcase. Published in 1869, it was a newspaper's account of a trial in North Carolina just after the Civil War. Most of the print was too small for her to read, but it was interesting to browse through the advertisements for that era. A jewelry store hawked, "Masonic and Odd Fellows Regalia by Pollard and Leighton." Duffy's apothecary sold drugs, paints, glass, stationery, garden seeds, and "Quinine Only One Cent per Grain in Ordinary Family Quantities." The Colonel would've been amused at Berry's Drug Store's offering: "Good Segars for Fastidious Smokers," and since he was proud to have been a Shriner, the advertisement by an agent touting "The Georgia Masonic Mutual Life Insurance Company."

Yes, Jefferson has turned out to be a good man. Thank heavens, my love of history rubbed off on the boy. I just hope I live to see his plans for restoring the old plantation house and grounds come to fruition.

When I stand before the judgment seat, I can say for a fact that I did the best I could. That I did everything I knew to raise Katherine's boy right when I got the chance. I listened when he talked about his mean daddy. Tried to comfort him when I saw the belt marks on his legs. Once, I even threatened to have Cleat arrested, but the child had protested: "If they put him in jail, I won't have a daddy."

"Grandmother, it's time for dinner," she heard the grown-up Jefferson saying as he came into the parlor.

"Good-bye for now," she whispered, looking up at the portrait, one more time making contact with the soul of her beloved. "I'll be seeing you very soon."

All of a sudden she felt weak. Heart fluttering. Vision blurry. Hands tingling. "Oh Jefferson my boy, I'm not feeling too well. Do you think everyone would understand if I go upstairs to rest a spell?"

"I'm sorry, Grandmother. Of course we'll understand." He helped her stand and supported her frail body as they walked across the foyer to the dining room. Stopping at the archway, Mrs. Campbell acknowledged her guests: "Y'all just go on without me. Enjoy your dinner now." Her breathing was getting constricted, but no one seemed to notice.

With the old woman leaning on the young man's arm, they slowly climbed the steps. Upon reaching the landing, she turned toward Katherine's room. "I think I'll rest in there."

Leaning on the bed post, Mrs. Campbell waited as her grandson pulled back the spread. When she was comfortably in bed, he asked, "Would you like for Nina Belle to bring you a dinner plate?"

"Not right now. . . . I'm too tired to eat . . . too tired to talk anymore . . . just too tired."

"Okay. Ring if you need anything." He turned and started toward the door.

"Jefferson."

He turned around. "Yes, Grandmother."

"I love you, son."

"I love you, Grandmother. I'll come up again before I leave."

As he walked out the door, Mary Katherine Delacroix Campbell closed her eyes . . . for the last time.

————————

When Jeff got down to the dining room, each person was standing behind his or her chair. Emily and the young folks, Matt, Carol, and Brad, were wearing Saturday-morning casual; Gladys looked dressed for church in a single-digit-sized knit cardigan and slim skirt; Cleat, drink in hand, was wearing khakis with that infernal CK monogrammed above the pocket.

The Hepplewhite table where Jeff had eaten many Sunday dinners was decorated with a centerpiece of dried autumn flowers and colorful gourds. It was loaded with a golden-brown turkey breast and the traditional Thanksgiving fare cooked up by Nina Belle on Wednesday: rice, green beans, creamed corn, cranberry salad, broccoli casserole, coleslaw, and Jeff's own favorite holiday dish as a child: scooped out orange halves stuffed with spicy creamed sweet potatoes topped with melted miniature marshmallows.

Assuming the head-of-house role, Jeff picked up the carving knife.

"Son, don't you think we should have the blessing first?" Gladys asked, looking toward Jeff.

"You go ahead, ma'am." He knew the protocol. His mother-in-law was the self-proclaimed religious leader of the clan.

"Let us join hands." More an order than an opportunity. Gladys looked around the table, making sure everybody had closed their eyes. "Lord, thank you for the opportunity we have as a family to eat together today. And for the many blessings you have given us, especially this bounteous Thanksgiving dinner. Keep us always, close in your loving grace. In Jesus' name, Amen."

"Amen," said the others in unison.

Slightly worried about making his daddy feel left out of the family circle, Jeff handed Cleat the knife.

"Good Lord! What happened to this bird?" Cleat snorted as he began to slice the white meat. The old man never laughed. He snorted.

"It was my idea," Emily answered. "I didn't think we could eat a whole turkey."

"Okay with me." Cleat winked at Jeff. "We're breast men anyway, aren't we boy?"

Ignoring the double-entendre, Gladys looked at her daughter. "Did *you* roast it?"

"Of course not, Mama. You know I don't have time to cook anymore," Emily said without apology. "I bought it at the A. M. E. Zion barbecue sale. They also made the corn bread dressing and giblet gravy."

"That's where that Rucker nigger goes, ain't it?" Cleat, hopefully unintentionally, pointed the knife at Emily.

"Granddaddy, why do you have to use that word?" Carol looked appalled.

"Well Sweetie, that's what she is. Tore this town all up with that false accusation against Dr. Bill. I've wondered some on who put her up to such a thing."

Again his remark seemed more directed toward his daughter-in-law, who picked up on it. "How do you know it was false? You weren't there."

Cleat looked up from his task, this time staring at Emily as if she were the archenemy of his soul. "That's what the prosecutor thought."

"But Ms. Rucker wasn't the only one," Emily argued.

"So what?" He set the knife on the table. "If you ask me, what I believe is that those pitiful poor women jumped on the chance to bleed a rich doctor dry."

"Excuse me." Emily stood up, grabbing the breadbasket as a foil. "I'm gonna go rewarm the rolls."

"Cleat, Phil tells me we're getting a shopping center," Gladys said, oblivious to her distraught daughter. Or perhaps deliberately ignoring her.

"So I've heard. They plan to anchor it with one of those Food Kings."

"We sure need something. When they changed from angled to parallel parking, our downtown died. Us old folks just refuse to park sideways." Gladys paused, as if waiting with baited breath for someone to dutifully play their part and say something like—

"Why Gladys, you're not old," Cleat took the bait. "Because if you're old that makes me old."

"Where are those rolls?" Gladys got off the subject.

"I'll go check on Emily," said Jeff.

He found her eavesdropping on the other side of the swinging door, rubbing her temples.

"I want this day to hurry and be over. My head's throbbing and my stomach's in knots."

"Why is it, any time you're around my dad, you get sick? I don't ask you to live with him for cryin' out loud! Looks like you *could* act halfway decent a couple times a year."

"I can't help it . . . I don't know."

"Well, your mother's not the most fun person to be around either. But please, for the sake of the kids, just try to be civil, will you?"

Emily and Jeff walked back into the dining room together. Before they even had time to sit down, Cleat asked, "Are y'all ever gonna build on this plantation?"

"Why should we?" Emily snapped, as she was pulling her chair up to the table. "I like where we are. And we certainly don't need anything larger for the two of us now that the kids are gone."

"Never," Jeff answered his father's question. "I want to develop it as a park for the public to enjoy. It's a very historic place, really. And anyway, who'd want tourists wandering around on their home grounds?"

"To each his own," Cleat scowled, "but I thought you might want to know . . . one of my real estate buddies has been contacted by an agent for a group of Japanese investors. They're looking for a large spread to develop as a business park." Leaning close to Jeff as he passed him the sweet potatoes, he whispered, "Your grandmother's plantation will be free and clear, as soon as . . . I know you'll be getting Mrs. Campbell's plantation before long . . . it'd be a great deal, son."

"You've always known how I feel about this place," Jeff whispered back, "so, no thanks." Loud enough so everyone at the table could hear, he added, "If it belonged to me, I'd look at it just like Papa Campbell did. He always said he never felt like he owned it except when he paid the taxes. Papa was always asking what right the king had to give away somebody else's land in the first place."

Undaunted, Cleat simply took another tact: "Okay then, would you be interested in investing . . . or loaning me some money to invest?"

"Like I said before, and I'll say it again. I just *ain't* interested in your deal."

This time there was no stuttering attempt to placate his father, Emily noticed, which made his angry defense of Cleat, only moments ago in the kitchen, seem incongruous. Which is it, Jeff? she thought. Which of his personas are you so afraid of: the daddy who once participated in hanging a man or the hypocrite who fixes up bikes for little kids at Christmas? What does the old man really mean to you—good or evil?

"How about your wife?" Cleat spoke as if Emily wasn't there. "Would she be interested in developing part of the old Lentz farm out there where y'all live?"

"You can ask me, you know. I'm neither deaf nor invisible." Her voice was iced with an antipathy no longer disguised. In the space of a single moment, something had changed. Cleat looked over at her, his eyes now an opaque veil: knowing something, telling nothing. Where had she seen that look before? "I'm sitting right here. And the answer is *no*. An unqualified *no*."

They finished the meal in near silence. When Gladys and Cleat had left, the younger folks went over to the parlor.

––––––––––––

Papa Campbell, in portrait, presided over the large room: a museum filled with lovingly-preserved cabinets and curios from a line of hard-working, skilled craftsmen; a library lined with glass-enclosed shelves built in the days before air conditioning to protect books from the hot summer humidity and the cold winter dampness; a music room with a grand piano where Grandmother Campbell had frequently played gospel hymns, Negro spirituals, and Broadway show tunes for anybody who wanted to listen or sing along.

In the center of the dimly lit room, stood an elegant, marble-topped table holding an oversized leather-bound family Bible, the repository of Campbell family records: the births, baptisms, confirmations, marriages, and deaths of over 100 years.

Matt opened the sacred tome and flipped through the pages.

"Careful son," Jeff said, "it might tear."

"How old is it?" Brad, the son-in-law of few words, asked.

"There's no actual publication date," Matt answered, "but look here, right across from this fancy page listing deaths . . . a 'Family Temperance Pledge' —" he laughed cynically, "but nobody signed it."

"Probably printed sometime during Prohibition then," Jeff said, looking awkwardly over his son's shoulder.

Matt moved aside so the whole family could examine the amazing picture of two angels suspended in midair who held up a banner proclaiming in large, bold letters:

Family Temperance Pledge
Believing it to be better for all, we the undersigned solemnly promise by the help of God to abstain from the use of all intoxicating drinks as a beverage.

"Where's Granddaddy Cleat when we need him?" Carol asked in jest.

Under the text, a group of biblical-looking characters were gathered around an ornate fountain. A naked toddler leaned over the edge of the pool with its hands in the water. At the bottom of the page underneath a place for signatures, the artist had printed, "He will bless all who walk before Him in a perfect way."

Matt carefully turned more pages. Somewhere over in the Gospels, he came to a loose, carefully folded piece of paper, yellowed and brittle with age.

"What's that?" Carol asked.

They all waited as Matt unfolded the paper and silently read it.

When finished, he answered his sister's question. "Good God Almighty! It's the oath of the Klan."

"The what?" Jeff asked.

"The oath of the Ku Klux Klan, I said."

"You've gotta be kidding!" Brad exclaimed.

"No, I'm not . . . it's right here . . . so help me." Matt moved to the fireplace and stepped up on the raised hearth; the better to give it a full melodramatic treatment, his impish grin implied.

> **I (name), before the great Judge of Heaven and Earth, and upon the holy evangelists of Almighty God, do, of my own free will and accord, subscribe to the following sacred binding obligations:**
>
> **1st: I am on the side of justice and humanity and constitutional liberty, as bequeathed to us by our forefathers.**
>
> **2nd: I reject and oppose the principles of the Radical party.**
>
> **3rd: I pledge aid to a brother of the Ku Klux Klan in sickness, distress or pecuniary embarrassment. Females, friends, widows and their households shall be the special object of my care and protection.**
>
> **4th: Should I ever divulge, or cause to be divulged, any of the secrets of this order or any of the foregoing obligations, I must meet with the fearful punishment of death, traitor's doom, which is death, death, death at the hands of the brethren.**

Matt's voice had risen in true thespian manner at the final phrasing of the death pledge.

Emily was first to react: "If members of any kind of secret society were to have to take an oath like this, it could surely explain why they never—"

"Tell? Let me see that." Jeff took the faded piece of history in his hands, a tidal wave of questions rolling into his mind. Questions he was afraid to ask, even of himself.

"Nobody ever told me my Campbell ancestors were in the Klan," Carol said disgustedly.

"This doesn't mean they were!" her father erupted defensively.

"But why does your grandmother keep the oath in the family Bible?" Emily asked softly.

"Nobody's perfect," said Matt, attempting a levity he probably no longer felt.

Jeff had wanted so much to believe that when it came to matters of racial integrity, of respecting their African-American brothers and sisters, the Campbell side of the family was pure. But in his heart, he knew there was only one answer to Emily's question.

Chapter 20

"T alking to the dead again?"

Emily jerked and turned around. "Good Lord, Jeff. You scared the you-know-what outta me."

"Sorry. Didn't mean to. Honest."

She had been waiting patiently in front of the tombstone of Hannah R. Lentz, her own grandmother's grave, while Jeff was raking, smoothing out Mrs. Campbell's final resting place in preparation for placement of the marker he'd ordered. "Have you done what you came to do?" she asked.

"Sounds like you *are* talking to the dead."

Knowing her husband was joking to cover the deep grief he was feeling, Emily tried to console. "You know what, I'm positive your grandmother did what she was put on this earth to do. And that was, in my opinion," she brushed her hands across his beard, "to raise the most wonderful man in the world. I miss her so much."

"Me too," he said, as Emily wiped a tear from under his eye. "Since we're here, why don't we walk down to the old section and check on my distant ancestors?"

"Fine with me," she lied. She'd felt antsy all day, maybe angry, and would've preferred being at home swimming laps on this warm Saturday afternoon when it was not quite spring.

They walked down the gravel road to Memorial Garden: a small oasis of beautifully cultivated and well-maintained nature; a sacred island of the dead where only Confederate War soldiers and their families were buried.

Admiring the tiny Johnny-jump-ups in a welcoming bed of flowers, she read the sign planted alongside them: "'These grounds are maintained through a generous trust fund bequeathed by the late General Jefferson Winslow Campbell, C.S.A.'" Slapping her husband on the back, she asked, "Just curious, where did the old boy bury his slaves? Surely it wasn't under any of these Clorox-clean white tombstones."

"For chrissake, Em. I didn't choose my ancestors. And I wish you'd get over it . . . whatever it is bothering you." With his handkerchief, he wiped the moisture from a granite bench and motioned for her to sit beside him. They sat on a knoll looking down a terraced walkway leading to the garden's centerpiece, an elliptical courtyard. Insects, and spider webs waiting to trap them, glittered in the high hedge of holly bushes forming its cloistered boundaries.

In this cemetery within a cemetery, the night's rain lingered in puddles on winding paths, leaving a fishy smell to compete with the delicious fragrance of hyacinths standing captive in the above-ground roots of a gigantic maple tree.

Jeff picked up one of the magnolia cones littering the brick patio and rolled it around in his hands, feeling the texture of the sharp woody petals, looking for seeds. "Used to pretend these were hand grenades when I was a kid."

"Is that a threat?" Emily joked. Knowing this wasn't the best time to bring it up, she did anyway, "I believe the Klan killed Fred."

"So you've still got that Crabtree guy on your mind? It's been a year now. He's dead, Emily. There's nothing you could've done. Just like J. D.'s dead . . . and Grandmother. That's life. And another thing, I wish you'd get off the damn Klan!" He threw the magnolia cone 'grenade' at the yard-tall statue of St. Francis with a lamb in his arms, looking serenely down over the little fish pond. "I just wish things were like they used to be. As it is now, all I do is teach my classes, acquiesce to the administration . . . and dodge bullets from you when I get home. Sometimes I wish you'd talk about something besides your bad memories or your work."

Although his last remark hurt deeply, Emily didn't say anything. She probably deserved it, as critical as she had been of Jeff lately. Instead, she went on with her day's agenda. "Do you believe that present-day evil cults exist?"

"Good grief! How many times do we have to have this conversation? You're always going on and on about secret cults with their secret oaths. Big deal! They've always been and always will be."

"Of course. That's everybody's answer. But I can't help wondering how many adults are out there who saw those cloth-covered faces with the red eyes looking through . . . I've never figured out how they made their eyes red."

"You can't save them all, Em. No one can. That's why there are churches."

"Okay preacher. What about the Nazis who 'churchified' themselves by using the word God? Or the clear inference of a God-ordained mission in so many of their public speeches while they went about planning the work of devils."

"Point taken." He picked up another 'grenade' and rolled it around in his hands. "If you remember, at the beginning of the war, Hitler replaced all the Bibles with *Mein Kamph*, his own rambling political philosophy. Hitler was religious all right but the god he worshiped was himself. And he was quite a student of mass psychology in his own twisted way. *Heil* Hitler! They addressed him *Heil* . . . Holy Hitler. Did you know he was reported to be heavily involved in the occult as a leader of a secret organization known as the Thule Society which believed in white superiority and hated Jews; that he and his Nazi followers were interested in astrology and the paranormal and engaged in secret rituals in one of those castles over there?"

"I've heard that. And I suspect some people considered him God, while others considered him Satan."

Jeff dropped the magnolia cone at his feet. "What I'm saying is, don't go overboard and take every piece of good sense or logic into the sea with you. Historically, every major religion in the world was a bona fide cult before it gained enough acceptance to be called a faith. When Martin Luther broke away from the Catholic church in his rebellion against its open corruption, and what we call the Reformation began, it was little more than a cult of—"

"You can't equate Luther's followers with a cult of the Devil."

"Why don't you come to my Luther lecture sometime?"

"Oh sure. That's just what I need right now, a lecture," and she promptly began one of her own. "What about those snake charmers up in the mountains who regularly trance themselves out, believing—so they say—the snakes won't bite them because it's all for God. Would you call that ritualistic? Would you call that a cult of some kind?"

"Maybe," he allowed, "but they're not hurting anybody but themselves, after all. And it's a free country, isn't it? People can believe whatever they want to. Besides, they're fascinating. Ask anyone who's seen them dance-in-a-trance on public TV. They're simply paving a path to the Pearly Gates in their own inimitable way; they quote scripture just like everybody else to prove it's a sign of their faith. God won't punish them for—"

"My mother quotes scripture to—"

"Your mother is a fine Christian woman who couldn't live one day of her faith if she didn't have somebody to forgive."

"Well it just so happens that she and I have different ideas about forgiveness. Personally I don't think God expects me to forgive someone who admits no wrong. And anyway, I don't want to talk about my mother right now." She stood up and walked over to the old fountain. Stepping on the foot pump, a geyser of lukewarm water spewed up her nose. She wiped it off with her shirt sleeve. "It's all very generational like the Klan was for so long. And may still be for all we know. 'No cults in Chestnut Ridge,' they say. So what about the KKK? We both know that in our town, some people, including Casey Paxton, are still proud and public about their Klan membership. Hasn't been too long since they marched in the Christmas parade."

He stood up and headed toward the gate.

"Wait just a minute," Emily followed. "I'm not quite finished with this conversation." She caught up and jumped in front of him, positioning herself with legs wide apart, planting them firmly on the ground like she'd done as a high school basketball player trying to draw a charge foul. "Under your liberal exterior are you secretly a racist? What else don't I know about you, Jeff?"

"That was a low cut."

"I apologize; shouldn't have said it. But right now I feel so angry about everything that's been happening. About what they did to Fred. About the burglary. About what my daddy did to me. About the way my mother reacted when I told her what he did to me."

"Not so loud . . . I started to say you might wake the dead, but even I'm not that corny."

"And what about the babies? What, pray tell, happened to China Doll's babies?"

"What does China Doll have to do with this?"

"People said she was always pregnant . . . but no babies. If there were black children or black babies, gone missing, who in God's name were those families ever going to report it to? The local law?" She was talking loud again. "What would ol' Casey Paxton have done about it? Arrest them for vagrancy?"

"It's a point; I'll grant you that. But please cut back the volume."

Emily ranted on, but a little softer. "For whole generations, people of color learned how to hide their children in the night when the Invisible Empire was on the move. They learned how to live inconspicuous in the day when the nightriders shed their hoods and walked around in broad daylight at their posts as pillars of the community. That's not hearsay, that's not imagination, that's not made-up stories: it's reality! The colored community learned how not to draw attention to themselves, how being essentially invisible was safer: Don't speak; don't let yourself be seen; don't let your presence be a reality in their presence."

She followed him to their parking place, still fuming. "Have they quit burning crosses to rev themselves up and terrify their prey? Have they put away the masks they hid behind? Or are they still out there just waiting for another acronym to peak through?"

When the Kleins had climbed into the truck, closed the doors, and buckled their seat belts, Jeff got the last word: "While you're still angry and so you won't have to get angry all over again, Dad wants me to fly him up to Slicky Rock tomorrow to help get the cabin ready for warm weather."

"I'm glad the old bitch is dead." Cleat was sitting in the biplane's passenger seat.

Jeff adjusted his earphone. "Wh-What did you say?"

"I said I'm glad the old bitch is dead. That old biddy. Snob. Ya shoulda seen the way she treated your mother after we got married. And with all the money the snotty Campbells had, she wouldn't give us one red penny to set up housekeepin' when I got back from the war. Stingy old broad. Now the Colonel wuz a little more generous. He wuz always slipping us a few dollars here and there. Enough to get by on. Keep us fed."

"I w-wish you wouldn't t-talk like that about Grandmother. She always took g-good care of m-me and I miss her a lot."

"She wuz almost a hundred. Everybody dies. Like my mama used to say, 'We all gonna live to we die, if a tree don't fall on us.'" Cleat snorted. "Oops, sorry. I wuzn't even thinkin' about that nigger . . . that black buddy of yours." Jeff would have liked to reach up and slap his daddy on the back of the head. "Really he . . . nobody deserved that," Cleat attempted to apologize. "What a way to go. Right there in your own bed. Least he wuzn't alone. I'd hate to die alone . . . especially with a tree limb stuck through my heart."

The pilot was trying to keep his mouth shut and his mind on flying. As they got closer to the private airstrip, he began to prepare for landing.

"If I should die," the old man's voice was back in Jeff's earphone, "when I die, tell ya what I want ya to do. I want ya to have me cremated and scatter my ashes out here across the rock. Will you promise me that? . . . ya know I ain't ever asked for much."

"Sure, D-Dad. If that's what you w-want." Jeff pulled his earphones off and threw them onto the cockpit floor.

After a rather rough landing, father and son hopped in the golf cart they kept stored in the small hanger and rolled over to the cabin. The mountain air was relatively warm for one of the last days of winter; warm enough to take their picnic lunch onto the porch. Except for the monologues in their respective heads, they ate silently.

Cleat was thinking:

Where did I go wrong? Raising such a pansy. But when you get right down to it, it's not my fault. Can't help I couldn't give him all the things the old woman did.

And now he's cryin' about losin' her. I hated the bitch from the first time I walked through that goddamn gold-plated front door. Always walkin' around carryin' that holier-than-thou attitude on her back. No wonder she wuz so hunched over.

That old lady, she didn't know the half of it. Thought the Colonel was perfect. But I knew better. The old codger was an oath-taker, too. That's what my daddy told me. And Daddy was a smart man. And he knew the right people; knew the right things about the right people. And the Colonel knew he knew, and I think that's why he pitched such a fit when me and Katherine ran off to get married. But would've probably killed me if we hadn't.

He couldn't have stood for a little bastard . . . white bastard runnin' around on the Campbell plantation. No way. For a fact, my daddy didn't get beyond the third grade, but he was plumb full of common sense. Raised me like a kid should be raised. Beat some of that sense into me like I tried to do to my own son. But his grandmaw always fussed at me; said I should've never used that belt on her precious little grandbaby. Why, my boy don't know what a rough childhood was like . . . my daddy taught me to be a "real" man. Jefferson didn't belong to that bitch. He was mine and Katherine's, and if my pretty woman had lived, I just know things would've been so different. Maybe my bride could've learned to love me as much as Emily Lentz seems to love Jefferson.

Jeff was thinking:

What an insensitive s.o.b. Having lost two of the dearest people in the world in less than six months, here I am drowning in grief and my old man defames Grandmother and jokes about J. D. Not concerned about my feelings at all. Worrying only about himself. Where he's going to be scattered, of all things. Dammit, I'd like to scatter him right now!

Ashamed of the thought, Jeff looked west across the Blue Ridge Mountains. Squinting in the afternoon sun, he imagined the roar of bi-planes doing their stunts and a mother squealing with delight: "Look Honey! It's going to come back this way really close . . . can you see it?"

Was that memory a lie too? God don't let it be a lie! Where were you Daddy? You're not there.

Jeff wiped the sweat off his forehead. He was so angry. Not at his mother who'd abandoned him a long time ago. Or his daddy. Of course he had reason to be angry with both parents, but what he was feeling now was anger at his wife. He was getting fed up with her all-fired hatred of his daddy and her relentless pursuit of the past. Why couldn't she just appreciate the present; get on with life the way it used to be? With this therapy she was getting herself into, she seemed determined to 'track evil to its lair.' And then what? Finish destroying their lives?

Chapter 21

"**H**e didn't talk about it.

Always said it was just too bad. He'd been through it one time and that was all there was to it." So said one of the last widows of a Confederate Army veteran with regard to her late husband in an interview the year before she died.

Emily disagreed.

One way to heal from trauma was to talk about it. And talk some more. And talk and talk until she had nothing left to say . . . if that time ever came.

Another way was to write about it, using a special kind of writing that she had discovered soon after her first psychotherapy session.

Indeed Emily — more specifically her unconscious — had figured out how to use that right hand she had raised during hypnosis. Her unconscious had picked up on Dr. Jacobson's challenge to use that tool to accomplish Emily's goal of redissociating, of accessing dissociated parts who could help her recover memories of traumatic experiences that were interfering with her present life.

She'd discovered that if she placed a journal, loose-leaf paper, motel stationary, index card, post-it notes, or even a napkin from the Village Diner in front of her and picked up a pencil, words came dumping out of her head like files on a hard drive downloading to a printer.

Automatic writing. Putting her unthought-thoughts — the mostly inaudible messages coming from outside her conscious awareness — on paper. Many highly creative men and women, even children, have given these dissociated aspects of themselves names, allowing them to take on separate identities, sometimes ostensibly losing control of their behaviors and getting diagnosed with a mental illness. Emily's voices, oral or written, had no names, only attributes: different ages, feelings, and thoughts. In some cultures they would be called guardian angels.

Emily's job, as she saw it, was to record the writings without censorship, trusting that some day, just as letters make words and words make sentences that have meaning, the once disconnected output from her unconscious would all come together in a logical coherent narrative.

For a little over a year now, Emily had religiously followed a self-created schedule set up to assure that she would not decompensate as she aggressively delved for traumatic memories. Monday through Thursday mornings, she saw clients. On the first Monday night of each month, she met with an MPD study group in Charlotte. Every Tuesday night, she ran a group for her own clients who were dissociative. She'd usually leave on Thursday afternoons for Charleston. At Julie's suggestion, she had participated for about six months in a therapy group of women with trauma histories run by the director of a new dissociative disorders unit at a for-profit hospital. On Friday mornings, she'd sometimes get a therapeutic massage before her afternoon psychotherapy sessions. Weekends were family time.

The psychologist had always tried to keep her professional life separate from her personal therapy, and those lives separate from her relationship with Carol and Matt. They knew she was in therapy, probably assuming that most therapists are in therapy from time to time, probably having remembered her saying, "A therapist who's never been in therapy is like a first grade teacher who never learned to read." Besides, with Carol and Brad expecting a baby in December, it wouldn't be fair to burden them with the problems of the excited grandmother-to-be. Now with Jeff, it was different. He'd pledged to live with her, "for better, for worse."

One morning after a particularly stressful group session with the psychiatrist, she'd told Julie, "I'm getting out. Last night I got down on the floor with a young nurse who had regressed to a little child. I began talking with her like I talk with clients. Dr. Nicholson, who with his scraggly white hair and beard reminds me of a mad scientist in a horror movie, got rather harsh: 'If you're going to fit into this group, you should keep your therapist-part at home.' Even knowing that I was in a power struggle with the authoritative group leader and that I was in the weaker position, I just couldn't keep my mouth shut."

"What did you say?"

"Something like 'that's part of who I am and if I can't be my whole self in here, I don't need the experience.'"

"What happened next?" Julie asked.

Emily described the experience in detail.

The psychiatrist had sneered, "Why Miz Klein, I believe you're angry with me. You do have feelings, don't you?"

"I never said I didn't. I've always said they're all-or-none. And right now, they're 'all.' . . . all over the place."

"She has every right to those feelings," a member of the group who was a dentist broke in. "And to show them once in a while."

"Thanks for your support," Emily nodded at her group mate. "As a child I was never allowed to act out my emotions. It was rare for me to cry. Apparently I learned it was better not to have feelings than to have them and not be able to express them."

The leader interrupted, "You might've learned not to feel, but you sure did learn to think. Too much, as far as I'm concerned. I've never seen anyone use intellectualization as a defense better than you."

"So what. Even if the feelings were conditioned out of me, I continued to think, and the perpetrators couldn't do a thing about it. And while we're talking about feelings, how do you feel about working with a patient, if that's what you want to call me, who treats the same kind of patients you do?"

"Well, Miz Klein, I don't know exactly what your expertise is, but you're in this group to be treated for your disorder and I will not be battered. I will set the limits.

He doctor.

Me patient.

Later that evening Emily had dreamed she was a little girl noticing blood around her cuticles. Terrified, she showed her short fingers to a man wearing a doctor's coat. He put his thumb under her chin, tilting her head upward. "You're very sick, little girl. You have to leave the group."

"What do you think it means?" Julie asked the next morning when Emily had finished telling her about the dream.

"I was not a good group member, never have been, never will be. In graduate school, I made a *B* in the experiential group course. The professor told me I didn't show good 'groupmanship' . . . that was a long time ago. Now it would be 'group-personship.'"

"The dream?"

"They told me in graduate school that I should become a public servant . . . not a private clinician. But I did my internship at the VA hospital and realized, without a doubt, I was not a team player; realized I couldn't make it in a bureaucracy."

"So what do you think the dream means?" It was the third time Julie had asked.

"To be honest . . . I believe I should get out of group."

"Why is that?"

"Because, although I like the other members, I don't see myself as a mental patient as Dr. Nicholson thinks I am. Sure, I had problems with the revved feeling and insomnia . . . didn't make me 'mental.' But that stupid psychiatrist tried to make me think I was crazy . . . that's not professional, is it? Calling him stupid, I mean . . . but he didn't treat me professionally, either. Then again, some good did come out of it . . . I learned what it's truly like to be demeaned as someone who has emotional problems when I'm only reacting normally to an abnormal situation."

"You don't have to stay in the group, you know. It's your choice."

"I know that. And know that as a child I had no choice about being in whatever group I may have been in, whether it was my family or even some type of cult as I'm beginning to suspect. But as an adult, I refuse to be controlled by any group leader; by group thinking, pressure, or programming."

Thinking about the dream, the client stopped talking and looked downward.

For a millisecond or two, she thought she saw blood on her hands.

Every morning when Emily was at home she would swim at least a mile in the pool or lake. At the beach, weather permitting, she'd swim in the ocean. Twenty minutes, twice a day, she practiced conscious relaxation techniques or self-hypnosis. Although there was no specific time for journaling, she continued to jot down unthought-thoughts, list images, and write about dreams to discuss in psychotherapy.

Cycling back into her denial state during one of the sessions, Emily had asked, "Is it possible all those things did happen to me? Was I really molested as a child?"

"You need more data, I think," remarked Julie. With her left hand, the therapist pushed back a few tufts of unruly black hair that had escaped from her tightly-drawn bun and were floating over her eyes; with her right, she continued to make notes.

"You don't get it, do you? What do you want? A moving picture show? Or is it that you think I'm delusional, and you're just playing along with me?"

The embers of a classic transference were nearing the combustion point.

Emily knew in her heart that she was angry at her mother. But by golly, she was angry at Julie, too: incensed by her therapist's seemingly degrading, slow-to-burn neutrality.

"You don't believe me, do you, *Doctor* Jacobson?" Emily aimed the title at her helper like a laser gun pointed at someone's frontal lobe.

"The important thing is not whether I believe you, but whether you can believe yourself."

"I don't expect you to accept things merely because I say them. Neither do I expect you to be like my mother and automatically discount the things I tell you."

"Will you do a little exercise for me?" asked the therapist in charge.

"Sure. That's what I pay you for."

"I want you to draw a map of your personality structure, a sort of self-portrait." Julie brought out a box of pencils and markers and chalks. "Use anything you want."

"I can't draw."

"It doesn't have to be a masterpiece."

Reluctantly, Emily reached for a pencil. Using the silver dollar in her change purse as a pattern—the last present her daddy had given her—she drew a circle and divided it into half. Next she colored one side black, then made concentric circles around the original circle until they ran off the page. "Okay Doctor, what do you think this means?"

"What do you think it means?"

How many clients had Emily asked to do this same exercise? Never before really knowing what it was like to be on the other side, to suddenly feel such rage toward the person she'd hired to help her find the answers.

Embarrassed at the way she'd just spoken to Julie, Emily considered her response for a long time before answering: "The inner circle represents the essence of my being. It's a split nucleus with two sides, the light and dark. Black hides the buried selves who can never come into the light unless I dredge them up myself. The concentric circles depict the layers, the shells around my inner self. Layers upon layers, protecting my very . . . soul," she said in realization. Smiling, the client risked a rare eye contact with her therapist. "I'm depending on you to help me stay centered here. Will you do that for me?"

Julie answered with a smile.

I'm on the vulnerable side now, Emily thought. And there's something humiliating about becoming the helpee. Like being seen as a mental-cripple in a world that expects you to 'get on with it.' I've always been the helper, the capable one. What I'm really wondering is, can I trust my own helper.

The client, a.k.a therapist, picked up the silver dollar and placed it in her palm. *E Pluribus Unum*, she read, now remembering the translation.

Covered by a white sheet, Emily lay face down on the table in the semi-darkness. Audiotaped ocean sounds flowed through the room. Trying to relax, thoughts surged like surf, as the fingers of the massage therapist palpated the deep muscles of her upper left arm in rhythm with the larger waves. In the blackness of her mind, an image of her daddy lit up over her, and she knew, somehow, where the pain was coming from. Struggling up to her elbows, she grabbed the edge of the big sheet protectively. "You won't believe what just happened."

Kristi rolled her stool around to the end of the table. "Try me. I've seen a number of powerful things happen in massage therapy." Although Emily couldn't see the young woman's face, she sensed a big smile. "The mind and body aren't nearly as separate as I used to think they were before getting massage training."

"Could you turn that ocean off, please? Maybe if we can hear ourselves think, you can help me figure this out." Twisting the ample sheet around herself, Emily sat up, no longer mistrusting her own experience, ready to do intellectual battle with the phenomenon trauma therapists were now referring to as body memories.

She pointed to an indentation in her left upper arm, faintly remembering Dr. Bill telling her daddy that it could've been caused by a mild case of polio. This explanation had always seemed implausible. "When you rubbed here, I felt a throbbing pain. You know, like the kind you get after a tetanus shot. And simultaneously saw an image of my daddy looming over me, his big hands squeezing both arms until I thought they'd break." She pointed to the other arm. "Look, this one has a smaller indentation. He must've been awfully angry at me for something."

Kristi examined both deformities. "Interesting. This one on the left feels like the large muscles were severed at some point in time. Was your father right-handed?"

"Yes, why do you ask?"

"Because it makes your explanation all the more logical. If somebody was facing you, putting pressure on both arms, it makes sense that more damage would be done with his dominant hand."

"But how do you think I could've been hurt, probably before I could talk, and just now call it up?"

"Well the way I see it, when I touched your arm, the molecules in the cells in your severed muscles were triggered to release the body memory they'd held for so long." Kristi, who had been a social worker, then trained as a massage therapist with all its emphasis on physiology, went on to talk about the mind-body connection. "Research has shown there are patterns of communication between the mind and body, involving something they've called messenger molecules."

Although Emily herself had done some reading in this area and had witnessed firsthand the power of the mind over physical processes in her biofeedback work, she listened intently to Kristi's explanation. "Things like sexual hormones, glucose, insulin, cortisol, and adrenaline. Physical sensations influence mind states. And thoughts release chemical molecules into the bloodstream, the nervous system, and even the tissues of our flesh which affect body states."

"So Kristi, are you saying that massage released the molecules carrying the message to my mind?"

"That's quite a mouthful, but a good way to put it."

"You know, I've often wondered if my ability to have a full range of feelings was knocked out even before I had a chance to feel. I recognize what probably did happen to me, but for the most part can't feel a thing about it. Unless I feel too much. All-or-none. Where are the feelings in between?"

"Still there I believe," Kristi answered. "Like damage in an old injured muscle waiting to be touched."

———

In session with Julie that afternoon, Emily described the arm-twisting body memory in detail before saying, "I've not been feeling well—"

"Sorry to hear that. What's the problem?"

"To tell you the truth, I believe it's all body memories. I've had a lot of sharp pains in my stomach and pelvic region. Sometimes it's feels like labor."

"How long has it been since you've seen a doctor?" Julie was playing the mother role again.

"Quite a while. Several years, actually. I detest doctors and medical stuff. And really I've been pretty healthy and . . . well, I'm pretty sure it's all psychological."

"Of all people, you, a psychologist, should know how important it is to rule out physical causes before determining that symptoms are emotionally related."

"All right, all right," Emily conceded. "I'll see somebody after I get back from the MPD conference in Chicago in a few weeks. Wouldn't miss that trip for anything, getting to meet up with my best friend from graduate school, and perhaps learn how to do what I'm supposed to be doing with my dissociative clients. Or maybe I'll wait till after the baby is born."

Emily stood up to leave. "I did tell you I'm gonna be a first-time grandma soon, didn't I?"

Chapter 22

As the first shot fired on Ft. Sumter had set off the War Between the States, so a single article in a professional journal had set off what came to be called the 'memory wars.' In an article published in the journal *Dissociation* in 1989, a psychiatrist had compared alleged satanic ritual abuse survivors to alleged UFO abductees. He reported that some sociologists had categorized these incredible accounts as 'urban legends' and questioned, ". . . to what degree do these vividly reenacted experiences represent purely factual accounts of multigenerational cult activities with actual human sacrifices as described, versus fantasy and/or illusion borrowing its core material from literature, movies, TV, other patients' accounts, or unintentional therapist suggestion?"

Only a year earlier at an MPD conference in Chicago, there had seemed to be a consensus that satanic ritual abuse of children was—in the past and present—a significant problem. And now at the 1990 conference, former ritual abuse survivors were being called 'alleged' ritual abuse survivors. It was as if some unknown force were attempting to traumatize trauma therapists; to split professionals into opposing camps, either believers or nonbelievers.

"Are they trying to tell me that the clients I've been treating for the last ten years, human beings whom I've sat with as they recounted minute details of their horrible experiences in evil cults . . . are they trying to say that I put those memories in their minds?" Emily asked her friend, Kate Stewart, who was sitting next to her at the luncheon table. If Kate answered, Emily hadn't heard. The voices of their colleagues were blending into a comber of white noise.

—Supposedly, a recent FBI study by a guy named Lanning showed a lack of evidence for organized satanic crime.

—But from what I've heard, that was actually a guide for investigation of such cases, not a scientific study. He must not have known about some of the cases that have produced convictions.

—Lest we forget, for fifty years the FBI said the Mafia didn't exist.

—That's true. When a client tells me, "I'm afraid that my father will kill my son," I know what to think as a psychoanalyst. Over the years, I've done some therapy with men who've tried to leave the Mafia network, and because of what I've learned about ritual abuse at this conference, now I know that it's possible they're simply speaking about reality.

—And they say there's no evidence. No convictions. That's false. What about the "Country Walk Babysitting Service" case a few years ago in my city, Miami? Our aggressive state attorney, Janet Reno, got convictions. Kids had accused the owners, a husband and wife, of making them eat feces, drugging and raping them with a crucifix, and teaching them prayers to chant to Satan.

—There was a case last year in my state, Georgia, where a teenager was convicted of a ritual murder of a woman and admitted on the stand that he had performed animal sacrifices, drinking the blood as a toast to Satan.

—What about historical evidence? Benko in his book, *Pagan Rome and the Early Christians*, wrote about the elements of a fourth century satanic mass described by an Egyptian monk, Epiphanius, who infiltrated a sect called the Phibionites. As an initiate, he participated in rituals such as sexual orgies, festive eating and drinking, and secret handshakes to check if a person belonged to the cult. He goes into graphic detail about some of the sickening things they did, things you wouldn't want me to mention while you're eating.

—But why did they do those horrible things?

—Presumably, they saw it as a way of communicating with their god, Satan.

—References on witchcraft show that in medieval times there were laws on the books to punish people who worshiped Satan, fines for people who ate human flesh or even carried the cauldron it was cooked in, excommunication from the church for people who made incantations or led dances to the Devil, and death to anyone who offered human sacrifice to demons.

—So we have to logically assume those things happened or there wouldn't have been laws against them. Something I have difficulty working through—is our all too willingness to forgive what these monsters do.

—I wonder if we have this need to forgive them because that's what we'd want them to do to us . . . in case our evil sides ever got out of control?

—There's other historical evidence for the ritual abuse of children. Do you remember the fairy tale of Bluebeard?

—Isn't he the one who murdered a bunch of wives and kept their remains in a locked room in his castle?

—Yes he is. Legend has it that the Bluebeard character was patterned after a real live monster, Gilles de Rais, who lived in fifteenth century France. That feudal lord, who practiced the Black Arts, was a contemporary of Joan of Arc. As a professing Christian, he built a chapel dedicated to the Holy Innocents, the children Herod slaughtered when he was trying to annihilate the baby Jesus. In what appears to have been satanic rituals, he slaughtered hundreds of children. At his trial, he confessed before the ecclesiastical judges that he and his accomplices had sodomized his victims' dying or dead bodies and had saved the most beautiful decapitated heads to kiss and keep. It is said that during sentencing, he broke down in remorseful sobbing, moving the witnesses to compassion and forgiveness. On the way to his hanging, he was accompanied by a crowd chanting prayers and songs and asking God to give him eternal life. Afterwards, de Rais was placed in a coffin and carried to the church for a Christian funeral.

—Of course.

—The skeptics are asking for scientific proof that cult and ritual trauma is real. You can prove something did happen, but you can't prove it didn't . . . you can't prove the null hypothesis.

—I'd rather believe it's not true than have to acknowledge that any parent would dedicate his or her child to evil.

—The ancient Greeks offered human sacrifices to the gods. Sometimes their own children.

—Probably, few people today realize that blood-sacrifice has been prevalent in many cultures with a type of generic belief that one who eats human flesh would acquire the power of the deceased through the consumption of the body.

—One of my clients talked about the Black Mass often performed as part of the Grand Climax at Christmas. Reportedly, she'd been forced to kill— or made to think she'd killed a baby. To a child it wouldn't have made much difference. Instead of celebrating the birth of a baby, her family's cult celebrated its death. Then they turned around and used its flesh and blood in a mock communion service to hype up the worshipers for sexual orgies.

—I've heard that, too. A child I worked with talked about magical surgery where she was told a bomb had been placed in her stomach and would explode and kill her if she revealed any of the secrets of the cult.

—If nothing's going on, why is it that people all over the world who've never met each other are talking in therapy offices about animal and human mutilations, about having been repeatedly subjected to sexual and physical assaults, hanging upside down, being buried alive, electroshock for punishment when they didn't do things perfectly, and drugs that made them forget what happened?

—Like that date-rape drug, Rohypnol or 'roofies' as the college kids call it.

—There's another one heading our way, Burundanga. It's a potent form of scopolamine used for years in Columbian ritual ceremonies and by criminals preying on tourists. They put it in gum, drinks, even dust it on paper. If it doesn't completely knock the unsuspecting person out, it makes him or her amnesic for anything that happened before the drug got out of their system.

—Part of the trauma itself is taking away the control.

—Unless someone has sat in our chairs and listened quietly, neutrally, professionally in a non-leading way, day after day to the life stories of these poor souls, and in silent mental privacy been forced momentarily to imagine the possibility of a hidden reality in it, there's no way they could understand what it's like.

—Or what it does to us emotionally, even physically. Sometimes I literally feel their headaches and backaches and earaches.

—Some people are claiming that patients get their ideas about MPD from books.

—How can a book implant memories? I don't see how reading about Sybil or Eve could make a person think she was multiple . . . any more than reading about Ted Bundy could make me a serial killer.

—Even if it were possible, why would therapists implant memories? For money? Good Lord! Nobody does this kind of therapy for money. We're tied in a double bind. Believe our clients and the parents may sue us; don't believe, and our clients may sue us themselves.

—Well, for your information, I'm keeping the names of all alleged perps I hear about in my safe. In case someone harms me or my family, there'll be a ready list of suspects.

—Good idea. Personally I'm about ready to get out of this business: the increasingly dangerous business of daring to help somebody.

—In this battle, therapists have a grave disadvantage. Accused parents can say anything they want to say about the therapists who treat their offspring, but unless the therapy notes become public in a courtroom, therapists are bound by confidentiality.

—And why in the world are those people so down on hypnosis? Their claim that it produces false memories makes it sound as if a person in a hypnotic trance has relinquished control of his or her thoughts and behaviors to the therapist. The way I use hypnosis—I don't make someone get up and walk like a chicken—allows people to tap individual creativity to find resolutions to whatever problems they bring to the table.

—That's a long way from the '50s when hypnotic methods attempted to condition and program subjects to do what the experimenter wanted.

—I must tell you folks, I don't believe memories obtained in a hypnotic state are any more or less reliable than spontaneous memories. Also, it's possible to have screen memories that shield a person from the knowledge of real events.

—You mean like making someone believe they were abducted by aliens so they don't remember what the earthlings did to them?

—Exactly.

—Do you want to hear why I believe they're so down on hypnosis?

—Sure.

—Because nobody wants what was deliberately covered up to be exposed, even to his or her own consciousness. Hypnosis, as we all know, is a mental state where deep healing can be done, but it's also a technique that's helping to unmask the dark sides of a lot of individuals, communities, and all kinds of organizations.

—How's that?

—Theoretically, it puts a person in an altered state, like the disconnection felt during the trauma, triggering memories of crimes committed when the child initially used dissociation as a defense in order to stay alive.

—I've been told there's a network of groups around the world affiliated with an ancient secret organization called the Illuminati whose objective is to create multiple personalities: human robots programmed to serve the elite as prostitutes, couriers of top-secret information, or even spies or assassins in a new world order or totalitarian state.

—But how could so many people from different countries or cultures plan anything of such magnitude? Why, in my neighborhood, we can't even get a few people to agree on the *how's* and *when's* of a block party.

—The U.S. Government's already done it. Created mutliples to be spies, that is. And a psychologist by the name of Estabrooks rather brazenly wrote about it in a 1971 *Science Digest* article—if I remember correctly, the title was "Hypnosis Comes of Age"—telling how, using hypnosis, he'd split a man's psyche into two separate personalities: one, a loyal American; the other, a card-carrying Communist Party member who was used, Estabrooks said, in military intelligence during World War II.

—Every one of my clients who alleges satanic ritual abuse or SRA also has memories of being used in pornography. It makes sense that pedophiles could use satanic elements and implements and rituals in the making of such films: a natural extension—by technology—of very old multigenerational cult practices.

—Ah! Kiddie porn. A pedophile's artwork; an avenue for perpetual gratification.

—Yeah, and as a bonus they can also make big 'tax-sheltered' dollars peddling their smut across the globe.

—Or a way to blackmail power brokers and politicians who get caught with their pants down on the wrong side of a two-way mirror.

—Raw evil, I'd say. Not a fit conversation at cocktail parties, Bible study groups, or neighborhood soccer games . . . even if law-abiding citizens knew what to say.

When they began talking about child pornography, Emily's mind had drifted away from the conversation. She would've much preferred to join the nonbelievers; to ratify their doubt; to turn back her life to the years before she'd become a therapist, the years before she'd learned that some so-called good people do heinous things to children on Saturday night and are perfectly capable of teaching their Sunday school classes the next morning.

Dr. Emily Lentz Klein had not put pseudomemories in her clients' heads.

Nor had she created their multiple personalities.

In fact, she could have written a book of case histories of clients who used dissociation, both adaptively and maladaptively, to defend against their traumas.

Charity

This forty-five-year-old protective service worker was referred by her family physician because she was experiencing symptoms of depression. Of average height, she weighed less than one hundred pounds. Successful in her job, married for twenty-five years, no financial problems, no problems with her four children, Charity wanted to die.

In answer to Emily's initial question, "What do you want to accomplish in therapy?" Charity had replied, "I'm unhappy. No one can get close to me. I'm sensitive and I've been hurt." She went on to say, "I was the oldest of six children. I was never allowed to be a child."

Charity wanted and needed to talk about her past and welcomed the opportunity to learn hypnosis. In one of the early trance experiences when Charity's eyelids began to flutter, Emily asked her to remember a time in her life when she had been happy. Tears rolled down her sallow cheeks as she spoke in a trembling weak voice: "I-I-I really can't remember a happy time."

"That's okay," Emily supported. "Just allow yourself to remember what you need to remember."

After a minute or two, Charity opened her eyes and looked around the room. She stuck a thumb in her mouth and began to whine.

"What's the matter?" Emily asked, drifting into the voice of an adult talking to a hurting child.

"My neck hurts."

"I'm sorry. Do you have a name?"

"I'm Little Bit."

"Do you know who I am?"

Charity's child part shook her head, no.

"I'm Charity's doctor. I'm here to help her . . . and you. How old are you?"

The regressed adult held up four fingers and spoke with a childlike tone: "The weal Chawity's dead. Auntie choked her with a wope. She told me I was bad. She told me to be Chawity." The person sitting in front of Emily closed her eyes and went limp, coming out of trance rubbing her neck. She stood up and walked over to the mirror. "My God! It looks like there's a rope burn." Putting her hands around her neck as if she were choking herself, she added, "It feels like there's a burn."

This was the first of many traumas Charity would remember. In about a year of therapy, she would discover an internal system of alters who protected her from her past and continued to shield her in the present from day-to-day pressures.

Charity's system was complex. Most of her parts didn't talk to outsiders. They had not talked with Charity until they began to appear in therapy. Some had no voices but wrote in her journal. The spy saw what he wasn't supposed to see. The recorder kept a mental record of everything that happened to her. The clown managed a group of alters created to make Charity feel happy.

Some names reflected traits of the alters. Unity's purpose was to keep it all together. Thanta wanted to die. "Charity's stupid," Thanta had once said. "She has to please everybody all the time. I'd like to blow her brains out. I did cut her wrist when she was a teenager." Roada, the persecutor, wanted to run away.

The mother in Emily was touched one day when Charity regressed and cowered in the corner. "Who are you?" Emily asked as she sat on the floor beside her client.

"Fraidy."

Without anticipating the poignancy of Fraidy's reply, Emily asked, "Do you have a last name?"

"Cat."

An image crossed Emily's mind. When she was four, Jimmy had taught her to be afraid of her shadow and when she became frightened, he would taunt her in a singsong voice, "Emily's a fraidy cat. Emily's a fraidy cat."

One Easter Monday, Charity anxiously began to tell Emily about a dream she'd had the night before. "I don't remember much about it. I saw a black pot, a black and white kitten, and an axe. My doll was in the dream. Crying."

She lay back on the couch, closed her eyes, and the part who called itself the recorder continued the description in monotone. "I see a lot of people. They march up the steps. They go in the church. Auntie's with them. They are screaming and yelling."

Another switch of affect and the client, putting her hands over both ears, screamed: "He's alive! Our Master's alive! Praise the Master!"

The spy came out to finish the narrative. "Everybody's jerking. Moaning and groaning. One of the men has on a dress. He's wearing a hat that comes down over his ears. They make her lie down on a little stage. Everybody touches her. They touch her everywhere."

"What is she wearing?" Emily asked, as a way of assuring Charity that she was with her in the moment.

"It's a white dress. They take her panties off. They make the sign of the cross on her chest. They use their mouths to make the sign of the cross on her titties."

Charity sat straight up, her face red, her fists clinched. "Auntie did that to me. She let them kiss me on my mouth, my breasts, my bottom. God damn everyone of them!"

In subsequent weeks, Charity remembered bits and pieces of other ritualistic activities: cats and chickens being slaughtered and sacrificed to the Master, and she, herself, being forced to drink their blood. Her grandfather, a traveling evangelist, appeared to her to have been leader of the group.

Some of Emily's clients had remembered abuse in the name of Satan. Charity had remembered abuse in the name of Jesus Christ.

Amy

Forty-year-old Amy had moved to town when her husband had been transferred to Syn-Tec. Believing she was possessed by demons, she'd requested Emily to continue with a religious ritual, the procedure called "deliverance," which her former Christian therapist had used. When Emily explained that she was not qualified to offer spiritual healing, and in reality did not believe the woman's alters were supernatural beings but that perhaps she had been made to believe they were by her perpetrators, the woman didn't reschedule.

The so-called demons Emily had talked with in a few clients appeared to be frightened kid parts who had been made to believe they were demons. Some of her colleagues, however, believed in demonic spirits. One called them critters. Another described them as energies.

Not that Emily doubted the existence of supernatural entities. How could she, given her own experience with the 'heavenly' entity that had literally touched and spoken to her in the middle of the night?

"It's a cultural thing," Jeff had once said. "If you believe in them, you will see them." Same thing some of her colleagues had said about multiple personalities.

Lisa

Previously living in a state where her Medicaid benefits allowed unlimited sessions, Lisa had seen her former therapist daily and, for a brief time, had actually lived with her. Before coming to see Emily, the patient had been hospitalized and aggressively encouraged to remember and relive as much as possible while in the hospital setting. Lisa had abreacted a flood of memories she couldn't seem to stop, causing her to decompensate.

Emily's treatment goal was to help her client pace the memory retrieval so that she could continue to function in the everyday world. The abreactions slowed considerably. Lisa found a part-time job and seemed to be making order out of the chaos in her life. One day she came in and said she was quitting therapy. Her reason: "I'm afraid you know what you're doing." This made no sense at the time, but later Emily decided that it could've been a compliment.

Kim

The most severely disturbed self-diagnosed MPD client Emily had ever seen did not have MPD at all. Kim played at being multiple. In her case, perhaps with good reason. Having been accused of abusing her three-year-old daughter and needing an excuse for her behavior, she had apparently convinced a judge that she was mentally ill. He'd ordered psychological treatment before making a decision on whether she would have to forfeit her parental rights.

"How did you find out about me?" Emily had asked.

"I called HelpLine to see if they had anyone listed who treated multiples."

In the first session, Kim had volunteered, "I have multiple personalities. Would you like to speak to everyone?" Something was wrong. Emily had never seen anyone whose switching behavior looked as contrived. The multiples she treated had always tried to cover their condition.

At her second session, Kim produced a notebook in which her so-called alters had written anecdotes using different colored pens. The handwritings looked the same, except for one that appeared to be an attempt to look like a secret code. Easily deciphered, it was signed "Satan."

Not overreacting, the therapist merely listened to the client's story. Kim didn't come to a third session.

In Emily's opinion, a person who, for whatever reasons factitiously presents as a multiple is likely to have more psychopathology than a person who has developed multiple personalities as a normal reaction to trauma.

Jennifer

This woman had decompensated in college and was diagnosed MPD in the university's counseling center. She dropped out of college, later cut her wrists, and was sent to the state hospital. After several years of wandering through the mental health system with varying diagnoses, including borderline personality, bipolar, depression, schizophrenia, and substance abuse, she'd ended up on Social Security disability, qualifying for residence in a group home for the mentally ill.

As soon as she became eligible for Medicare, she sought private treatment. Since the woman was also seeing a private psychiatrist for medical management, Emily agreed to work with her. The psychiatrist concurred with the overall dissociative diagnosis and didn't interfere with psychotherapy.

For about a year, Jennifer worked diligently in therapy. Her IQ was in the superior range and the state's Department of Vocational Rehabilitation paid her expenses to enroll in a university. She made A's in her classes until she met a student who was heavily involved in drugs. Jennifer began using drugs herself and was arrested for possession. Fearing that she would fail a drug screening test and lose her place in the group home, she slashed her arms and got admitted to a psychiatric hospital, one that had a policy of not serving patients with MPD.

After leaving the hospital, Jennifer called Emily, tearfully asking for an appointment. "I'm sorry I lied to you, Dr. Klein. I don't have multiple personalities. I'm sure my mother didn't molest me as I told you. In the hospital they said I was borderline and put me in a chemical dependency program, but I want you to be my primary therapist. My new psychiatrist said that it would be all right for you to treat me for my borderline personality."

Emily declined the offer.

Jennifer, who had never worked to develop a responsible adult response to life, was destined for a future of turmoil.

Besides seeing dissociative individuals for therapy, Emily had evaluated for various agencies, other persons who presented posttraumatic stress symptoms along with other mental disorders such as anxiety, depression, bipolar disorder, and schizophrenia. From medical reports and psychiatric histories, she surmised that many incapacitating mental disorders have a trauma-based etiology.

George

This twenty-nine-year-old man was trying to get disability benefits because he had uncontrollable seizures. Medical reports showed no organic problems, and the neurologist called them hysterical seizures. During the psychological evaluation, the patient described the experience as feeling as if he were being electrocuted. While he was doing a drawing task, Emily noticed that a little finger was missing. When asked how he had lost it, George, looking puzzled, answered, "I don't remember."

Emily speculated, but of course didn't tell him, that George had been a cult initiate who was unable to dissociate as a defense against trauma. He'd never acquired coping skills for the real world. His seizures could've been physiological re-enactments of electroshock treatments he received when he was being conditioned to be a slave of some type of coercive group. But he was a failure. Perhaps, for punishment, or to show others what happens when they do not obey laws of a secret society, his finger was chopped off.

Ricky

A three-year-old child of hard-core drug addicts, Ricky was already in the mental health system. He had been referred by the Department of Social Services for psychological evaluation. The fact that the toddler had been physically abused and neglected had been proved. Social Services wanted every kind of rational evidence possible to support their attempt to save this child, even if it required a court-ordered termination of parental rights.

In the foster home, he had hit another child with a hammer, used a cigarette lighter to set fire to curtains, and smeared feces on the bathroom wall. The foster mother said that he was fascinated with knives and that she had to keep them hidden. The child's behaviors were overly sexualized, causing her to wonder if he had witnessed violent and pornographic movies. A health department doctor had diagnosed him as having attention deficit disorder.

At the beginning of the testing session, the little boy got down on the floor and crawled around, barking like a dog. Later he changed from being a passive shy child to a distractible, hyperactive child who could have destroyed the office in two minutes if given a chance.

Testing showed average intelligence, although Ricky had been described by a pediatrician as retarded. When Emily had shown him a picture of a man's face, a neutral stimulus, he called it a devil. She suspected the little boy could've been deliberately traumatized, but had no proof. In her report, she'd documented his behaviors and responses and stated that his symptoms were consistent with those of severe abuse.

If the psychologist had written in her report that this three-year-old child had multiple personalities, including a shy alter, an aggressive alter, and an animal alter who barked like a dog, and that he may have decompensated under the pressure of being severely mistreated by someone who looked to him like a devil, she sincerely doubted that the report would have had much credibility with either the social worker or the judge.

Ricky was severely disturbed, and his feet were now firmly planted in the mental health system. If by chance, when he became an adult, he reassociated his presently scattered memories of—perhaps—being ritually abused as a young child, no one would believe him because he would be considered delusional: "He's been in the system since he was three, you know." Emily could already imagine how easy it would be to destroy whatever was left of Ricky if he made it to thirty or thirty-five.

Lester
Diagnosed psychotic, Lester was a teenage version of Ricky. His parents were trying to get him into a group home for mentally ill children and needed a current psychological evaluation. Medical history showed that for unknown reasons, the boy had been hospitalized in a children's psychiatric unit when he was five or six years old. Of average intelligence, he was enrolled in special classes at school because he was considered emotionally disturbed. At eleven, he'd told a counselor at a mental health center about some bizarre things he'd witnessed, the nature of which was not discussed in the report. His father found out, said it was all lies, and made him recant. A psychiatrist admitted Lester to a children's ward because of reported delusions. While there, the teenager disclosed that he often heard voices inside his head and visually hallucinated evil shapes and colors.

During the interview with Emily, Lester's speech was logical and reality-based, although he claimed that voices often told him to hurt himself and that babies screamed in his nightmares. Obsessed with the Holocaust, he liked to read and watch movies about the subject.

Lester hadn't been believed at eleven when he told someone about "bad things." Probably no one would believe him as an adult if he ever told of his personal holocaust. If he had been traumatized, terrorized, as a child, he would likely never know his truth. He was convinced he was crazy. He was fourteen years old.

And of course there was the client old doctor Bill had referred to Emily shortly after Fred had been murdered and just before he had surrendered his medical license because of the molestation charges by Maggie Rucker.

Brenda

"How ya doing, Miss Emily?" The voice was friendly and folksy. Although he didn't identify himself in the early morning call, Emily knew it was Dr. Bill. "Are you still doing hypnosis?"

"Well . . . well yes I am. Why do you want to know?"

"Oh, I just hoped you could help me with my golf game," he laughed. "No really, I got a young lady I'd like you to see. She can't get her migraines under control and had to quit her job out at Syn-tec because of blackout spells."

Emily thought it was unusual that the doctor himself had called to set up the appointment but really had no reason not to see his referral.

"How can I help you?" Emily asked when Brenda had come in later in the week.

"Dr. Wilhelm said you could help me get rid of my headaches. I'm so tired of them. They get so bad that I often pass out, and sometimes I apparently don't pass out because my friends tell me that when I have them, I do all sorts of things that I don't remember doing." She held up her right hand. "That's what happened to my little finger. I must've passed out in the factory and it got stuck in a machine. It got cut off right here at the first joint. At least that's what they said. So they won't let me work any more."

During that first session, Emily learned that Brenda's father had died when she was fifteen and that she had gone to work in Earl Elliott's drugstore to help take care of her mother and younger brothers. Brenda had been out of work for over a year, yet she lived alone in an upscale apartment and drove a late model sports car. She was quite evasive when Emily asked her how she was supporting herself.

Before the first session was even over, Emily was suspecting that Dr. Bill had sent this naive young woman to spy on her, to learn exactly what went on with clients who had been victims of the local pedophiles. Nevertheless, she saw her three more times and taught her some biofeedback techniques to help control the headaches.

The therapist's suspicions that Brenda had been sent as a cult plant were given validity when, after Brenda's fourth and last session, Emily found a note the woman had left on the sofa. She had written:

Here I sit listening to you talk
Wondering just what makes you tick.
I listen carefully to the words.

Perhaps Brenda had been programmed to remember those words so that she could repeat them around a campfire some night.

"I wish the writer of that article that showed no evidence for satanic ritual abuse had been in on a session with one of my shelter's residents, Joan, when she remembered having been 'dedicated' to Satan in the basement of her Catholic church."

Hearing Kate's voice, Emily tuned back in to the table conversation. "Once and for all, I'd gotten her to give up the irrational belief that she's Satan's child, so I thought. But a couple sessions later, she was talking about the same thing again. I got so frustrated, I raised my nice, nunny — pardon me, ex-nunny — voice: 'In the name of God, they can't hurt you anymore. To protect themselves, they made you think they would if you talked.' In the next session, when I'm apologizing for losing my cool, Joan says dryly, 'I've heard about scream therapy, but isn't it supposed to be the patient who does the screaming?' And I thought, right in that moment, she's starting to get well."

Amidst laughter, Emily heard her own voice as if muted under water: "If these kinds of crimes against children aren't real, how can I explain a client identifying my own father as her rapist in what clearly appears to have been a cult of pedophiles masquerading in old Ku Klux Klan costumes?"

Everyone at the table became quiet as Emily continued to speak. "Would that my memories of that moment were false, that I had picked them up from the media or from some therapist." Looking down, Emily slowly lifted the cloth napkin from her lap and placed it over her mouth as if trying to absorb the bile rising in her throat and the rest of what she wanted to say: "And I could get down on my knees in front of my mother and beg her forgiveness . . . for having destroyed *her* delusion that my childhood was safe and good."

Trying to cope with an assortment of feelings: pains shooting through her pelvic region, anger, anxiety, mostly embarrassment, but also shame for having admitted to a group of colleagues that she was one of *those people* they were treating, Emily skipped the afternoon session and went up to her room. Leafing through a packet of convention handouts, she found and read an article by a therapist, Kathy Steele, titled, "Sitting with the Shattered Soul."

Waiting for the icy chills to melt away, she re-read the conclusion:

> So how do you sit with a shattered soul? Gently, with gracious and deep respect. Patiently, for time stands still for the shattered, and the momentum of healing will be slow at first. With the tender strength that comes from an openness to your own deepest wounding, and to your own deepest healing. Firmly, never wavering in the utmost conviction that evil is powerful, but there is a good that is more powerful still. Stay connected to that Goodness with all your being, however it

manifests itself to you. Acquaint yourself with the shadows that lie deep within you. And then, open yourself, all that is you, to the Light. Give freely. Take in abundantly. Find your safety, your refuge, and go there as you need. Hear what you can, and be honest about the rest: be honest at all cost. Words won't always come; sometimes there are no words in the face of such tragic evil. But in your willingness to be with them, they will hear you; from soul to soul they will hear that for which there are no words.

When you can, in your own time, turn and face that deep chasm within. Let go. Grieve, rage, shed tears, share tears. Find those you trust and let them be with you. Know laughter, the healing power of humor. Trust yourself. Trust the process. Embrace your world, this world that holds you safely now. Grasp the small tender mercies of the moment. Let you be loved. Let you love. The shattered soul will heal.

And she re-read the paragraph about therapists who are also survivors:

Therapist-survivors are the crucibles from which emerge a terrible blessing, a gracious curse. This is the blessing: that they intimately know the way of healing, that they choose this precious gift for themselves and then share it. This is the curse: that they intimately know the way of anguish, that their own shattering is the price exacted from them, their own soul wrenched for a time into wretched darkness.

The blessing . . . it *was* possible for Dr. Emily Lentz Klein to "know the way of healing . . . and then share it."

She could sit with clients as they told their stories but couldn't pull them from the pits of their private hells. She could show them some ways to get out but couldn't force them to use her suggestions.

She could teach them to access the dissociated states who had saved them, allowing each client to choose the way: writing, painting, sand play, self-hypnosis, dream analysis, mapping the system, free association, deprogramming, just talking.

She couldn't rescue them from the grips of their perpetrators, external or internal. If they wanted to confront their abusers, she couldn't stop them.

She couldn't stop them if they chose to go public with their stories. She could share her concerns about their decisions but wouldn't attempt to control them.

She couldn't save them from self-destruction but could help them understand why they were compelled to hurt themselves.

She could be with them as they discovered ways to tame their inner tormentors, to rewrite their destructive programs.

She could be a companion on the spiritual journeys of those who, consciously or unconsciously, had defected from the ways of evil and were trying to restore their shattered souls.

Drinking ginger ale and munching on pretzels in the bar, Emily and Kate waited for a table to become available in the hotel restaurant. It was the final night of the conference and they'd decided to skip the banquet.

"I wonder how many therapists will go home with PTSD as a result of what they've experienced at the conference," Emily was saying.

"Count me in," Kate responded. "You think you've heard it all—the ultimate in evil ways—and then you hear some more."

"The thing I've found most interesting," Emily said, "is how few of us are talking about the spiritual component of trauma. Perhaps it's because we're afraid of offending others who don't believe like we do."

"You're right. In graduate school, we learned all about the diagnosis and treatment of psychopathology, but not much about the dilemma of good and evil. Not any ways to answer our clients'—and our own—questions like: Where was God when I was being tortured? Why did he let it happen?"

"Well sister, we could give them the pat answers: God doesn't abuse. People do. I can tell them what I believe: that it's all about free will, that their perpetrators chose to be evil. But to tell you the truth, I feel a little hypocritical here because I really don't know how much choice perps—or anybody—in dissociated states have. Also, I often wonder if abuse victims who blame God are really projecting onto him the blame that should go to their parents or other caretakers."

"Good point, Emily. In a similar vein, I believe some people who devote their lives to serving God are really trying to gain approval from a heavenly father that they didn't get from an earthly father. To be honest, I don't always understand God either. In my opinion, the people who believe they do have likely made the entity conform to their own needs."

"So, using that logic, the people who don't believe there's a God, don't need one. Is that what you're saying?" Emily asked.

"I've never thought of it that way exactly. But I do have respect for the few atheists I know personally. In fact, a colleague of mine who claims to be a humanist is one of the most 'Christian' persons I know, especially as he relates to clients."

"When you think about it, Kate, the whole 'God thing' must result in mass confusion for severely dissociated individuals. Some of them have different personalities with different images of God and different religious practices. One of my clients had an alter who converted to Christianity, but while she was being baptized, a New Age alter who had been abused by a priest came out, panicked, and ran down the aisle, straight out the church door with water dripping all over her face."

The maitre-d' came over to announce that a table was ready.

Emily looked at Kate. "I'm not feeling very well. Really, I think it'd be best if I go on up to my room."

"I'm sorry. You should've told me earlier."

"To be honest, I was hoping the pain would go away so we could talk into the night like we did in graduate school. It used to be so much fun in the wee hours, especially when we got silly."

"We'll just have to get together another time real soon. As always, you know you have an open invitation to come to Santa Fe. But for now, you need to get a good night's sleep. Have a safe trip home and be sure to call me when that new grandbaby gets born."

"Definitely I will, and you have a safe trip, too."

"And one more thing," Kate said before they hugged good-bye, "perhaps you should think about seeing a doctor for a checkup."

Chapter 23

T here *is* life outside therapy, thankfully, gratefully, new life, Emily was thinking as her son-in-law placed Winslow Emily Amato, less than ten minutes old, into her arms. Brad, grinning like a . . . like any proud new father, had just described the whole birth process in minute detail. After a few minutes of doting, Emily passed the tiny cherub with a head full of orange fuzz to her other grandmother.

"Where did she get that hair?" asked Brad's mother. "You can be sure it didn't come from our side of the family."

"From my mother," Jeff answered, pensively looking out the tenth floor window of the same hospital in Atlanta where he'd been born in much different circumstances. He'd been told his daddy was in Germany at the time. The only family member present was the aunt with whom his mother had spent her pregnancy. Jefferson Winslow Campbell Klein had supposedly been born two months early, a nine-pound, six ounce preemie.

"And my handsome daddy," Carol glanced at her in-laws. "Comes from their Scotch-Irish heritage."

"My turn," Jeff said, after the other grandmother had held Winslow a reasonable amount of time.

A nurse came into the room. Looking at Brad, she said, "Time for weigh-in. You can come with me. Bring your camera. The rest of you can watch from the window. And Mrs. Amato, somebody'll be right in with your breakfast."

"Thank you. I am a bit hungry. An all night's labor is pretty hard work."

"I'll stay with you, Honey," Emily said, chuckling at Carol's play on words.

"Me too," the new Granddaddy Klein chimed in.

"Thanks," Carol said, as the other relatives followed Brad and the nurse out the door. "I want you both to know something. I pray that Brad and I will be as good to Winslow as y'all have been to me." Without giving them time to react to this honor above all honors, she went on: "There's something I've been wanting to talk with you both about. Brad and I have decided," Carol raised the birthing-room bed to a sit-up position, "with being parents and all, we've decided that Winslow needs to grow up around an extended family, around grandparents. And since neither one of us wants to live up north, we're planning to move back to Chestnut Ridge if—"

"Wonderful!" Emily interrupted.

"Wonderful!" Jeff parroted. "I've been thinking about asking you to come up and look after restoring and managing the plantation and asking Brad to take care of all the other family businesses and investments. With his background in tax law, I can think of no one better qualified."

"Wow! This is too much excitement for one day." Carol lowered the bed and lay supine, smiling at her father. "I'll talk it over with Brad, but I'm pretty sure what his answer will be."

"Great. As your Granddaddy Cleat said at your engagement party, 'What this family needs is a good lawyer.'"

Slipping easily into the role of grandmother, Emily spent the first week of Winslow's life in Atlanta: cooking a little, cleaning a little, mostly rocking the baby and trying to ignore the sometimes shooting, sometimes cramping pains in her right side and pelvic region.

More body memories, she assumed, remembering labor pains from long ago . . .

"Get them out of here," Emily whispered to Jeff upon seeing Cleat and Amanda Jarrett come bursting through the door of the private hospital room on the third floor of Campbell Memorial Hospital during her twelfth hour of labor.

"They just came to see how you were doing."

"But it's embarrassing," she said, so low her visitors couldn't hear. For some reason Emily had felt ashamed during the whole pregnancy with Carol. Happy, although for some reason, ashamed. She'd had morning, noon, and night sickness, throwing up so much she'd actually lost weight.

Her father-in-law made some asinine comment and Emily turned over, pretending to sleep.

A few minutes later Gladys came into the room carrying a bud vase with a single red rose, saying, "The girl must not be having too hard a time if she's asleep."

Emily 'woke' up. "It's been rough, Mama."

Gladys didn't bother to sympathize at all with her daughter's travail, rather she described in vividly boring detail how difficult Jimmy's birth had been: "Had him right there at home in the hot summertime with no air conditioning, and the windows were wide open . . . it was so embarrassing. And when he was born, Dr. Bill wasn't even around. As I remember, he and your daddy had gone downtown to get a bite to eat. If it hadn't been for old Lossie Mae standing by my side, don't know what would've happened. Oh my, it was much worse in those days. I'm sure everybody up and down Main Street could hear me hollering. Now they just give you something and put you to sleep."

While Cleat, Amanda, and Gladys were still blabbing, an orderly and a nurse came into the room. "It's time to go now," the nurse said.

"Go where," Emily asked. The nurse ignored the question, concentrating on getting the patient lifted onto the gurney: "One . . . two . . . three . . . lift."

"Can't my husband come with me?"

"No ma'am. That's against hospital rules."

Jeff kissed his wife good-bye and they wheeled her away.

All alone on that cold gurney, Emily spent the last six hours before Carol's birth in hard labor surrounded by three or four groaning women just as terrified as she, awaiting the unknown.

But Emily Lentz didn't groan. She didn't cry. No sir-ree. She was a good girl.

At one point they gave her a hand-held ether mask to use during contractions. One whiff of that cold, sickening gas and she cussed a little and threw it on the floor.

The last things she remembered were feeling the top of the baby's head between her legs, and seeing another mask coming toward her face.

A quarter of a century later, they made Emily drink something awful; strapped her to a table. A man in a white coat came in the room saying, "This won't hurt a bit," stuck a needle in her arm, put her in a big machine, told her to lie still, and took about fifty pictures of her private parts.

When it was over, Emily asked the Charleston gynecologist, "Are you gonna have to cut me open?"

"If you want to know what's there, ma'am." In the tone of an auto mechanic describing the problem with a car's transmission, the doctor went on to describe the risks and procedures of the surgery. "We'll prepare your bowels in case there's a problem and target the sites for chemotherapy—"

Her blood turned cold.

"Could be you have ovarian cancer."

Her blood turned colder.

"The CT scan shows a large mass in your pelvic region. We won't know if you have cancer till we take it out and get a report from the pathologist. You also have several gallstones. I'll get a general surgeon to take out the gallbladder while we're at it. We need to get you in here in a hurry."

"Why? You got a vacation coming up?"

The man looked at her like she was a nut.

As she was putting her clothes back on, reality socked her in the belly.

Emily Lentz Klein—not quite fifty years old, two weeks a grandmother—could die without seeing Baby Winslow take her first step.

In preparation for the surgery, using what she taught clients, Emily practiced self-hypnosis, reminding herself to use the pre-op shot as a cue to go into an altered state of consciousness, a willful attempt to block out the trauma.

There was one problem. When it came time to be taken to the operating room, she was so relaxed, according to blood pressure and heart rate, the doctor skipped the shot. The orderlies loaded her onto a gurney and wheeled her to a room with a big light overhead where people were standing around getting ready to mutilate her body.

The last thing she remembered was the mask coming toward her face, learning only later that the surgeon had been about to make the first incision when the anesthesiologist yelled that the IV had not been started.

Dissociation at its finest. Classical.

The next thing she saw was the doctor standing over her head mouthing the word, "Benign." Surely he must've said more when she was in the recovery room but that was all she saw. Selective attention?

The patient would live.

The body was back in her hospital room but Emily was out of her mind.

"Over there." She pointed to a huge magnolia tree outside her window, its leaves glistening in the winter sun. "Do you see those witches and fires?"

Saying nothing, Jeff followed her line of vision.

The patient looked around the room. The wall was covered with faces. "Don't you see them, Jeff? They're laughing at me." To Emily they were as real as the pictures on the wall at Cricket Cassidy's beauty shop except they were moving.

"Who's laughing?" her husband asked, compassionately.

"Don't know." A part of her realized she was hallucinating because of the morphine, but another part wasn't sure.

Alone in the room after Jeff had left for the night, Emily heard her mother talking—a clear distinct conversation—to someone in the hall.

But her mother was not there.

Early in the morning, a nurse came in to inspect the electrodes attached to her abdomen. Fiddling with the TENS unit, an electrical device used to block out pain, she turned up the current; turned it off and back on again.

"Shut that damn thing off." Literally shocked out of her delirium, Emily cried out, "What are you trying to do? Electrocute me?"

"I was just trying to see how this gadget works," the nurse said meekly.

"Well, in the morning you can explain it to the CEO because I'm going to call him right now and tell him how you hurt me and—" Suddenly, Emily realized she was getting out of control and began to feel sympathy for the woman who had tortured her. "I'm sorry. I won't call him but I do think I should tell your supervisor so you can get the proper training in how to use that thing."

"Guess I had a few body memories cut out." The morning after surgery, Emily sat in the recliner smiling at her therapist. "Thanks for stopping by. The whole ordeal was quite an experience."

"Tell me about it."

"Routine surgery, it was. Like my mother said when she called me earlier this morning, 'Glad it was nothing serious.' Said it'd probably do me good to get a rest."

Uninhibited by the drugs in her system, Emily opened her hospital gown to show Julie the incision that ran from between the breasts to the pubic area. "They took out a grapefruit-sized tumor, a Fallopian tube that looked like an overripe banana, and a gallbladder filled with stones that looked like blackberries."

"Sounds like they extracted a fruit salad and you're angry with your mother. Glad you could separate the past from the present."

"*Now* I can, but I'm not sure if I did when it was going on. I've been doing a lot of thinking—"

"And?" When therapist and client met together, it was hard not to do therapy.

"Vaginal examinations, food deprivation, forced drinking, drugging, taking pictures of my private parts, strapped to a table, bright lights overhead, masks, electroshock, hallucinations, mental confusion, needles."

"Triggers?"

"Yes ma'am. It was quite an adventure." While giving a play-by-play account of the previous twenty-four hours, emphasizing the 'electroshock treatment,' Emily suddenly felt severe abdominal pain and clutched her stomach.

The world turned black.

"What's happening?" Julie's voice seemed far away.

"I'm not sure."

"Do you want me to call a nurse?"

"No, I think I'll be okay, but would you please stay a few more minutes." She reached for Julie's hand. "I'm remembering . . ." Realizing it was present time, Emily described what she was remembering: "I'm lying on a table, feet in stirrups . . . a woman over me is saying, 'Start counting backwards from a hundred' . . . 100, 99, 98, 97 . . . "

"How old do you feel, Emily?"

"About eleven."

"Where are you?"

"Not sure . . . now I see . . . walls with rusty ripples . . . mask coming toward my face . . . don't . . . don't . . . it's over my mouth and nose . . . a few whiffs of gas . . . chloroform . . . ether. I don't know what it is. . . . I breathe in darkness." Emily was wiggling, as if trying to get out from under straps on her wrists. "Now it's light . . . the doctor . . . what's he looking at? . . . bloody, red, tiny . . . in the palm of his hand."

"Emily . . . Emily." She heard Julie's soothing voice. "You're safe in this place. Do you know where you are?"

"In the hospital," whispered Emily, "I feel woozy." She pushed the button to bring the recliner up straight. "At one point I thought it was happening right now."

"What do you think was going on?"

"Can't be sure, but it must've been an abortion." Emily rambled on, "I know this sounds weird, but all the time I was hearing Christmas music . . . or perhaps it was the 'doctor' singing."

"What was he singing?"

Emily shook her head incredulously, trying not to laugh because it would hurt too much. "Somebody was singing 'Here comes Santa Claus.' It had to be a record. Roy Rogers? No, it was Gene Autry." She began to sing the last line: "Bells are ringing, children singing; all is merry and bright . . . " She stopped singing and screamed, "Where was Mama? Where was she when they pulled that life from me?" Covering her mouth with her hand, she managed to say, "Gotta go—"

Reeking with pain, the patient struggled to get up from the chair and into the bathroom. She got down on her knees in front of the toilet bowl and heaved up about a gallon of dry anguish from a stomach that was supposed to be empty. Feeling as if both her stitches and her heart had been ripped out, she stood up and turned around slowly. Her body wouldn't bend and she wet all over the floor.

In a frantic panic, Emily pulled a towel from the rack and wiped herself clean. She took a few deep breaths, then went back into the room to talk to her therapist acting as if nothing had happened.

Nothing at all.

"Is it possible that the stress of remembering trauma could have triggered a disease process in my body?" Emily was sitting in Julie's office a little more than three weeks after the surgery.

"That's an interesting question," commented the therapist, predictably. "As we've talked about before, some research has shown that gynecological problems are more prevalent among incest victims than non-victims. But I believe we should be cautious in attributing all discomfort to body memories."

"You know, Julie, when I was a child, I wasn't allowed to get sick. My mother didn't even have a thermometer. As far as I know, I was healthy, but somebody—either my mother or daddy, I guess—was always giving me medicine: mostly paregoric. I thought all kids had to take paregoric at night. They told me it was to help me sleep. It was an opiate and back then they didn't need a prescription for it. One of their friends, whom I called Mr. Earl, was a pharmacist—they used to call them druggists—was probably a ready supplier."

Emily looked up and noted that her therapist was yawning. But that didn't seem to deter her from rambling on. "I've often thought that's why I've had so many dental problems. Too many drugs. A dentist once told me I had soft teeth. Too many cavities. And another thing, somebody was always pouring eye drops in my eyes. I haven't figured that one out yet."

Without realizing it, the client had positioned herself on the couch with her feet on the backrest. "You know what . . . what I hated most was the smell of ether. They gave it to me when I was seven and had my tonsils taken out and during labor with my first child."

"Have you had any thoughts about the abreaction you had in the hospital?"

"Yes I have. To the point of obsession. I'd like to believe my imagination was out of control that day."

"Isn't it amazing, you've never had an abreaction in here, but you had one in front of me in the hospital? Why do you think that is?"

"I don't know, Doctor. You tell me."

"I'll give it a try. Perhaps the memory was state-dependent and because you were in a mental and physical place like they would have put you in during an abortion—drugged and in a medical setting— the memory was triggered."

"Or is it possible the nausea that usually goes with my abreactions would make me unable to drive home after therapy, and my unconscious knows it and won't let me have one? Anyway, you've said you don't think they're always necessary for recovery. Hope you're right. Although I've only had two other major ones— the preverbal molestation and the ritualistic-type abuse in the church basement—it'd be nice if I didn't have to go through any more."

"I can understand that. An observation I've made is that my clients who aren't recovering the memories want them, and those who are getting the memories don't. There's another theory about your not abreacting in therapy . . . related to the transference. You protected your mother from knowing what happened to you. Are you protecting me for the same reason?"

"Not at a conscious level. You're a professional and can take care of yourself. Thank goodness, you've kept things at a pace I can tolerate and never overreact to anything I say. Neither have you tried to downplay how it's affecting me. I suppose if I haven't decompensated after learning that people who were supposed to love me, hurt and betrayed me, I should be able to make it through therapy. About the abortions that a lot of ritual abuse survivors report, I'd like to know if they're done to procure a sacrifice to the Devil or only to get rid of the evidence."

"Good question. What was going on in your life when you were eleven?"

"I would've been in the sixth grade. I remember my mother telling me I was too fat, and she put me on a diet that spring . . . made me wear blouson blouses to hide my stomach. . . . Oh my gosh, she knew!"

"When did your first period start?" Julie didn't seem to have heard Emily's last comment which was just as well because Emily didn't want to talk about that possibility anyway.

"A few weeks before I turned eleven. It's like it was yesterday."

"Why so clearly?"

"Because it was the day the new town pool opened and Mama wouldn't let me go. You weren't expected to live normally during that time of the month. And something else . . . I remember saying to my mother when I showed her the blood, 'Don't tell Daddy.' A strange comment at the time. But now, knowing what I do, it makes perfectly good sense."

"Did you miss any periods?"

"Not that I recall. But I do remember having strong sexual urges. Didn't know what they were at the time. How could I? In a house where no one talked about sex. I was in the seventh grade or eighth grade before finding out where babies come from."

"No wonder you didn't know you were pregnant . . . if you were."

"It could've been possible, couldn't it? That I was pregnant and was aborted. Because if my father or anybody else messed with me, it's likely they didn't think about a condom—if they even had them in those days."

"There's some research to suggest early sexual stimulation can cause early puberty." Julie said.

"Mine was early all right. With big boobs already in the fifth grade. It was so embarrassing, especially when I went to summer camp and had to undress in front of other girls."

"What else do you remember about your eleventh year?"

"I was so afraid of thunder and lightning storms and so afraid I was going to die—so revved."

"When did you first learn about death?"

Emily thought a long time before phrasing the answer. "The first dead person I ever saw was my mother's mother, Grandmother Keller. But when I saw her in that copper casket, I didn't believe she was dead. I remember my brother and I touching the glass over her head, just to watch her hair fly up. Static electricity, I suppose. We thought it was funny. At any moment, I expected her to sit up and tell me to 'act like a little lady.'"

"She'd said that before?"

"Somebody did. Then there was my friend Jane who got run over by a school bus. She died. They dressed her in a frilly pink dress with a matching hair bow, painted her face with rouge, pasted her eyes closed, and took her home to rest. When I looked into that big shiny wooden box, I didn't believe she was dead and kept waiting for her to wake up so we could play."

Emily positioned herself flat on the couch, closing her eyes.

It was at least ten minutes before she spoke again.

"Death was a game . . . until I was eleven. I know something terrible must have happened that year. It could've been an abortion, couldn't it?" The client really didn't expect her therapist to answer the question. Wouldn't have been neutral. So she went on talking. "With each flash of lightning and crack of thunder, I cowered in fear. With every train whistle, I thought they—"

She interrupted herself in mid-sentence.

"Why in the world would I have been so afraid of trains? I thought they were coming to get me. Another thing I remember was being scared of sunsets. Every evening during my eleventh summer, the sky would turn orange, and I was afraid it was the fire at the end of the world. But I never told anyone, not even my mother."

She opened her eyes, closing away the memories and ending the session. "Death was a game . . . until I knew I would die."

Chapter 24

"Do something!"

Emily shouted. But in her heart she knew there was nothing her husband could do. After a year and a half, the cottage had been completely restored from the ravages of Hugo, and the family—Jeff, Emily, Matt, Carol and Brad and their four-month-old daughter—were at the beach on Easter Sunday.

Sitting in lounge chairs near the water, Jeff had been bouncing Baby Winslow on his knee when suddenly her tender gurgling and cooing changed to squeals, then open-mouthed silence. Her face was turning purple.

Rationally, Emily knew the baby was angrily holding her breath like babies sometimes do, and that Winslow would eventually breathe again. But all she could see at the moment was the helpless face of a little child who was dying.

"What do you want me to do?" Jeff handed their granddaughter over to her mother. He stomped up the boardwalk toward the cottage. Emily, close behind, didn't stop until she was in the upstairs bedroom—alone.

A face frozen in eternity.

Lying in bed with her eyes closed, a net of images appeared with the ocean sounds and breeze coming through the window: the smell of ether, tiny Christmas lights, tinkling bells, a baby in a manger, a huge hand over a little hand. A knife—

Nothing made sense till she saw the baby's dark, curly-haired head. Someone was systematically removing its skull.

Talking to herself—to the child ego states—like a therapist might talk with clients immediately after they'd just remembered atrocities, she said, "It's 1991. Those things happened a long time ago. It wasn't your fault. He made you do it."

As it seemed to be happening all over again, Emily felt as if she were boiling in a cauldron with the inner kids who had gone through hell for her when she was little; who had just turned over their once dissociated guilt, revulsion, horror, and grief at being forced to commit murder. When the abreaction was over and her focus was on present-time, Emily's automatic switch, which usually turned off her feelings when they were too intense, failed.

All the wounds—behavior, affect, sensation, and knowledge—she had pasteurized, homogenized, and stored for more than four decades seemed to be splattering all over the place.

It was a gift, in its own way—those feelings.

Emily Lentz Klein was reclaiming her soul.

But at a price.

All uncertainty toppled. The huge left hand that had forced little Emma Wee Wentz to commit murder was missing its little finger.

By the time the sun had set, Emily's heart was beating normally again. She walked downstairs and lifted Baby Winslow from her crib and carried her up to the top deck where she stood for a while, looking out over the ocean.

In almost darkness, she remembered the exact moment when Emma Wee Wentz was sitting on the little wooden chair in the Blue Bird Reading Circle in the first grade, and for the first time the letters on the pages of the big book hanging across the teacher's easel became words . . . and the words became sentences . . . and the sentences told a story that made sense.

Taking a deep breath, Grandmother Emily sat down in the chair at her back. Lovingly holding Winslow over her heart. Rocking the infant gently into the night.

Chapter 25

Humans cannot be programmed like robots, Emily had believed. But that was before she began working with Sandy Witherspoon. During the winter of 1991 when people all over the world were being entertained by the Cruise missile show, that massive attack of weapons launched from air and sea during the Gulf War, the tiny woman with blue eyes and long straight blond hair had begun psychotherapy.

"This is embarrassing." Sandy positioned herself on the couch with her feet resting on opposite thighs. "I woke up last Saturday night in my hotel room with a strange man on top of me and . . .. "

So vivid was her description of the experience, Emily almost felt as if she'd been there with the woman. "After it was over," Sandy continued to speak as if she were reading a book report in front of class, "he left without saying a word. As I lay in bed like a stunned deer, blood streaming from my vagina and nose, the phone rang and another man who seemed to know a lot about me told me that I'd done a good job. After taking a long shower trying to scrub the dirt away, I walked down to the Battery. Overlooking the harbor, I could see myself living a whole other life. For months, I'd been going to Charleston on weekends to peddle my artwork . . . and always had dinner in my room and went to bed early, I thought. What's happening in my life, Dr. Klein? Could I have another personality out working the streets?"

"Do you have a history of mental illness?"

"So you do think I'm crazy?"

"I just want to know more about you, that's all."

"Me too," said Sandy. "And no, I've never been treated for mental problems, but the physical side is another story. I have these uncontrollable migraines, severe pain in my knees, asthma, chronic sinus infections, and you can see I'm way too skinny. Probably bulimic. Or is it anorexic? Most of the time when I am able to get food down, something comes over me and I make myself throw it up."

"Why do you think you do it?"

"Helps me feel better. Isn't that weird? And while we're playing true confessions, there's something else I do. This I've never told anyone . . .I can't stand the feel of hair around my pubic area and when one comes in I pluck it out."

"Trichotillomania."

"You mean there's a name for it?" Sandy asked with more emotion in two seconds than she'd shown in the previous forty-five minutes. "I've always done it, even as a kid."

"What else do you remember about your childhood?"

"Just that it was horrible and I've always tried to forget it. My mother had a brain tumor; died when I was five. Daddy was a chaplain in the military and dragged me all over the country—New Orleans, Tucson, San Antonio, Houston . . . we stayed in Houston a long time . . . Colorado Springs, Los Alamos, and somewhere in Nevada—when he wasn't on a secret assignment."

Emily wondered why a Christian minister was involved in covert operations with the U.S. Government, but refrained from asking.

"And there's something else I've never told anyone . . . too ashamed . . . but he would use me . . . like a . . . a wife . . . but sometimes I stayed with my maternal grandmother in upstate New York. She was wealthy and had a summer home in Chestnut Ridge, so I spent a lot of time here, too."

"What brought you back?"

"Several things. After college, I took a job in Boston as a commercial artist. Married a coworker who was the kindest man I'd ever met, but it only lasted a few months. Turned out he was gay, which didn't surprise me after the few times we tried having sex, but it was devastating. About that time my grandmother died, leaving me her house, and . . . I suppose you'd call it independently wealthy. So I moved to Chestnut Ridge and set up a studio where I do some free-lance work, but mostly I do what I want to do. I'm pretty much a loner. Learned to be that as a child. We were never in one place long enough for me to make any close friends."

"You mentioned headaches," said Emily who had been listening intently for hints about her primary problem.

"I've had them checked out and my knees too. One thing is really strange. A few months ago, I had sinus surgery and the doctor said my cavities were covered with scar tissue and wanted to know if I'd ever had surgery and I told him not that I remembered. My scan was normal, of my head anyway."

"That must've been a relief, since your mother died from a tumor. Any other physical problems?"

"They did a bone scan and it showed my bones were covered with some kind of film. One doctor said he'd never seen anything like it before. Also I have a chronic low-grade fever and they can't tell where that's coming from. Another doctor said I have some symptoms of the onset of multiple sclerosis. But I'm not a hypochondriac. The problems are all real and documentable."

"Do you have any social life in this town at all?"

"Not really. As I mentioned earlier, I'm pretty much a loner. Sometimes though, when my father comes in to visit we have dinner with some of his old military buddies."

"But didn't you say he sexually abused you as a child? It must be tough being around him."

"I try not to think about that. He's the only family I've got and as I told you, I spend most weekends in Charleston . . . which brings me back to my reason for coming here. Do you think it's possible I've been doing things I don't remember doing?"

"Possible? Of course. True? You'll have to figure that out for yourself. There was a case reported in the professional literature of a woman who studied medicine by day and worked as an exotic dancer by night. And for a time, neither personality seemed to know about the other."

"How could that be?" asked Sandy. "And how could I be prostituting myself? But from the memories that have gushed out over the last few days, someone must've been—or is—making a bundle off me. Please Dr. Klein, please help me find out what's going on. Help me find out who's controlling my body and mind."

In the first few months of therapy, Sandy had become immersed in her expedition to find the buried clues about her other life. Fortunately she had the intellect and financial means to chart her own course. The disconnected aspects of herself began to relinquish the messages and memories they had been charged to keep. And Sandy continued to remain emotionally unaffected—until faced with the memory that she had been used in child pornography and the possibility that the pictures were still floating around somewhere in the universe.

One morning, she'd found a typed communication on her dresser.

To Sandra from Marilyn,

Let me first say that I understand I am not a real person, that I am only the remnant of a little girl who lingers in your mind. But there was a time when I was very real, when you created me to do what you couldn't do. What I am about to say is something that nobody in the world wants to hear, but I think it is time that you and your therapist know exactly what happens when little children are used in making dirty movies. Perhaps you and she can find a way to make the details of such horrible crimes against children known to people who can do something to stop them.

You were six or seven when your daddy handed you over to another soldier. Then you turned things over to me. It was I who went into a big metal building holding the soldier's hand, and he took me into a little room where a woman with bleached-blond hair and dark brown false eyelashes cleaned me all over and brushed my hair and put makeup on my face and took me out to a stage with lights and cameras all around.

A big man lifted me up to a table that was very close to the floor. About a foot, probably. He took off all his clothes, and took mine off too, and carefully folded them and laid them on the floor. I waited stiff as a board as he put some kind of cream on his you-know-what. I remember hearing someone say before they turned the cameras on, "Be sure and get a close-up of his manroot." I suppose they were talking about his you-know-what. Once I looked up manroot, but it's not in the dictionary.

Well anyway, the bright lights came on and I heard someone say, "Shoot." I remember thinking that somebody must have a gun, but I was very little and hadn't yet learned much about being in movies. The big man squatted over my face. "Lick it off," he said. "It's ice cream." And I was afraid that I would be shot if I didn't, so I began to lick his you-know-what and it swelled up like a funny-shaped balloon, you know like one of those that looks like a hot dog, like the kind the clowns at the Shriners' Circus blow up to make little children laugh, and it tasted like almond flavoring.

After that first time, you would leave as soon as your daddy said he was taking you to the movies. That's where you must've thought you were going. I suppose he was trying not to lie to you because we both know that preachers aren't supposed to tell lies, and you *were* going to where the movies were being made.

For the next year or two, I was in lots of movies. First, they took pictures of big people sticking things like pencils, then candles, then flashlights in me, getting me bigger and bigger down there. Getting me ready to be the special star, they said.

Sometimes they brought dogs and monkeys to be in the movies too, but I didn't stay around. If you ever want to know about that, somebody else will have to tell you.

By the time you were nine, I was big enough to "act like a grownup," they said, and they made me do all the things that big girls do with big boys. Sometimes with the big boys taking turns in different places.

One day the woman who was primping me up at the time noticed some fuzz accumulating around my private parts.

"Oh no," she said. "That's not good. They won't have that. You have to look like a little girl." She made me sit still while she rubbed some kind of hot wax over the area. Made me wait for a long time, then took a rough rag and rubbed it and the fuzz came off. After that I always kept the new hairs pulled out so the big man wouldn't get mad at me.

Don't feel sorry for me. It never hurt a bit.

After reading the letter from the alter her unconscious had designated to take care of the pornographic abuse, Sandy had panicked and overdosed on prescription pills. Just before passing out, she had called a friend who took her to the emergency room.

———————

"The doctor said you're going to be okay." Emily, whom a nurse had called at Sandy's request, gripped her client's hand. "You're a survivor."

"I hope so," Sandy responded, still groggy. She pointed to the letter on the bedside table. "Will you please read this? So you will understand what got me here."

While the therapist was reading the letter, the patient got out of bed and moved to the recliner. When Emily had finished reading, Sandy said, "Last night, thinking about being used in those horrible ways and the possibility that the pictures are still floating around out there somewhere. . . well, I just didn't want to go on any longer. But when I woke up this morning, I made the decision once and for all . . . this last year has been kinda like riding a roller coaster. Every time a new memory was about to surface, I'd get all wired up. The antsy feeling would grow in intensity, peaking for a time until I couldn't stand it any longer, then

I'd cut myself or binge-eat and make myself throw up, and that'd make me feel better for a while . . . or pull the hairs out around my pubic area."

Emily said nothing; she didn't need to. Sandy had already made the connection. The therapist sat quietly, listening intently to the rest of what her client had to say.

"Thanks, Dr. Klein, for coming by. What I wanted to tell you is that when I woke up this morning, I made a decision once and for all."

"What was that?"

As if all the weakness Sandy had been experiencing suddenly evaporated, she spoke assuredly, "I want to live. And I don't care what those assholes—whoever they are—told me. I will remember and I will not die!"

A year and a half after Sandy had first come to therapy, Emily, so as not to be a distraction, settled on the sofa as the client created a three-dimensional picture in the sand tray.

The therapist noted that the young woman was stopping frequently to count to five over and over. Sandy had said that she had been taught to do this to keep herself from telling something that she had been programmed to keep secret.

Watching her client, the mind of the therapist was racing through a catalog of comparisons she would have never wanted to have to make.

It had been only a few weeks earlier in June of 1992 when Emily and her friend Kate had attended a conference in Alexandria, Virginia, where they'd heard therapists from all over the country discussing patients and clients who were remembering what could only be understood as mind control and other programming techniques. Everyone, without exception, wanted another explanation. Another kind of answer. Emily, most of all. But there had been no other intellectually viable answer from anyone. No therapist was making this up and perhaps they were beginning to realize, neither were their clients; the ones Emily had begun to call "unwitting initiates into organized evil."

One presenter talked about a possible connection between the CIA and Satanism, stating that toward the end of, or immediately after World War II, the U.S. government in an operation called Project Paperclip, in addition to recruiting German rocket scientists, had smuggled out Nazi doctors who'd been conducting mind control research in the concentration camps, and who may have been involved in Hitler's brand of occultism. The psychologist believed that some of the Nazis had continued their experiments in U.S. military hospitals and/or had gone to the already existing satanic covens to get their pool of subjects—children who'd already learned the lessons of dissociation. He reported that declassified documents on secret mind control research had proved that the CIA did, in fact, fund experiments in the testing of brainwashing techniques.

Speakers and attendees discussed techniques involving projects like MKULTRA and Bluebird and Artichoke, Oz-programming, primal dissociation, psychic-driving, remote viewing, and Alpha, Beta, Delta, Omega, Gamma, and Zeta programs. They talked about individuals who reported, but couldn't actually prove, they had deliberately been structured to be multiples so that they would unknowingly carry out covert activities for the government.

A social worker from Florida mentioned that one hypnosis exercise, using the elevator image, had seemingly been used to create alters who could then be exploited in orgies, pornography, prostitution, blackmail, drug running, assassinations, and about any other criminal purpose one could imagine.

During a break, several therapists were discussing the idea of primal dissociation. According to this theory, preverbal children were purposefully conditioned to dissociate as foundation for later programming. Could it be that Emily's frequent sensation of pins sticking in her feet was a body memory of her having been tested for her ability to dissociate pain?

A type of programming using physical spinning along with other mind control strategies, such as cognitive and imagery training, was reportedly used by experimenters to spread physical pain, confusion, inappropriate sexual feelings, and all sorts of emotional havoc through an experimental subject's personality system. Because Emily had often felt out-of-context sexual urges when she felt threatened or made a mistake, she wondered if she had been subjected to such conditioning.

Someone said that parents often cued their grown children, who had entered therapy and were disclosing cult abuse, with the phrase, "I'm praying for your full and complete recovery." Supposedly, the purpose of this was to bring the wayward child back under control.

While one speaker was describing the suicidal program, "If you remember what happened, you will kill yourself or go crazy," Emily remembered—how could she forget?—jumping off the pier into the black ocean water. What about all the times when she'd tried to talk in therapy or write about taboo topics and she'd feel a drugged-like feeling come over her?

Someone mentioned *The Book of Torture*, which contained recipes for all sorts of sadistic activities including forcing children to hold out heavy objects on outstretched arms for long periods of time. Miss Amanda Jarrett, with her geography books as tools, must've owned a copy signed by the Devil himself.

Reportedly, rhythmic dancing and chants were used to put children in states of highly-focused attention and concentration so they could learn their lessons better. Teaching children to write backwards was possibly done as an experiment to develop the right brain, not necessarily as part of satanic training. Some initiates had been instructed not to be hypnotized by anyone but their programmers.

She heard about children being forced to maim or kill other children or animals, of little boys being taught to practice sexual acts on siblings.

Another common programming technique, the reversal of meanings, was highly significant. Now she had a feasible explanation for her unexplainable, horrified reaction when Jeff had first said, "I love you" on the pier at Windy Hill beach when they were sixteen years old. Some lingering ego state could've heard it as "I hate you."

There appeared to be a correlation between the era in which a person was initiated into a destructive organization and the sophistication of programming. Pretechnology methods seemed to have worked better. Emily had read nothing in the professional literature about people in her mother's generation seeking therapy for aftereffects of ritual abuse. If Gladys were a product of deliberately inflicted trauma, as Emily suspected, she'd likely used dissociation to escape conscious knowledge of her own persecution, and also any remembrance of things which happened to her children.

Declassified documents had indicated that drug experiments were conducted in prisons during the war by the OSS, the forerunner of the CIA. Henry Kiser had said that he was a subject of some type of experimental program while in the POW camp in Chestnut Ridge. Government agents could have conducted those procedures—German prisoners weren't going to tell . . . who was there to tell?—and stayed after the war to keep the lab operating.

Was it possible that the POW camp, and later the military academy where Cleat was 'keeper of the keys,' could have provided facilities for the CIA experiments on children? Linda Lou had talked about electroshock in what sounded like the infirmary out there. And right there on the grounds was a train track and an airport to ferry kids in and out.

As the therapist was making all these connections in her own mind, Sandy had begun to sob like a fearful child. From the shelf of toys, she'd just taken a few pieces of doll house furniture and other assorted props, including three tiny tables on which she'd placed three finger-sized dolls. A male figure in a doctor's uniform stood next to one table. Beside another was a little bundle made from gauze. She picked up a wad of black modeling clay, shaped it into a cube, and placed it next to the third.

"Black box . . . that will hurt you," Sandy whined, but kept on working. For the other scene, she picked out a little red plastic coffin that had held Halloween candy in the real world. Making the best black robe she could from modeling clay, Sandy used it to dress a male figurine. Next, she rolled a snake from a piece of green clay. Then she picked up a tiny baby doll and placed it and the snake in the coffin together. She used the robed man to bury them in the sand. To complete the sand picture, she turned a tiny gold cross upside down and stuck it on top of the grave.

"Something stinks." The client coughed and gagged until the therapist suggested, "Try to relax, if you can. Take a deep breath."

"I'm okay," the grownup Sandy responded. "Just a little surprised at what one of my alters just told me."

"What was that?"

The client stood up and walked over to the dry-erase board. With a red marker, she made two columns:

Woods	Laboratory
Altar	Gurney
Moon	Bright overhead light
Graves	Isolation tanks
Ropes	Straps
Goats	Dolphins
Cross	Scalpel
Blood	Drugs
Symbols	Computer codes
Snakes	Electroshock

"Same rituals, different technology," Sandy said, insightfully.

Chapter 26

From the moment they'd first walked

into the room in 1992, it was obvious Betty and Franklin Griffin hated each other. Divorced for two years, they shared custody of their daughter and had come together again, only because their child was exhibiting learning and behavior problems in class. The teacher at the Christian school had suggested a psycho-educational evaluation, noting on the referral form:

> Crystal Griffin is seven years old and is repeating first grade. Her group IQ score is average but she's not doing grade-level work. I'm concerned about the inconsistencies in her academic performance. For example, on a recent math test she missed two thirds of the questions; repeating the test a day later, she missed only one. She takes Ritalin for attention deficit disorder, but I don't think that's the whole problem. She often stares into space unaware of her surroundings as though she's in a world of her own. Frequently she makes self-deprecating remarks. At times, she sucks her thumb and exhibits other quite immature behaviors.

Emily didn't know the parents personally but had often seen their names in the paper. An executive at Syn-Tec, Franklin Griffin was a man involved in many of the community's organizations. His ex-wife was a volunteer with the Arts Council.

Her long straight prematurely gray hair framing a sun-wrinkled face, Betty wore jeans and a plaid flannel shirt. Franklin was dressed in a three-piece suit worn over a stiff white shirt which he'd accented with a hand-painted silk tie decorated with heads of African animals.

The mother spoke first without any prompting. "Crystal's such a bright child. She's been in beauty pageants all across the country and has never had problems learning routines." Reaching into the side pocket of her large handbag, Betty took out a small portfolio. "I just happen to have these with me. Want to see what a beautiful child she is?"

The psychologist politely shuffled through the studio prints, amazed that the heavily made-up subject was only seven years old. "They're very nice," she said.

"Give them here." Franklin grabbed the folder from Emily's hand.

"I think she's capable of doing first-grade work when motivated," Betty went on talking, ignoring her ex-husband's rudeness. "The biggest problem is math. Sometimes she recalls math facts; sometimes she doesn't."

"You're wrong." The father looked up from the pictures, hatefully. "Her biggest problem is not concentrating. The pediatrician says it's attention deficit disorder but I'm not sure I agree. She just lives in a . . . a lollipop world."

"Tells lies all the time," the mother offered helpfully.

"Come on, Betty. She doesn't always know what she's saying. For crying out loud, she's only a little kid whose imagination runs away with her sometimes," Franklin now countered, contradicting his own earlier remark, apparently for the sole sake of making his ex-wife sound foolish.

"How do you discipline her?" Emily interrupted their clash, thinking this was not the purpose of the meeting: to referee two squabbling estranged parents.

Franklin was quick to answer first. "I guess we're . . . a little inconsistent, maybe. I never spank; spoil her rotten," he grinned, "buy her anything she wants. If you ask me, Betty uses a hickory stick way too much. Anybody knows it doesn't do any good to whip her. She just kinda wings-out; doesn't even know you're doing it."

Betty faced Franklin. "Well you try to make her act like a little soldier and not do anything wrong." Then she turned to address Emily. "She's got, like two extremes. Nothing else. I'm telling you, sometimes she's passive; sometimes violent. Moody, she is. I think she's trying to hurt someone and I don't know if it's me or her daddy. And another thing, since about the age of three, maybe almost four, there've been times when she's so sensuous that I—"

"At least I don't let her use foul language around me." Franklin was in the driver's seat again. "The other day when she was sitting on my lap and I was picking, just playing around like, she yells, 'You're not gonna get my ass!' Now I wonder where she hears stuff like that. Unless it's from one of those sissy men you've been hanging out with. I tell you one thing—"

But he didn't get to finish. "Why do you buy all those provocative clothes then?" Betty hurled the attack like a rock through a plate glass window. "She's a little girl, for Pete's sake, and you make her dress like a slut."

"A lot of room you have to talk . . . with that closet full of all those glitzy pageant costumes you order from New York." He looked satisfied with the return missile.

"In either of your opinions, has she ever been hurt in any way?" Emily asked.

"You could say so," Franklin glanced spitefully at his wife, "if her mother trying to abort my little sweet pea in the third trimester would count."

Emily glanced at Betty for verification or denial.

"Yes. I did. I was having a hard time. Real depressed. Didn't think I could take care of a child . . . so I drank some quinine. Made me awful sick with a lot of bleeding. . . . but it didn't hurt the baby, she got born okay."

"It's hard to tell the possible effects of prenatal injury," Emily commented, matter-of-factly.

"There was an incident with sexual overtones once in a day-care center—"

"Oh Betty, come on. There was nothing to that."

"Tell me about it anyway," Emily nodded at Franklin.

"Well, she and some of her little friends came home with some wild tale saying the day-care owner—who happens to be my good friend, mind you—had made all the children take off their clothes and dance around the room and play doctor with each other . . . kids do have wild imaginations at that age, don't they?"

The parent interview was over before Emily had time to learn much about Crystal, other than the fact that she was the product of a very disturbed relationship.

The following week during the videotaped observation and examination, Crystal obtained IQ scores in the slow-learner range, but appeared much brighter. Achievement scores were at grade level, suggesting that the IQ scores didn't give a valid estimate of her academic potential. There were many inconsistencies in test responses, very much as the teacher had reported. Sometimes the little girl would miss questions, then be correct on items at a higher level.

After the testing was completed, Crystal eyed the dry-erase board in the corner. "Can I draw something?"

"Sure."

"Tell me what to draw."

"How 'bout a picture of your family?"

Crystal drew three ghostlike figures on the board and captioned them "Dad," "Mom," and "Star." In the Griffin family was a child named Star—but not herself. "You know what," the little girl looked under her shirt, "I can push my bellybutton and make Star come out."

"What does she look like?"

"She's cute and has short blond hair and blue eyes."

Crystal had long brown hair and dark eyes.

"Star's happy. I like her. You know what, she always tells me math answers."

"Would Star talk with me?"

Again the child looked under her shirt; this time pushing on her tummy, calling, 'Star, come here.'"

Her facial expression changed to a more mature-looking child. Body language shifted to a childlike representation of a sensuous adult. "Hi. I'm Star."

"Where's Crystal now?"

"Up there." The little girl pointed to a corner of the ceiling. "Can't you see her up there?" The child was apparently experiencing depersonalization, a phenomenon in which a person feels detached from his or her body.

Eyeing the camera on a tripod, Crystal picked up a microphone, stood up, and like a tiny actress pretended to sing and dance.

Without warning, she threw herself down on the floor, kicking her legs in the air, moaning, "No. No. Don't make me." Putting her hands over her mouth, she curled into a fetal position.

Later playing the tape for the parents, Emily had explained, "I don't have to make a formal diagnosis, but I believe your daughter has created at least one imaginary friend, perhaps a different personality state, to help her cope with something she couldn't tolerate."

"What could that be?" Betty asked.

"I can't say, but it's possible that it could be something like the day-care experience you mentioned, or anything traumatic."

"Like the attempted abortion—"

"Just shut up, Frank."

Things were getting out of hand, and Emily was beginning to suspect that either of these two people was capable of inflicting the kinds of mistreatment that would cause a child to dissociate, or—as Crystal's teacher had aptly described—to escape into a 'world of her own.' Unfortunately, there was not enough evidence of wrongdoing to report anything to Social Services.

"In my opinion," Emily said, "your daughter definitely needs to be in therapy. Probably structured play therapy."

"What's that?" both parents asked at the same time.

"Well, if she's experienced trauma, some of it may have been before she was verbal. The behaviors you've been seeing such as the regressions could be unconscious re-enactments of experiences she's actually had and doesn't know how to communicate or is consciously afraid to communicate. Play therapy using the toys in my office may give her a way to tell without talking if, in fact, she has anything she wants to tell."

Apparently having already decided that Emily was getting too close to the truth, Franklin jumped in to say, "We certainly want to find our daughter the help she needs. My company has a private jet and I can fly her to an expert anywhere in the country."

Betty also appeared eager to take Emily off the case. "I think we should at least get a second opinion," she said. "There's a child psychiatrist in Charleston who's supposed to be good."

The therapist's hope of being able to help the little girl vanished. Franklin and Betty Griffin both agreed that Crystal was disturbed and needed help; clearly, they didn't think Dr. Klein, small-town psychologist, was the professional who could provide that help.

On the other hand, they might have been afraid she could.

———————

Emily never got to say good-bye to Crystal . . . or Star.

Several months after the last session with the Griffins, Franklin's attorney had called saying that Emily would be receiving a subpoena. Crystal had told the new psychiatrist that her daddy had made her do bad things; that he had made videos of her and other children without their clothes on. The doctor had reported the accusation to Social Services.

In a three-hour deposition taken in the presence of the prosecuting and defense attorneys and the guardian *ad litem* for Crystal, Emily made it clear that the child had made no verbal disclosures of abuse and had been taken out of therapy when the possibility of trauma as a cause for her dissociative behaviors was suggested.

Later Emily had learned that the father had been cleared of all charges. Crystal, the judge had ruled, was an emotionally disturbed child who was fabricating horrible stories merely to get attention. She'd been ordered to a treatment center. It was doubtful that her memories would ever be credible because she had already become a certified mental patient, stamped with stigmata that would follow her forever.

"Crystal's an enigma," the new therapist, calling to get copies of the test protocols, had said. "We don't seem to be making much progress. The kid's always getting in trouble then denying she's done anything wrong. Sometimes she whines and pouts like a baby. At other times she's overly mature. Unnervingly so."

"I believe she's mentally constructed a number of alternate expressions of—"

Emily was quickly interrupted by the man. "Oh, we've seen no evidence of that."

"Are you going to allow visitations with the father when she's released from your facility?" she asked.

"I see no reason why we shouldn't, Dr. Klein. Mr. Griffin appears to be a decent caring man. If you ask me, both of her parents spoiled her rotten. They tore her apart."

Chapter 27

"Well child, 'pose I can tell
ya now about ya mama since she don't know she's in de world no more."

"What, Aunt Beatrice? Tell me what?"

"Whatchu been askin' about. Who ya pappy wuz."

Putting her random thoughts aside, Maggie was "all" there at her mother's bedside as she listened to the story of her conception.

Later that night, January 3, 1994, the older Miss Rucker passed on and the younger Miss Rucker made the decision to close out psychotherapy as she had no other choice.

Maggie came walking—walking—through the front door. Emily went over to greet her with a warm embrace.

"Told you I'd do it," Maggie smiled. "I feel like I've sprung loose. My muscles are stronger, I rarely feel pain and, thank God, no more seizures."

"Terrific. I'm impressed. You've certainly added new meaning to the term 'mind-over-matter.'"

"But I couldn't have done it without your help. Thank you so much." Maggie sat down on the waiting room sofa. "I still have to rest a lot. If it's okay, could we wait till my fiancé gets here before we start the session? I want you to meet him."

"Fiancé? You never even told me you had a boyfriend."

"I haven't? Sorry, I forgot . . . no that's a lie," Maggie argued with herself. "To tell you the truth, I just wasn't sure it was for real; if every part of me was really in love." She glanced out the front window at the short stocky bearded white man coming up the walk. "Here he comes now."

When the groom-to-be came into the waiting room, Maggie made the introduction: "Emily, this is Wayne Volz. He knows all about you and . . . all about all of me."

"Congratulations," Emily said, shaking his hand.

"Pleased to meet you, Dr. Klein. Your husband is a colleague of mine. I teach at Wesley, too. Sociology."

After several minutes of superficial conversation, Maggie looked at her watch—it seemed like she was always looking at her watch. "Gracious, my time is half gone." She caught Wayne's eye. "I really need to talk with Emily alone."

"Fine. If it's okay, I'll just wait for you out here." He offered to help Maggie stand.

"I can manage." Refusing his gesture, she stood up and kissed her lover lightly on the lips. "See you after while, Honey."

When Maggie and Emily were both comfortably seated in the therapy room, Maggie said, "I'm happy and I think I'm making the right move, but this falling in love with Wayne thing has me sorta worried."

"What do you mean?"

"To be honest, I'm afraid that our biracial relationship is going to cause some problems here in Chestnut Ridge."

"Surely Maggie, the administration at Wesley won't care."

"That's probably true, but did you know that the constitution of our great state still prohibits interracial marriages? It hasn't been enforced in years, but it might be interesting if I can't get a license and have to challenge the law. Especially since I'm apparently as white as I am black."

"Oh Maggie, nobody in the legal community will harass you. You, of all people, they're not going to violate your civil rights."

"It's not them I'm worried about. Whites pretty much leave us alone now. It's not like it was when I was little and we lived in fear the Klan would attack and burn our houses to the ground."

"Then who are you worried about?"

"It's the black community. Many of the older generation just can't stomach the thought of a white man with a black woman. I think it goes clear back to slavery."

"But things have changed."

"Have they really? You can say that with a straight face after all the recent church burnings in the South? If our churches aren't safe, what is? Sometimes I wonder if the fight for freedom was worth it. And then

I think about what it must've been like in the days before the Civil War when Whites rationalized slavery by saying Negroes didn't even have souls." Maggie wiggled around on the couch as if posturing herself for something she didn't want to say. "There's one more thing . . . I've decided to close out therapy because—"

Emily gasped. This time she didn't even try to cover it with a cough. She wanted to shout: No! No! No! You can't do that. Quickly she got back to neutral, detached, hoping that the client hadn't seen her reaction. Probably not. Maggie's eyes were fixed on Emily's hands.

"You're ready to close out your therapy?" Emily reverted to Counseling 101 and the reflection technique.

"Yes I am. I'll want to see you occasionally, but since I feel as good as I do now, I don't care about processing—God I hate that term and what it means to me—any more memories. There are other things I'd rather do. Wayne and I are even talking about moving somewhere else. The way I look at it, if they do come . . . the memories . . . I'll see them for what they are. With your help, I've learned to separate the past from the present. Although there may be lots more memories in that proverbial closet you talk about, I believe I can handle them now. It's like I've seen the movie and know how it ends. I don't have to go back and replay all the scenes I missed."

"I really do understand what you're saying, Maggie . . . more than you'll ever know."

Client and therapist stood in synchrony and walked to the middle of the room: each giving; each receiving a single embrace.

In another time and place, Margaret Rucker and Emily Klein could have been friends.

Chapter 28

The professor sat in a circle with members of his senior seminar at Wesley College. He opened the week's topic, "Destructive Cults," by reading:

> Thus ended the third day's examination, and what does it tell? Simply this. That if the evidence is to be believed, there is a state of affairs in this State, which sends a chill of horror over everybody, and every man, without regard to political principles, should have an earnest desire to have the thing fully investigated and sifted to the very bottom. If these charges cannot be sustained the people should be relieved of the terrible suspicion, and if the witnesses told the truth, and there is, as yet, no reason to doubt their word, the law- abiding citizens should wish to have the perpetrators of the horrible crimes punished, and their diabolical organization rooted out of the county. It is to be hoped, not only that the courts will investigate the affairs before an impartial jury, but that the people of this section who love order, and detest crime, will render all means in their power to have the truth vindicated.

"Would anyone venture to guess what diabolical organization this writer is describing?" the professor asked.

"The Ku Klux Klan," answered everyone but the other white member of the group.

"Correct," said Dr. Klein. It was a subject dear to his heart. A subject he'd become obsessed with since finding the "Bull" costume and KKK oath. In fact, he'd taken the robe and headpiece to a museum curator who had identified them as the regalia of the early Klan in South Carolina. "But what I just read could be a description of any destructive group, any cult that can provide a secret place for criminal activities."

He held up a little brown book that was smaller than his hand titled, *The Testimony of Witnesses in the Preliminary Examination of the Lenoir County Prisoners: The Secrets of the Ku-Klux-Klan, &c, &c, &c, 1869,* which he'd recently found among some of his grandmother's books and papers. "This is a journalistic account of an incident up in North Carolina where some Klan members had been charged with murdering Negroes. I use that term, which some of you may find offensive in present time, because it's the term used in the book. They were imprisoned; however, some of their fellow Klansmen broke into the prison, releasing them by force. When the alleged murderers were brought to trial, three former Klan members turned State's evidence and on the stand revealed some of the secrets of the Klan."

"For real, Dr. Klein? What were they?" one of the students asked. "I've heard that they believed in a white man's government, but I've never heard any specific secrets."

"I'll tell you some of the things I've read, but if y'all would like, I'll have my secretary make copies of the whole book. It's too old for any copyright to be in effect. Who all would like to have one?"

Everybody raised their hands.

Jeff handed the book to the student nearest him to pass around the class.

"As I was saying, they talked about guarded meetings where they plotted to kill Negroes. Each initiate took an oath to obey all officers, even if he had to kill his brother or father, and was told he'd be killed himself if he disobeyed orders or talked with anyone about the secret organization."

"Listen to this," a female student who'd been leafing through the book interrupted: "On page 42 it says one Klansman had testified, 'When I joined the organization, the sign of recognition given was to put your right hand on the breasts, the sign of distress is the hands behind the head, the grip is a shake of the hand with forefinger doubled in.'"

"A secret handshake. Don't the Masons have those?" asked the white student.

"I think so," answered Jeff, "but I believe that it's quite common in all secret groups. As are oaths."

One of the students offered: "From what I read in a local history book, the Klan around here actually began in 1865 under the name 'Slickers.' It was similar to other secret societies, such as the Knights of the White Camelia, White Brotherhood, Constitutional Union Guards, Invisible Empires, Invisible Circles, and who knows what else. Eventually, they all united under the KKK moniker. Whatever they called themselves, they were a sort of terrorist organization attempting to overthrow Reconstruction from within."

"Like guerilla warriors," added another student.

"Yes, but there's another side to this controversy that's not politically correct to talk about in this day and time," the white student said.

"Oh yeah. What's that?" asked the woman at his side.

The white student defended: "From what I've read, the radical government leaders used former slaves for their own self-interests to plunder the land."

"Whatever it's purpose," continued the young man who'd mentioned the Slickers, "it was organized by an ex-sheriff from a neighboring county."

"Must've been an ancestor of the Paxtons." Tyrone, who was always late to class, had come through the door and jumped right into the discussion. "All us local black folk know that in the days before the civil-rights movement, Sheriff Casey Paxton was big in the Klan. But you gotta give him a little credit. At least he wasn't a hypocrite like some of the other town leaders who probably went to their graves denying any involvement in it."

Thinking once more about the Klan oath in the Campbell family Bible, Jeff had the urge to crawl under the table.

Tyrone sat down directly across from the professor: "Sorry I'm late Dr. Klein, but I was downtown making a child-support payment. And would you call this coincidence—or what—given our current class topic?" He held up a flier he'd yanked off the courthouse bulletin board announcing a Klan meeting at the Smith farm in the eastern part of the county on Halloween night. "Anyone care to go?"

———————————

When Jeff arrived at the Smith farm wearing jeans, a flannel shirt, cowboy boots, and a red bandana wrapped around his head, the dusty cow pasture was alive with men, women, and children. Some wore white robes, probably ones they'd borrowed from choir rooms in their regular churches. Holding Bibles in their hands, many of the older folks were sitting on wide wooden planks supported by five-gallon buckets, twanging out, "The Old Rugged Cross," as if they were at a camp-meeting revival. Up front was a wooden trailer still attached to a John Deere tractor. It held a pulpit built of orange crates stacked on top of each other. Two flags, slightly blowing in the cool autumn breeze, stood on either side of the trailer: one a Christian; the other a Confederate.

He looked for a spot to stand, ending up behind a little girl wearing double pony tails. She was waving her own tiny battle flag that was attached to a pencil-sized pole.

After some warm-up testimonials and the singing of a few gospel songs, the leader introduced the speaker for the evening, a visiting 'dignitary' from Alabama. Wearing a white robe and a playing card-sized gold cross around his neck, the middle-aged man began preaching a message of hate, peppering it with put-downs like, "America is a white man's country and if the niggers don't like it, load them on a rowboat and ship them back to Africa."

Near what he hoped was the end of the sermon, Jeff smelled kerosene misting up from the bottom of the field and began to feel sick. It was one thing to have read about this diabolical group, quite another to pretend, even for an hour, that he belonged.

The preacher was stumbling over a few verses of the *King James Bible*, interpreting them to mean that races shouldn't mix and that Blacks are cursed. Ranting, raving, and misquoting scripture for another twenty minutes, he suddenly stopped, reached out his hands to the flock, saying reverently, "Let us now go."

The followers left their pews and stopped by the stage to pick up torches which they held in front of the leader to light with his own torch. Everybody got in line and marched to the bottom of the field down by the creek where they formed a large blazing circle.

What must those little children be thinking? Jeff was wondering as he joined the procession . . .

The ritual begins. From out of the darkness, a robed figure carries his torch inside the circle and ignites the tall cross in the middle announcing, "Christ is the light of the world." He continues in a deep voice. "We light this cross as a symbol of hope. It is our duty to save America. We must preserve the white race for our children."

Jeff smiles at the Klansman's pastoral voice—actually more pastural: i.e., full of manure.

In response, worshipers slowly move their torches up and down chanting, "God, Country, Klan . . . God, Country, Klan."

With the cross still aflame, the service ends and the party begins. A concession booth like those at the county fair has been set up on a hill where women are putting together burgers and barbecue. Kids line up to buy syrupy snow cones. One man has set up a table of Klan memorabilia: silver rings with a Klan insignia, KKK engraved knives and belt buckles, Confederate flags in all sizes, and T-shirts printed with the flag.

Apparently sensing a new convert, the leader walks over to shake Jeff's hand. "Glad to have ya with us tonight." He turns his head sideways and spits out a mouthful of tobacco juice. Turning back around to face Jeff he says, "Hope you come back again, Mister . . . what did ya say your name is?"

"Paxton," Jeff, thinking fast, lies. He is positive that this open naive group of people is not related to the secret group that flourished under the reign of Casey Paxton—unless they were planning to hold a meeting after the meeting at which only a select few pedophiles would be privileged to attend. Anything was possible, but he hoped this was just an ordinary run-of-the-mill hate group.

"Well Mr. Paxton. It's a fine bunch of folks. We'd be mighty proud to have you as a member. If you ask me, it's the only hope for the white race."

Jeff feels like saying, "Your claim of superiority is really a claim of hate," but he is on their turf and keeps his mouth shut.

Walking up the hill to the parking area, Jefferson Winslow Campbell Klein felt like a bomb of betrayal was rolling around in his gut. Betrayal by bigots; by his daddy; even Papa Campbell—a man of his word as Grandmother Campbell had once described her husband.

Chapter 29

"That's how they got me to comply as a child, I think. My mother sang to me, rocked me, and stroked my head. Sometimes she counted backwards until I swam away to a safe island in my mind."

Julie responded, "Your mother must have been a natural—"

"Hypnotist?" Six years into therapy, Emily was certainly relaxed enough to say whatever came into her head without stopping to analyze or hedge every statement. "Lately it seems as if I've been flooded with . . . insight, let's call it."

"All right, let's call it that. Tell me about it."

In the natural style of all self-analysis, Emily continued talking. "You've said we need more data. Here goes. I'm going to try to get a perspective on it from the beginning. First came the revved sensation. Looking back, I see a lot of repression that forced me to take action. I suppose that poltergeist show I told you about was just a little added entertainment. At any rate, everything together forced me to get myself down here to see you."

"Revved—it certainly got your attention," said Julie. "Go on."

"In here . . . at times when I've tried to talk, my tongue feels like something caustic has been put on it. Often when I try to write, a drugged feeling comes over me . . . ."

Slipping into self-hypnosis, Emily lay flat on the couch.

"Tell me what's happening."

"A single drop of blood . . . eyes . . . a hunting knife . . . a child hanging by her feet . . . people wearing white robes and conical hats marching up a mountain to the cross on top. And the storms of sin are raging." Emily sat straight up. "Where in the world did that come from? Am I making these things up?"

"Why would you make up something like that?" the therapist asked. "It had to come from somewhere. Any interesting dreams lately?"

"That's about all I do at night," the client quickly answered, chuckling at the absurdity of her response.

"Tell me about them."

"In one, I'm a little kid about six or seven getting ready for my wedding . . . that's weird . . . upset because no one will help me get my makeup on."

"Interesting. How about your mother? Was she there?

"No. My mother just wasn't there. And the child parts wanted her to care."

"What do you think that means? Do you see anything you've carried over into adulthood?"

"Even adult children want their mothers to care," Emily quickly answered. She lay down again and went back to the point she wanted to get across. "I think I've told you about the secret family I used to imagine. Well, there's got to be a connection between the way I was traumatized and my fantasy life as a child. By the way, one of the people in that family was a grandmother who loved and protected me."

Oh my goodness. Was Hannah around when I was little, telling me everything was going to be just fine? she asked herself. *Or was it God she was asking? Or was it God who was telling her everything would be okay? Or was it her unconscious?*

"Your inner protector, perhaps," Julie said. "How do you think all this relates to your image of the cross and the storms of sin raging?"

"That's easy to see. The storms of sin are blowing, raging like storms at sea. And it's like I'm jumping back and forth between ships: one is good, a safe ship that carries the cargo of my happy childhood, wonderful family, and all that; the other is probably sitting at the bottom of the ocean and even after this long period of searching for memories, I still don't have any idea about some of the dark and evil things it's sheltering."

"Any other dreams?"

"Well yes. It wasn't really a dream, but last night before I dropped off to sleep I saw a kaleidoscope of faces: Miss Jarrett, my sixth grade teacher; Uncle Phil; Dr. Wilhelm; the Oz-like face of Mr. Earl, the druggist; Reverend Miller, the minister who baptized me and taught me in

Catechism that telling dirty jokes is committing adultery and that God loves you like a father."

Emily sat up again, slowly this time. She faced her therapist, stretching her arms. "It's a wonder I didn't become an atheist when I was eleven years old."

"Those images really seemed to open you up. Is there anything else you want to say about them?"

"Let me think . . . yes . . . there was one of my daddy. I know it was him because he was wearing white buck shoes, you know the kind popular in the fifties." Emily took a sip of the diet soda she always kept by her side during therapy. "So Doctor, what do you think all this stuff means?"

"Em-i-lee." Julie sounded like a mother disappointed in her daughter's lack of self-confidence.

"I know. I'm the one who has to figure it out. If you want to hear it, this is what I wrote immediately after waking up this morning."

"Of course I do."

Emily pulled a pink index card out of her pocketbook and read a single sentence written in cursive:

> Jeff's daddy was there but no one would believe it and Jeff is scrunched in the corner whimpering.

She turned the card over and read the large print.

> Snow Force. Who was she?
> The princess. She knew how to turn men on.
> She had them in the palm of her hand.
> Jeff's daddy did not like her.
> He was mean.
> I HATE Jeff's daddy. He is a turnip.

"Looks as if you've redissociated—to use your term—and you've gotten back in touch with those parts and they're talking," Julie interpreted.

"Wide open, aren't they? But I don't especially like what they have to say. And there's something else I need to tell you."

"Go ahead."

"Well I went back to sleep again, but at daybreak I heard an audible voice—and I rarely hear those—saying, 'Cleat, the little girls are beginning to remember, do you?' Thank heavens I know a little about dissociation and auditory memories or I'd probably have myself committed."

"Emily, you are *not* crazy. As I've heard it described, you're just having sane reactions to insane situations."

"Thanks. I say that to clients all the time, but I needed to hear it . . . for me."

"It would be impossible to say whether the dreams and images and automatic writings are purely symbolic or whether they represent concrete events or—"

"But which is it?" Emily interrupted, her eyes searching for some absolute in the therapist's facial expression. "You don't think Jeff—"

"I don't believe we know yet," Julie paused, "but I don't think he would have shown up in some gruesome montage stimulated entirely by your having listened to the traumatic experiences of your clients."

Silence sat between them like a third person in the room.

A little later, Emily thought she heard wind . . . in sails, but didn't make mention of it.

Chapter 30

Something was telling her to go back to the old hotel. A few days after Cleat and Jeff had walked clearly into her graphic memories, Emily dragged Jeff on a field trip, as she'd come to call her return visits to possible crime venues.

Acadia, home of the Gray Nun Ghost and social center of the town for a hundred years or more, was now, thanks to Mary Katherine Delacroix Campbell's generosity, home to the living ghosts of Chestnut Ridge: parents whose children had forsaken them, retired winos, schizophrenics who had given up the streets, and Vietnam vets who were still fighting the war in their minds.

A woman standing behind the old registration desk looked up from filing her nails. "Good morning. How can I help y'all?"

"We just want to take a look in the attic," Jeff answered. "My grandmother used to own this place and I think she might've stored a few things up there . . . if that's okay."

"Fine with me." The woman went back to her nails.

Walking past the cloak room, Jeff pointed out the original oak telephone booth in the corner. "That door beside it leads to the tunnel."

"Tunnel?"

"Yes, when I was little Papa Campbell used to send me through it to carry the hotel's deposits to the bank. In those years, all the merchants on the street had underground connections."

They probably still do, Emily started to say, but changed her mind. "Must have been scary for you down there all by yourself."

"Not really. I thought it was fun. During the Cold War, they turned the bank basement into a fallout shelter that was accessible from about every building on Main Street."

"Yeah Jeff. Sounds like the good ol' boys' network was looking out for itself, if you know what I mean."

He didn't respond.

Cutting their way through heavy cigarette smoke spilling out from the ballroom, they walked up the steps to the mezzanine. Except for a TV set in front of the fireplace where residents were sitting around watching "All My Children," not much had changed in the six years since the final charity ball. The same round tables and straight-back chairs were scattered around the room. Faded gold brocade drapes hung over dingier sheers. Dusty artificial palm trees filled up the corners. The Rotary Club banner hanging over the mantle was still asking, "Is it the truth?"

Seeing the old elevator with its door open, Emily said, "Let's ride up to the top. Can you run it?"

"Should be able to. I saw J. D. do it enough."

They stepped inside. Jeff pushed the red button for light; the black for power. Nothing happened. "We'll have to walk up," he said.

Climbing the stairs, Emily's knees buckled. Using the hand-carved railing for support, she noticed her heart racing and began to talk to herself. "What you're experiencing may be a body memory of something which happened a long time ago. Breathe deeply and relax." This time, her prescribed treatment for her clients' stress didn't help her at all. On an intellectual level, she knew she was not in harm's way. But her body, probably responding to some unconscious knowledge, was telling her something else.

Upon reaching the third floor, they stepped into a hallway floored by black and white asphalt tiles. Tongue-and-grooved walls, long ago painted white, were splotched with dirty hand prints. They went through a door at the end of the hall, up a few more stairs and found themselves in the attic. A few feet in front of them, an old chimney protruded through the floor to the roof.

Across the way, Emily saw it: the oval-shaped, stained-glass window in her vision. Chills washed over her like a breaking wave as it all came together in her mind . . .

Strapped to the table. Above her looms the huge Oz-like face of Mr. Earl. Beside him is someone wearing the horned hood. She smells roses.

Candlelight flickers in the window. Palm trees all around. Painted green ocean on the wall. Lights. Bright lights come on. They bring the little boy from the corner. Put him —

Little girl, don't cry. Not now . . . You can cry when it's over . . . Swim to the ship.

"Em, are you okay?" It was Jeff in present-time.

"No I'm not. Get me outta here!"

Floating in the middle of Lentz Mill Pond on the pontoon, Emily was eventually able to verbalize the images of Acadia. "In that room there was a boy on top of a little girl and somebody was running a movie camera."

"Are you sure you weren't remembering a dream?"

"When it was happening, it's like I was a little bird perched on one of the rafters."

"Did you see any faces?"

"One. Mr. Earl. He looked just like the Wizard of Oz in the movie. He was the one who gave me something to drink, probably some kind of drug to make me not remember. The others weren't clear. But I'm pretty sure one was wearing the horned hood . . . and we both know about the hood. Somebody else was standing behind an old home movie camera on a tripod." Emily gagged. Her stomach was churning and she got down on her knees with her head over the side of the boat still talking. "Jeff— you were there, too."

"What are you saying? What are trying to tell me?" he asked from the driver's seat.

"I'm not trying to tell you anything except what I saw."

"Come on Em, you had to be dreaming."

She turned around and sat on the boat's floor by his side. "I was wide awake. It wasn't a dream. And there was a wedding . . . and they had you on that table with me. And . . . and you don't believe me, do you?"

"I believe you, Hon. It's just that I don't want to. Maybe I'm a little afraid that if I have to go through what you're going through—if I re-member what you're remembering—I'll lose my mind."

"Perhaps you should see a therapist."

"Why? To confirm your memories?"

"No, but maybe to assure me I'm not as crazy as my mother thinks I am."

"But you're trying to prove the unprovable! Why, Em? Why? What good would it possibly do you to know that . . . that we . . . that we were more than childhood sweethearts? You can't unring a bell—"

"Or ever be a virgin again? Is that what you're saying?"

"No. But for God's sake, leave it alone! Our life's good enough as it is. What if they do come after us?"

"It's too hot," she said, ignoring his question, "I'm feeling better now. Think I'll swim back to the shore." She stood up, kicked off her shoes, pulled the pontoon's door open, and still wearing street clothes dived into the pond. Upon surfacing, she yelled back, "See you there."

Gliding over the water, her thoughts went back to the days before she began her plunge to the past; to the nights when she craved her husband's touch. Emily was yearning to experience that feeling again. Whatever was happening, they were in this together; had always been. There would be time to figure out why she'd once pulled away, but today she wanted to be loved—physically.

When she reached shore, Jeff was waiting on the dock. As if hearing her thoughts, he pulled her close. "I'm sorry Hon. I'll do anything I can to help you except please don't make me dig up any of my own old bones."

"But Jeff—"

"Come on. It's been a rough day. Let's play a little in the hot tub."

Letting the water jets massage her aching shoulder muscles, the hot ice in her cells seemed to melt away. Surprised, she felt herself feeling amorous.

They climbed out of the bubbling water. He pulled a towel off the hook and began to slowly dry her body. For a long time they played together on a plush sunroom rug. Laughing. Teasing. Caressing. Starting at his toes, she massaged each of his muscle groups as if she were kneading a ball of dough. When she touched the inside of his thighs, her fingers felt a roughness she'd never noticed, had never wanted to acknowledge. Hidden beneath thick coarse clumps of hair, she saw three long narrow scars on each leg near his groin.

"You've been cut," she said, trying to hold back the scream lodged in her larynx.

"Must be stretch marks," he said without bothering to look.

Not wanting to spoil the moment, to stifle the normal erotic feelings cascading through her body—the first in a long, long time—she turned over on her back.

"Your turn," she said. Not flinching or pushing him away, she guided his hand to places aching for relief.

He waited until she was ready—until she pulled him to her. And their bodies entwined in a passion she'd thought was lost.

Chapter 31

Was that her mother's voice she heard above the crowd? Emily noted that the pastor and the congregants were chanting responsively Psalm 130.

Out of the depths have I cried unto thee, O Lord.
Lord, hear my voice:
 *let thine ears be attentive to the voice of my supplications.
If thou, Lord, shouldest mark iniquities:
 *O Lord, who shall stand?
But there is forgiveness with thee:
 *that thou mayest be feared.
I wait for the Lord, my soul doth wait:
 *and in his Word do I hope.
My soul waiteth for the Lord more than they that watch for the morning:
 *I say, more than they that watch for the morning.

"Blessed are the dead . . . " a man in a black skirt overlaid with a white cassock began to read the committal.

A whiff of rose fragrance floated up from the casket spray triggering an embarrassing sneeze under the canvas tent in Mt. Hermon Cemetery. Rose water. Now she remembered. Her daddy's cologne. The scent carried her back to 1955, the year she had turned thirteen . . .

Her daddy was talking into the mouthpiece of the black pedestal phone that sat on the half-moon table in the middle of the long wide hallway of their home on Main Street. Emily was in her bedroom eavesdropping on one side of the conversation:

"I ain't gonna bring her. Can't. Saturday's the day she'll be gettin' back from camp, and I won't be able to get her ready in time."

. . .

"I know, Cleat. That's the rule, but I don't believe they mean it."

. . .

"They ain't gonna do nothin' like that. They only wanna keep us all scared. Let me handle it. I'll explain it to Phil."

. . .

Forty-one years later, Emily was now suspecting that she had missed her thirteenth birthday 'party' where she would've stood before the 'sacred' group to officially become one of them—the big initiation.

Loyal to the end, they'd pledged. *Death to the traitor.*

They all took the oath seriously.

Except her daddy. He hadn't delivered his daughter. Perhaps he had not accidentally fallen off the trestle; perhaps he had been judged a traitor and had received the sentence of death.

Today, if she chose, Emily could believe that her daddy had given his life for her, that he died rather than taking her to a ceremony designed to tie her to the cult forever. One thing she believed: with Jake Lentz' death, she had been freed from physical entrapment in a destructive cult. When she became thirteen, her ego states were relieved from active duty and she had led a normal life—until that day Linda Lou Lackey had walked into her office shouting, "The Bull. The goddammed Bull!"

"Into your hands, O merciful God, we commend your servant, Gladys Keller Lentz," the young minister of First Lutheran Church was saying as he cast the red clay dirt of Campbell County over the polished oak coffin.

Earth to earth . . .

Ashes to ashes . . .

Dust to dust . . .

Emily kicked off her sandals, grabbed a pillow, and sat down at the end of the sofa. Crossing her legs over each other, she waited for the question.

"What's been happening?" Julie asked.

"Nothing in particular. But I'm not the same person who first walked through that door wondering only if I had been sexually abused; not knowing that I had been a victim of organized criminal abuse. It's like the time I went looking for a tiny sand dollar and a huge conch shell washed up at my feet."

"Tell me about that different person."

"Let me think . . . perhaps I feel like the first astronauts who went to the other side of the moon must've felt when they got back to earth. They, and the people here on this planet who cared for them, worried that they might not come back around after going into that unknown dark space . . . I know Jeff is relieved I'm about through with therapy."

"Really? Are you telling me you're ready to close out?"

"Did I say that? When I first came here—good grief, has it really been seven years?—I was afraid I'd get stuck on that dark side. But believe it or not, it's been worth the struggle. I discovered what was there, grieved it, at least for now, and am ready to move on. But I gotta say that there still are times when I question if it happened."

Julie smiled.

Emily smiled back. "Like a writer who has to step outside herself to edit her own work, I had to step outside myself to understand what was happening to me. When I walked into Mt. Hermon's children's church, when I climbed to Acadia's attic, when I found the snow blocks and the robe and the bull's horns, and when I remembered the abortion, I knew truth."

"Do you feel a need to know more?" Julie asked.

"Maybe. Maybe not. I now understand why I was revved. It's funny, but that awkward word is the only one that's come close to describing an otherwise indescribable feeling . . . to you or to Jeff . . . even to myself. I hope I never have to relive the torture of overstimulation again. However, I recognize that as long as I continue to treat clients who've been deliberately traumatized, my own fragmented memories will sometimes be triggered. The container which served as a repository for forty-seven years was just too loaded to be emptied in six or seven."

Julie nodded, agreeing.

They were two therapists talking about the terrain now; two professionals walking together.

"Each time I hear a tale of horror, a part of me will cower in fear and shame. Another will rise in moral indignation at the crimes perpetrated on children. And the—that well-trained, deeply caring part of me—will sit with shattered souls as long as they want me to."

"How long has it been since your mother passed away?"

"About six weeks."

"You've haven't said much regarding your feelings about losing her?"

"I suppose that's because I haven't had many. When I think about it, I believe that grief process—the one from losing her—began the day I told her about the preverbal abuse memory and ended the day I showed her the Klan costume. I couldn't even cry when they called from Whispering Pines to tell me she'd suffered a stroke while playing bridge and died at the table, nor did I cry at the funeral, and I haven't cried since. It's not that I try to hold back the tears. It's just that they haven't come. Anyway, if there's any truth to what the preacher said in the eulogy, my mother whose world was always beautiful in her eyes has passed on to an even more beautiful world."

"What's happened to the anger toward your mother?"

"What anger?" Emily smiled. "She once said she'd do anything to help me. But she'd never let me help her. Let me help her see the real world. Perhaps that was best. What right did I have to destroy her defenses? . . . Here comes the guilt again. Maybe the reason it's difficult to get to the anger is that I get too stuck in the guilt."

"That's an interesting thought," Julie commented, before changing the subject. "So what's it been like on the other side of the couch?"

Emily assumed her best position for free associating: flat on her back focusing on the recessed light overhead. "Thinking about the therapy experience, I'm now beginning to understand how important it's been as a professional to be, for a time, someone else's client. Before, I don't think I fully realized where all the residuals are for clients like me.

"My automatic writings exposed the real me. Looking again at them, I saw the 'me' I didn't see in the mirror—or bring to your office—or even my office for that matter. What I saw in my own words was the hidden me, and to some degree, the 'hidden' in so many of my own clients who, like me, were forced to defend themselves and their emotions against outrages no one could comprehend."

"It's good you could dissociate or you may not have lived."

"Yes, but I believe that somehow after my daddy died, I put the pieces together and lived a normal life. Perhaps if I'd never treated a ritual abuse survivor, I might never have needed a therapist myself. You've helped by just listening, by letting me talk it out. I'm very grateful that you never tried to push me to remember . . . or not to remember."

"As I've said before, I'm just an old-fashioned therapist."

"Me too. One thing I want to say is that the most conflicting thing for me as a therapist working on my own goals is the problem of neutrality. How can you be neutral when you know it's real? Experience is not neutral. As I heard some of my clients' stories, at some level, I must've known they were also telling my story."

"Perhaps that's why you were able to sit with them and listen to their horrors. You'd been there, too."

"To be honest, Julie, even today I'm not absolutely positive it was my own experience . . . but I'm not at all sure it wasn't. Neutrality versus human experience: I don't know, versus I do know. It's as if I'd gone to war but strictly as a dispassionate observer—wearing, say, the universal neutrality of the Red Cross, the symbol of the unbiased helpers of humanity—only to find that War didn't care and I'd be hit, too. Like the others. And once having been fired upon and injured, how could I remain dispassionate, professional, neutral?"

Silence.

Thank goodness her therapist knew when to listen and wait.

"The bottom line is: I have to be neutral with my clients so I can handle the countertransference without further splitting myself. But I don't have to be neutral with me and the dissociated parts of myself who saved me. To discover that my good childhood was a delusion was devastating. Although telling the story to you made it more bearable, I'm not sure the wounds will ever heal completely."

"What would it take to heal completely?"

"That's easy. Proof. Absolute proof that what my unconscious told me really happened. Absolute proof that my soul was raped, that my virginity, physically and metaphorically, was ripped away from me even before I understood what innocence was."

Again, silence.

"There's one goal I haven't attained. Although I learned to ask questions of my unconscious and accept the answers it gave in images, voices, dreams, writings, and body memories, I haven't yet learned how to regulate my emotional responses to that knowledge. My inability to modulate feelings when they become overwhelming is the most damning . . . I mean damaging—or perhaps I mean both—element of the aftermath. It's the all-or-none syndrome again. When I'm in the "all" state, the feelings are often too intense to tolerate. I immediately cross over and get into the feel-nothing state. I've accepted that the damage done when I was taught to suppress feelings may be permanent. So I continue to try to cope with the injury."

"Emily, that all-or-none feeling is described by almost every trauma victim I've ever known. It may be that the way a person handles this feeling determines functionality. Self-mutilators cut or burn themselves; alcoholics drink, and smokers use nicotine to regulate feelings."

"I guess everybody has his or her own way to self-medicate," Emily said. "I eat, although not as much as I used to. And exercise, swim, work, write, or use self-hypnosis. You know, I'm still not sure I understand why Jeff and I reacted so differently to similar experiences. In my opinion, he's lucky. He refuses to allow himself to know what happened; therefore, he is able to go on feeling normally. Me, I recognize what probably did happen, but for the most part can't feel a thing about it. Unless I feel too much. All-or-none. Where are the ones in between?" Emily couldn't help smiling. "I asked you that once before, didn't I?"

Julie made her final interpretation. "Because you've been angry so long at feeling unable to directly tell anyone — or because you were never able to get an explanation for your mother's revision of your childhood — you've almost ceased to believe in your capacity to feel. But I believe that capacity is like memory, it's still there, if you want it."

"Maybe. An interesting thing has happened, though. Since my mother passed away and I was forced to turn loose of my need to have her validate my feelings and memories, I don't seem to have the need to talk with you anymore."

"I think we'd agree, as professionals," Julie smiled, "it appears that the client has worked through the transference. The validation came from within yourself . . . not from your mother or from me."

"At least I'm no longer obsessed with the need to recall what they wanted me to forget. Neither am I afraid to keep the window to my unconscious open so I can see what's on the other side."

The client stood up. She walked over and sat down beside Julie's sand tray. There was something still nagging her brain, something she'd not yet been able to disclose, even to herself. Following only her intuition, she picked up the tools for telling and arranged them in the sand.

A fence divided the landscape. On the right was a village with a church in the center. Children played in the yards of the houses. A train, cars, animals, flowers, and trees depicted this side as a busy, active, pleasant place. On the left was a wooden block. In front of it were three figures dressed in monks' robes standing over an infant who was stripped and strapped to the altar. Five little girls of different ages — three, five, seven, eleven, thirteen — waited their turns to be sacrificed to the Evil One.

Studying her creation, Emily saw that it wasn't complete. She picked up a figurine of a bearded old man wearing a black robe and cap over his long white hair and placed it beside the altar.

God — or the nearest thing she could find that represented God — had been with this child in her time of tribulation.

Still, something was missing.

She picked up a hard rubber mother-figure with a painted-on purple dress, rolled it around in her hands, scrutinized it, then carefully placed it straddling the fence.

"Tell me about your picture," the therapist said.

"I don't really want to." The client paused, rubbing her forehead, studying the montage for a few minutes. "I don't want to believe it: that my mother reigned over both worlds. On an intellectual level, I know she betrayed me; at the same time I was cared for and nurtured. It's hard to accept the reality of having grown up in two different worlds with two different mothers. I don't want to believe she allowed me to be tormented in a world dedicated to Evil. I want to believe the things she taught me about Good."

Emily looked at her therapist who had sat down on the floor by her side. "Now I understand why it was so important for my mother to teach forgiveness. At perhaps an unconscious level, she knew that some-day she'd want to be forgiven."

Chapter 32

The null hypothesis.

Ten years the Kleins had spent trying to prove that the stories were false; the symptoms, benign. However, like barnacles on a pier post, the data had kept piling up—evidence from their minds, their bodies, their histories. The thought that you can't prove the null, that you can't prove that something didn't happen, had trickled into Emily's mind, somewhere on the air route between Charlotte and Boston.

Just as nobody knows what triggers a hurricane, what causes the initial spin on the winds to spiral faster and stronger as it moves through time and space gathering up energy and finally devastating everything in its path, it was difficult, at first, to understand exactly what made a healthy successful professional person become an overweight fright-ened, almost manic therapist seeking help for her own problems.

It could've been menopause coming on. But since the hysterectomy at thirty-two, she hadn't paid much attention to hormones or to any-thing else going on in her body.

It could've been secondary PTSD from the trauma of working with traumatized clients like Fred Crabtree and Linda Lou Lackey.

But it wasn't.

More than anything, Emily had wanted to believe that the memo-ries and images from her unconscious were pure imagination; that finding the old Klan costume in the *Mona Lisa* was coincidental with Linda Lou Lackey's memory of the Bull; that the 'dedication' service in the basement of Mt. Hermon was mixed up with her Christian bap-tism; that there was no abortion; that no three-year-old child was ever forced to participate in a baby scalping; that her mother had loved and protected her.

More than anything, Jeff had needed to believe that his chronic joint and muscle pains were caused by bacteria, a virus, anything but the wear and tear of having been perpetually tense under the controlling hands of a morally weak father; that his physical scars were really stretch marks; that his mother had not willfully abandoned him.

In the time since Emily had become a psychologist, twenty years now, her own world, like the miniature village encapsulated in the crystal globe the Weaver's had given her when she was little, had also been turned upside down. Most of the old town leaders—excluding her Uncle Phil who still had his hands in a lot of things, and Cleat who was as independently mean as ever—had moved on to retirement centers, nursing homes, or Olde Towne Cemetery. New industries were moving in. Big corporations had bought out the hospital and local newspaper. Outsiders and Blacks were being elected to local government positions.

Race was still a hot topic. At the national level, lawmakers were arguing about giving African-Americans an apology for slavery; at the state level, lawmakers were fighting over if and where to fly the Confederate flag; at the local level, most churches and even some children's baseball teams were still segregated.

On the Internet, an implant traceable by satellite systems and small enough to be injected into the body was being marketed as an economical way to monitor and control, even disable, convicts. "There will be no abuse," the advertisement said, "because it will be under government supervision."

The 'memory wars,' ignited in North America in the early nineties, were spreading across the globe. In May, 1998, a British newspaper had reported the case of a young woman who killed herself two weeks after having been told that her mental anguish was caused by false memory syndrome.

At a trial in Charlotte held during the summer of 1998, a psychologist and a psychiatrist were cleared in a malpractice suit involving claims that they used hypnosis, suggestive questioning, and drugs to make a patient falsely believe she'd been abused by Satanists. In a *Charlotte Observer* article, one of the defense attorneys described the expert witnesses who testify at repressed memory cases: "It's like a Broadway show that travels. They sing the same songs, they give the same lines." Another, referring to the plaintiff's plea for at least three million dollars in damages, stated: "This isn't about the search for the Holy Grail. It isn't about the fight to stamp out false memories. It's about money."

According to an article posted on an Internet list in February 1999, a district court judge had ordered an alleged perpetrator of satanic ritual child abuse to pay $1,000,000 in damages to victim Paul A. Bonacci from Omaha. Emily wondered why she'd never seen anything about this significant story in the mainstream media.

Several mental health professionals in Houston had been tried by the U.S. Government on charges that they intentionally created DID and implanted false memories in their patients in order to reap large sums in insurance payments. The case had resulted in a mistrial in March 1999, ending with a dismissal of all charges against the defendants before the defense was ever heard.

Emily knew of colleagues across the country who were no longer treating trauma survivors for fear of being accused of implanting false memories in their clients. Although expert testimony in civil trials against therapists was routinely used to show how therapists could be making clients believe things that didn't happen, nobody in the court system seemed to be considering the fact that so-called recanters—those who'd first claimed they'd recovered memories and were now saying the therapists were responsible—were influenced by accused perpetrators.

The plane began its descent. Emily directed her thoughts to the logistics of picking up her luggage, finding transportation to the hotel, and getting up with Kate Stewart and a few other colleagues who were meeting at the 1999 Annual Convention of the American Psychological Association.

Four days of fun and freedom where she didn't have to worry about what to cook for the family's traditional Sunday dinner or get angry because Jeff was doing something or other for his daddy or try to figure out if any of her clients' (or her own) memories were true or false.

In a room two stories below Emily's, Leslie Roberts, fresh out of journalism school, listened to a tape her boss had made of a recent discussion by accused perpetrators of sexual abuse.

—A bunch of crazy witch hunters, they are. We've got to stop those shrinks from tearing up families, from convincing our offspring that recovered memories of incest and other horrible things are true when they're really false. It's an epidemic. A plague. The cruelest hysteria ever to pass through our society.

—My dear husband . . . God rest his soul . . . went to the grave denying any improper behavior toward our two daughters. After he died, the younger one recanted, saying a therapist made her believe all that garbage.

—One self-proclaimed Christian counselor convinced our ex-daughter-in-law not to let us visit the grandchildren. It's been six years now and I doubt if I'll ever see those babies graduate from high school or college or get married.

—Thank the dear Lord, my husband and I are lucky. Our daughter took back everything bad she'd ever said about us and is suing the psychologist, the psychiatrist, and the hospital where they gave her high-powered drugs and implanted those horrible nightmares. More than a few times, they tied her to a bed kicking and screaming until, to use psychobabble, she abreacted. They forced her to remember and relive something that never happened. Fortunately we've found an aggressive lawyer who's told us how easy it is to win these cases without ever going to court. Because of his roster of trusted expert witnesses who'll testify in depositions that there's no scientific evidence for repressed memories, he predicts a seven-figure, out-of-court settlement. Another point in our favor is that the doctors never got informed consent for their controversial unproven treatments.

—In my opinion, we should get the last of those hell-holes they call "Dissociative Disorders Units" shut down. The doctors, who would have to be mentally ill themselves, diagnose our kids with severe mental conditions so they can keep them hospitalized a long time and make a lot of money. And when the insurance maxes out, patients are pushed out of the wards like dirty linen.

—The only way we're going to run the recovered memory therapists out of business is to completely discredit what they do.

—That shouldn't be too difficult. Why would any intelligent person believe their wild tales of human sacrifice in devil-worshiping ceremonies? Where's the evidence? The bodies?

—Some madman brainwashed my daughter into believing she was a high priestess in a satanic cult. After a year in psychotherapy, she decompensated and went on Social Security disability. Now recovery from satanic ritual abuse permeates her whole life. There's recovered memory therapy, group therapy, massage therapy, art, music, even aroma therapy. She reads every book about incest she can get her hands on and is always going to some kind of survivor conference or spiritual retreat.

—Well, get this: my daughter is now alleging that I sold her to the government to be used in Cold War medical and mind control experiments. She'd better watch what she's running around telling everybody. High level people in government will never allow such heresy.

—Some people say it's impossible to implant memories . . . seems they just don't know the early hypnosis research. As a matter of fact, I published some of it myself.

—To me, what's really awful are the therapists who claim they, themselves, were victims of cult and ritual trauma and are drawing our children into their delusions. Just the other day I heard of a so-called therapist/survivor treating another therapist/survivor who's treating another therapist/survivor.

—What about their making our daughters believe they have multiple personality disorder? But to keep it from sounding sensational, they've changed the diagnosis from MPD to dissociative identity disorder, DID. Even have their own 'dissociation association': the International Society for the Study of Dissociation—ISSD for short.

—So, if their 'magic' works and a patient gets well, are they going to make her a DIDn't?

—It's not funny, what they're doing.

—Does anyone in this group know about that silly sandbox technique? I can almost see my three-hundred-pound, forty-year-old daughter down on the floor playing with dolls and toys. Or EMDR? I don't even know what the letters stand for, but it's where the therapist wiggles a finger in front of your eyes and makes you come up with a memory to—what is it they say?—reprocess.

—And now the Christians have come up with something called theophostic prayer. From what I hear, they actually try to make the patient believe that Jesus is talking to them right there in the therapy room and telling them that everything we told them is a lie.

—Nothing surprises me anymore. First, my daughter claimed recovered memories of me penetrating her with a finger before she could talk. How can anybody remember what happened that early? The latest accusation is that I passed her around to my friends and used her in kiddie porn. Next thing you know, she'll be saying she was abducted by aliens.

—As a priest, my life and career were ruined when not one, but five, young men came forth saying I'd done terrible things to them. What we need is a concerted effort to warn religious organizations about the dangers of false memory syndrome.

—We've got to educate the court system, especially about the unreliability of repressed memories that come up in hypnosis. And another thing, how can anyone distinguish true from false memories unless there's physical evidence?

—I took my child to a mental health center because of bed wetting and night terrors. Two days later, I was being interviewed by protective services as a possible child molester.

—How did it turn out?

—Okay that time. They found no evidence whatsoever, but my ex-wife turned all my kids against me and moved out of the state.

—Three children accused me of crimes against nature: six-year-old Susie and four-year-old twins Luke and Lucy. Problem is, these three—whatever they are—all say they live in one body with a grownup who stands to make big bucks, ruin my medical career and, if a jury believes her cock-and-bull story, maybe even send me to prison.

—We'll just have to hit them where it hurts most—in the pocketbook.

—But malpractice carriers will bail them out. As an attorney for damaged patients, I'm looking at criminal intent such as mail fraud because of insurance claims sent through the mail for bogus diagnoses and untested treatments. Other antiracketeering laws might also apply. Basically, I'm looking for something that would send those psychos to jail for a long time.

—Criminal intent may be hard to prove. For what it's worth, I believe we should keep on tackling their professional pride. Paint their fannies as the quacks they are. Picket their offices. Go after their licenses.

—We need to continue to inform the media, appear on talk shows, and write articles for newspapers and magazines.

—And to get this new documentary produced and see that it gets aired.

The documentarian turned off the recorder and looked over the presentation she planned to make to interested persons on the last day of their convention. Her assignment was to find one or more therapists who would emerge from the mysterious therapy setting and naively demonstrate how false memory syndrome is created.

What better venue to find a guilty therapist than in a crowd of partying psychologists?

Chapter 33

Doing the best she could to keep her mouth shut, Emily took the last bite of hotel-flavored cheesecake, wondering why she had responded so impulsively to the bulletin board invitation for a free lunch and discussion of the topic: "Memory and Truth." Perhaps it was because she was angry at a society whose tendency to deny ugly reality is overwhelming.

Perhaps; perhaps; perhaps. Emily was sick of the word; sick of the reasonable, logical, professional, ethical need to use it; sick of the language of ambiguity. Perhaps . . . maybe . . . conceivably there is no evidence confirming survivors' stories about the terrorization of infants and children.

But there is, she thought; there *is* evidence in the human mind.

And there is other evidence all over the world. In small towns and big cities, the tracks of organized evil have been found in the computers of pedophiles and pornographers masquerading as teachers, preachers, scout leaders, business persons, doctors, nurses—about any group of people you can think of.

Above the tinkling of crystal and clanging of pots coming from the kitchen, the suave city-girl was presenting her Yankee-accented spiel: "My goal is to produce a documentary for cable or network TV which will provide an objective journalistic view of RMT."

"Recovered memory therapy. Hogwash!" The man looked old enough to be her grandfather. "That's a made-up term and doesn't describe at all what we do to help patients who're struggling with physical problems, profound spiritual dilemmas, and blocked memories and feelings."

"Making sense of memories is just one aspect of healing," added a woman with Kate Stewart Ph.D printed on her name tag. "In the shelter where I work, my role is to help women who've been subjected to extreme human cruelty; to help them overcome its aftereffects by listening to their stories in whatever way they choose to tell them: art, music, poetry, drama . . . mostly just talking. In my opinion, healing comes through their own words and images."

"Thank you." Leslie looked down at her notes. "I'd like to demonstrate how this therapy movement evolved from focusing on incest in the '70s, to the epidemic of therapists creating multiple personality disorder in the '80s, to all the current problems with FMS—"

A bearded man from Atlanta interrupted, "For your information, false memory syndrome is a term that has absolutely no scientific basis as a clinical diagnosis. It's a pejorative term used to attack therapists whose clients are remembering things they were supposed to forget. And Ms. Roberts, I'm just curious, who's funding your project?"

"Uh . . . uh . . . I can't divulge names but will say they're a group of parents who've been falsely accused of horrendous things; poor victims enraged at therapists for assuming their children's reported memories are all true, causing families to be destroyed, reputations and careers ruined."

"That figures," the man said under his breath.

"But won't such a sponsorship affect your objectivity?" Dr. Stewart asked.

"Of course not. Unlike the recovered memory therapists—"

"Please quit using that term." It was Grandpa again.

"—unlike therapists I've heard about who believe everything they hear, I've been trained to be neutral and present all sides of a controversy so viewers can decide for themselves what the real truth is," Leslie countered.

Dr. Klein, antsier than a smooth southern drawl revealed, could no longer remain silent. "Psychologists are trained to be neutral, too . . . and scientific . . . much different from parents who're conjuring up false diseases to account for natural posttraumatic stress reactions."

Stuffing her mouth with a piece of leftover hard roll, she refrained from truly speaking her mind: *My dear Ms. Roberts. You look all grownup. And may be well informed about FMS, but I for one, know the difference be-*

tween information and knowledge. How would you—some preppy idealist out to save the world from the evil therapist—know what it's like to sit week by week with those shattered souls?

A chunk of crust skittered down her windpipe, blocking the rest of her grievance. Not able to stop coughing, Emily left the table. Somewhere on the way to the atrium, her airway cleared.

At the bubbling fountain, a lone little girl with long brown hair and dark eyes was tossing pennies, one by one, into the shallow pool.

Crystal?

What a silly thought. Crystal would be almost grown by now.

Savoring the soothing stream of water spurting upward toward the glass ceiling, Emily felt a tug on the jacket of her teal pantsuit. It interrupted her reverie but not her worry about the other little girl with an imaginary playmate named Star.

Two days before the psychologist had left for the convention, Crystal Griffin had gone missing.

"Are you a grandma?" asked the little girl at the fountain.

"Yes I am," Emily answered, suddenly having the urge to return to the days when she was just Mrs. Klein: devoted wife, proud mom, good daughter, respected member of the plantation-porch crowd, and the PTA.

No one could possibly know how much she had hurt; how much energy it had taken to close the inner closets, concealing the agony— for the good of her husband, children, clients, even herself at times.

———————

When Emily returned to the table, Ms. Roberts was passing out business cards. "I want to thank each one of you for coming today. You've certainly given me a different perspective on this topic. If anyone's interested, or if you have clients who'd be willing to be interviewed for my documentary, please let me know."

Dr. Klein took the card and dropped it into her canvas convention bag.

Chapter 34

"Honey, I'm home,"

Jeff called from the kitchen. No one answered. He knew where she'd be.

Kate Stewart was talking on the answering machine in his study. Something about a documentary producer and unethical therapists. Not particularly wanting to talk with Emily's friend and eager to see his wife, he hurried through the family room to the deck.

He saw Emily dripping up the path and trotted down to meet her, enfolding his arms around her waist.

She spoke first. "I need to talk with you about something." Her tone was deep, serious.

"Can't it wait?" Hands now on her shoulders, he slowly slipped off the wide bathing suit straps. "Why don't we do it in the Jacuzzi?"

"Je-eff." Apparently not ready for their favorite prelude to love-making, she stiffened, pushing away.

"Talk. That's what I meant."

Pulling the swimwear back over her chest, she hurried toward the house, her husband tagging along behind.

"There's a message on the box from Sister Kate," he said, but the words seemed to fall onto the stone walk.

"Have they found the Griffin girl yet?" she asked.

"Not that I know of . . . so that's what's bothering you. I'm really sorry, Em. Last night they were interviewing her mother on the local news. The woman was hysterical—"

"The old pervert. I knew it a long time ago and there was not a darn thing I could do."

"Knew what?"

"That Franklin Griffin was using her in pornography."

"You don't know that for sure and whatever happened, it's not your fault. Why do you have to blame yourself for everything?"

"Because I was more concerned about my own credibility. And now if Crystal's not dead, she'll probably end up in some mental hospital or out working the streets doing what they trained her to do. I could've saved her . . . if only I'd been more persistent."

"Or if the gods have been good, maybe's she's found a therapist just like you who can help her put herself back together."

As they walked into the sunroom, the grandfather clock in the corner struck twelve times.

"Want some lunch?" he offered.

"I'm not hungry," she said. "I'm gonna go upstairs and try to take a nap."

Too much to think about. And her feet were feeling like someone was pricking them with pins and needles. Emily went back downstairs where Jeff had prepared a salad.

"It's just too hot to cook." He poured two glasses of iced-tea. "Weather reporter said it might reach a hundred today . . . here, have some salad . . . said things should cool off later this afternoon. They're expecting a thunderstorm . . . even mixed up some of our house dressing," he winked, "especially for my bride."

"Thanks but I'm not hungry."

"Maybe you could use a chocolate fix." He took the lid off the pink depression-glass cookie jar on the center of the table. "Care for a day-old brownie?"

"For the third time today, I'm not hungry. But I still need to talk. I can't get Star . . . I mean the Griffin girl off my mind."

"Okay. Talk."

"The Crystal I evaluated looked much older than her years in some of the pictures I saw . . . with globs of makeup and a sophisticated hairdo. Only seven years old and the parents had already taught her to be a sexual object: for applause, for approval. They'd put her in beauty pageants all across the country. And I do happen to believe, but obviously can't prove, they used her, perhaps sold her into outright child pornography."

"Why would a man sell his own daughter into pornography, if he did?" Jeff asked. "When the child is no longer worthwhile, the money would surely stop. I can halfway understand people doing brutal rituals in the name of religion, whether it be Christianity, Satanism, or even Masonry, because there's a belief system. But in pure pornography, there is no 'religious' observance."

"I have no idea. Another thing I don't understand is how any of this criminal activity can be kept so secret."

"If you ask my opinion, it's because that as long as people stay involved in such things, they're not going to tell anyone. And even if they're too old to participate, they still won't tell because of secret oaths. 'Death, death, death to the traitor.' Remember, from the Bible."

"That's not in the Bible," Emily laughed.

"You know what I mean. The family Bible."

"Jeff, more than anything I'd like to believe that memory repression and recovery are myths, that no little child in the whole wide world was ever hurt in such horrendous ways. Wouldn't you think the general public would wonder what happens to kiddie porn stars when they grow up?"

"Some turn out all right." He reached across the table, covering her hand with his. "I know that for a fact."

"And some grow up to be wrecks," she countered. "Dissociative wrecks. Or perpetrators themselves. Even toward their therapists, like all those people out there who're recanting claims against parents and suing therapists for putting the ideas in their heads."

As if unaware of what her hand was doing, she slid it out from under Jeff's and put it in the cookie jar. Grabbing a brownie and taking a bite, she rambled on with food in her mouth—something her mother never would have allowed.

"I forgot to tell you, a few weeks ago I got a letter from a professional liability carrier who wants my business, but only if I don't treat false memory syndrome or repressed memory disorder or—and this is hard to believe—multiple personality disorder, or use hypnosis. As we both know, the first two are bogus diagnoses making you wonder what kind of medical knowledge the insurance guys have. And hypnosis. For heaven's sake, it's such a powerful technique in helping people control life-threatening habits such as smoking and overeating, and helping people cope with chronic physical discomfort, or get a good night's sleep. I could go on and on."

Jeff reached into the cookie jar. "Hell, it's empty. Okay, let's get back to the kids. Not taking advantage of children in one's care is a relatively new phenomenon. In fact, the further back you go the more likely they were molested and/or murdered by their parents. The whole idea of taking advantage of children is an intergenerational response. It isn't any certain culture or people, not only one country or another, who commit and/or deny atrocities. And I'm sure I don't have to tell you the psychology of it."

"Nor do you have to tell me how children have always been used to contain the anxieties and guilty feelings of their parents; how they've been sacrificed to appease the gods under the guise of religion, even medical experiments and national security."

"National security?"

Emily paused, chewing the last of her brownie, before explaining, "That's what I said. At the convention, I met a psychologist from Raleigh who gave me a copy of the transcripts of a therapist from New Orleans and two of her patients who testified before the President's Advisory Committee on Human Radiation Experiments in March of 1995. Both patients claimed they were victims of radiation and mind control experiments during the Cold War."

"Really? Something that sensational should've made the news and I don't recall hearing a thing about it."

"But it didn't. Makes you wonder why, doesn't it? And it makes me wonder why there's a concerted effort to discredit them. Who knows what's behind it? What's the motive for this denial by denigration?" She slammed the lid back over the cookie jar. "How far will they go to cloak their shame? The destruction of careers? Of psychology itself?"

"You didn't mention murder."

"I don't want to go there right now."

"Well Em, the way I see it, very few people who see horrible things going on in front of their eyes want to say anything. They'd rather float along in their states of chloroformed consciousness—"

"Wow! I like that term. Sorta like the numb feeling described by my clients with posttraumatic stress disorder. Wish I'd thought of it."

"As I was saying before you so predictably interrupted, they'd rather float along in their states of chloroformed consciousness, sublimely unaware of the things you've been hearing for years."

Emily stood up, stretching her arms. "I'm so angry . . . and so tired. Maybe I *could* use a romp in the tub."

"Fine with me." Grinning, he followed her into the sunroom. "We can boil together. Can I undress you again?"

"You bet. This time I'll really try hard to keep my mouth shut."

It didn't work. Slipping into the bubbling water, she laid in: "Look what happened when no one responded to the Jews during the Third Reich. Might be the same thing will happen if we don't believe people who remember things just as horrible in our time. What Hitler did could have happened anywhere . . . and almost did in America. And what about Saddam Hussein? The Persian Gulf War was just a slap on his hand. Who knows what he's up to now? Somebody's got to take a stand, sometime. Whole societies have developed a way of pretty much pretending bad things never happened, that destructive cults don't exist. What about Jim Jones and the People's Temple? David Koresh and the Branch Davidians? The mass suicides of the members of the Order of the Solar Temple? . . . if they *were* suicides. How many generations will it take before the story of Jeffrey Dahmer eating his prey becomes a myth? How soon will everyone forget Susan Smith, the young mother who, not too far from here, willfully buried her babies alive, rolling them into a watery grave, not even giving them a chance to dissociate their traumas? And of all things, created a fictitious story of a black man to blame. Back to Crystal. Where is she?"

She stopped long enough to take a deep breath, but not long enough to give Jeff a chance to answer her question.

"Somewhere. On the street, I imagine. That's where they end up. How old would she be? Thirteen or fourteen? If she ran off, wasn't abducted and being held captive by some sexopath, she's likely changed her name, on the way to becoming a grown-up star. Or maybe she's taken off with the gutter punks, the latest in a long line of rebellious teenagers . . . "

"Kids have always rebelled." Jeff was able to take advantage of one of her infrequent pauses. "Remember Enoch?"

"Enoch who?"

"Never mind. We had rebels in our day, too. The beatniks, later the hippies preaching peace and love and better-living-through-chemicals," he spouted the old saying, hoping to slow her down a little.

But she hammered on. "Runaway kids today are different, choosing a dark urbane dangerous world. And sticking safety pins through their eyebrows and sniffing glue—not seeking visions, but just what it's always been, seeking oblivion."

"I wouldn't call it that. I believe they do that crap to get the attention they're sorely lacking from their parents."

"Could be, but from the psychological point of view, they may inflict physical pain on themselves to override their emotional pain, consciously trying to set off the natural painkillers, the endorphins, in their brains. Wherever Crystal is, by now she's likely dyed her hair purple, pierced her nipples, and blacked out on drugs—the best way she knows to escape the nightmare of her life."

"But Em, she's not the only one."

"Exactly. So what about all the others? Where are this country's or any country's missing children? Because you're right. She's not the only one. So where are the utterly-vanished, the kids who've gone up in thin air? The ones who're just nowhere. Societies don't produce cults, only a few serial killers, an occasional cannibal, a thriving worldwide child-prostitution industry and now and then the uncovering of a child pornography ring in somebody's old run-down warehouse."

She paused for a moment. Jeff offered to massage her shoulders which she readily accepted, positioning her back at his front.

"What are they told, I wonder? The young ones. That it's all right with God? Or that God is in the camera or on the scenically-staged altars on which they've unknowingly—through artificially-created alters—sacrificed their privacy of body and mind . . . oh Jeff, that feels so good . . . can you get a little deeper?"

"Your muscles are awfully tense. I'll do the best I can."

Her almost-manic chatter was exhausting, but she couldn't seem to let up.

"These days, kids probably don't ever hear, 'You're so special, we want you to be our high priestess.' Rather they're told, 'Welcome to cyberspace . . . where you'll be a star on the World Wide Web!' The pedophiles don't even have to hide their perversions behind robes any more. They just use the new-and-improved anonymity of the Internet."

"Em—"

"Please let me finish what I have to say." He stopped the massage. "There's never any evidence of foul play. Never any trail to follow; no bus or train ticket to the city recorded anywhere; no hitchhiker reports; no sightings of any kind. And no response to most of the thousands of posters, milk cartons, television pleas, missing-children registries, or to the efforts of computer bulletin board networks. People everywhere looking for them. And they're not there. They're just gone. No clues, no witnesses . . . precious little continuing investigation of any real meaning . . . no bodies ever found, no remains of any kind. Jeff . . . it's too hot in here. Let's get out."

"Good idea." Playfully, he cupped both hands on her bottom, shoving her up the steps.

Looking back over her shoulder, she said, "One more thing. What about those radiation experiments our latter-day Department of Energy admitted to? They were—what, accidental? Some of the subjects were children, you know . . . and some were aborted fetuses." Stepping onto the floor, she pitched her voice in disgust: "Our government once killed unborn babies . . . just to test their thyroids!"

Reaching for a towel, she took a deep breath and in a lower, slower tone, concluded her diatribe of the day. "And what about the men of the cloth; wayward priests or pastors who've hidden, sometimes for years, behind childhood's taught-trust in their robes and rituals in order to assault that trust clear down through the soul for their own purposes? But no one would define that—or the protectors of such important personages afterward—as in anyway cultish, would they?"

Jeff took the towel from her hand and wrapped it snugly around her body, holding her tightly till the shivering stopped.

"Now I think I can get that nap," she said softly.

"Later. First I want to know what Kate was talking about."

He led her into the study and replayed the message: "Hi Emily. Hope you got home safely. Have you thought about talking to that documentary producer? If there's anybody in the world who could contradict her belief that we're all unethical therapists, it's you. Just wanted you to know you're in my prayers."

"What's this about a documentary?" Sitting down behind his desk, he motioned for Emily to sit on a black leather wingback across the room.

"Uh . . . it was at the convention. A woman named Leslie Roberts who's producing a documentary on false memory syndrome invited a group of us for lunch to talk about the reality of memory—"

"Did you blab to her about—"

"No I didn't. Not yet. But for your information, I have decided to volunteer for the project. Maybe I can get her to realize that we're not in it for the money or whatever else those jerks think; help the general public understand what trauma therapy is all about. Somebody needs to speak for those afraid to speak for themselves."

"So why does it have to be you? What if they figure out that—" The man couldn't even say the words. "Look at how many lives you would affect . . . and even destroy . . . what about our kids and grandchildren? And think about all the lawsuits to follow . . . we're not exactly shallow pockets, by any means." He stood up and walked over to the window, turning his back toward his wife. "Surely my dear, you wouldn't tell anyone about us" — then turned around to look her in the eye, "would you?"

"I don't plan to. But if the woman talks to any of my former clients who claim to have been ritual abuse/mind control survivors, she'd have to come away with a much different point of view than the one her investors tout."

"Don't fool yourself. We both know the mainstream media's reporting misinformation right now. Em, I can't let them bring a bunch of cameras in this town. Asking questions. Making a mockery of all the things my ancestors stood for. You can't have some carpetbagger coming down here tearing up the decency in this town . . . what there is left of it."

"Well, Mr. Klein. Mr. Blue-Blood son of a Red-Neck. What does that make you? A blue-neck or a red-blood?"

"Very funny. I do feel pretty red-blooded right now."

"Maybe so buddy, but as I was about to say, you have no right to tell me what to do. If I want to tell the whole world the whole truth, I most certainly can."

"Of course you can. But the world might think you're a certifiable nut case."

Abruptly the yelling stopped.

And they talked calmly for a few minutes—

Through a form of silent communication like that between two people who've been dancing together for a long time, Jeff knew exactly what she was going to do next.

Emily walked over to the rolltop desk. Nodding at Grandmother Hannah, she opened the laptop and set her hands to the task.

AFTERMATH

Chapter 35

*N*ow *I lay me down to sleep* . . .

Stealing a smoke, Leslie Roberts peered through her office window overlooking Central Park, trying to recall the original words of the child's prayer and trying to digest the mind-shattering information in the thirteen page letter received that morning from a Dr. Klein in South Carolina:

Dear Ms. Roberts:

I am a psychologist who was present at the luncheon you recently hosted in Boston. After careful thought and deliberation, I have decided to volunteer to be a participant in your documentary. For almost twenty years, I have worked with clients, some who always had memories of abuse, some who recovered them before coming to therapy, and some who recovered them while in therapy.

To give you a brief perspective on why I would welcome the opportunity to participate in your project, I am including a vignette about one of my former clients. I also offer documentation to show you why I believe there is truth behind the accounts of some individuals who claim to have been unwitting initiates into the dark sides of families, even religious, fraternal and/or governmentally-connected organizations.

In 1990, long before I had heard anything about the deliberate creation of multiple personalities in government-funded mind control experiments, Nora, a former X-rated movie actress who carried the shame and humiliation of having been used in child pornography, and only God knows what else, had come to her weekly therapy session with a severe headache and a poem titled *Hidden People*:

When you look at me what do you see?
Do you see the HIDDEN PEOPLE inside of me?
They can see you, but you can't see them.
They live in my mind where they've always been.
Some doctors call it Mental Illness.
But it's not you see.
It's survival because they came to save me.
They saved me from him because I was too small
    to let my mind endure the pain of it all.
I broke into pieces and out of that came
    the people who keep me alive Night and Day.
Each one has a purpose for being in me.
And Oh! so much pain they had to see.
He beat them, and raped them, and tortured them, too.
But they could endure much more than he knew.
Each one of them holds a memory inside of them still,
    and at nighttime it gets them.
It seems so real.
Sometimes I hear them as they cry and scream.
One likes to cut to watch the blood stream.
How much more are they expected to take
    before it's they who are forced to break?
Integration is what I'm told they need.
But how can we become one when I still need
    separate parts of me?
Without them . . .
How will I ever survive?
The lesser of two evils . . .
To *Live* or to *Die*?

"Oh, Dr. Klein," Nora had begged, "could you please hypnotize me to help me deal with the pain?"

"We can try," I answered. "Exactly how would you describe the sensation?"

Nora placed the fingers of her right hand over her left eye. "It feels as if something's been burned into my brain."

With the client lying flat on the couch, I used a classic induction: "Close your eyes if that's okay and take a real—ly deep breath and picture yourself stepping into an elevator on the top floor of a tall building. Let's say it has thirty stories. I don't know . . . and you may not know how far down it is to a place where you can learn to control your headaches . . . but your unconscious knows. And when you're deep enough in trance to do the work you need to do, the elevator can stop and you can step out." I began a slow countdown. "30-29-28—"

"Stop it!" The panicky young woman opened her eyes. "Now I see it. That's what the doctor did when he wanted one of his little girls to come out."

"Doctor?"

"Yes, there was a doctor . . . a Dr. Greene . . . the name on his white coat. And each one lived on a different floor and they would come out when he called their number."

"Number?"

"Each one had a number . . . like a code."

In subsequent sessions, what appeared to be artificially-created ego states began to relinquish behaviors, emotions, physical sensations, and knowledge that Nora's authentic self had apparently been conditioned, or programmed, to dissociate.

Sometimes she brought pages and pages of writing, each section signed with a different number.

"How can my hand write things I don't know?" she asked. "It's as if a secretary is taking dictation for the people who live inside my body."

"Automatic writing," I interpreted. "Writing for the unconscious."

My role, as I saw it, was to gain access to those dissociated aspects, to educate them—educate Nora—about the malevolence of such conditioning and to convince my client that the parts didn't have to work alone. Hopefully, they could learn to work together like sailors on a ship to forge a tranquil passage through life.

On the day Nora missed her first appointment ever, I received a note in the mail:

"Now I Lay Me Down to Sleep" is supposed to be a prayer that all children say at bedtime so God will protect them and their souls in case they don't wake up. For me and a lot of children like me it was:

Now I lay me down,
But sleep it will not be
Because they are coming in here—
If I should die before they're done
My soul will have no home.
They will make sure of that.
No peace will ever come.

I cannot live in this body any longer. My bones are breaking; lungs, drowning; blood, rotting. My brain is like a computer breaking down, crashing. Dr. Klein, thanks for everything you ever tried to do for me but, when you get right down to it, there was really nothing you could do.

Love, Nora

Ms. Roberts, I ask you. Can you tell me how I could have possibly implanted false memories of rape and torture in my client's mind?

Below are some of the things that I have come across in my search to understand the relationships among multiple personality (dissociative identity) disorder, incest and other sexual abuse, cult and/or ritual trauma, child pornography, unethical mind control and medical experimentation, and false memory syndrome.

For information about legal proceedings involving allegations of satanic crimes, I direct you to the *Satanism and Ritual Abuse Archive* on the Net. To find corroborated cases of recovered memory, check out *The Recovered Memory Project* website hosted by Ross Cheit. The most comprehensive website I have found that shows possible connections between secretive organizations, ritual abuse, and mind control is S.M.A.R.T.'s *Ritual Abuse Newsletter.*

Early next year, James Randall Noblitt, a clinical psychologist, and Pamela Sue Perskin, Executive Director of the International Council on Cultism and Ritual Trauma, will be coming out with a revised edition of their 1995 book, *Cult and Ritual Abuse: It's History, Anthropology, and Recent Discovery in Contemporary America.* The authors discuss their professional contacts with individuals who suffer the consequences from having been subjected to ritual abuse which they define as "traumatizing procedures that are conducted in a circumscribed or ceremonial manner."

Other books you might find helpful as you delve into this material are *Out of Darkness* by Sakheim and Devine and *Painted Black* by Raschke.

Ritual abuse—which I define as "deliberately inflicted physical, sexual, psychological and/or spiritual trauma designed by perpetrators, alone or in groups, to exert control over the thoughts, feelings, behaviors, and memories of their victims"—is an international phenomenon.

If you happen to read German, you might want to look at Fröhling's *Vater unser in der Holle* (Our Father in Hell). This book, the first in-depth case study of a German DID patient with a background of ritual abuse, made the German government aware of the existence of ritual abuse. For a UK perspective, I recommend Sinason's *Treating Survivor's of Satanist Abuse.* Fraser's *The Dilemma of Ritual Abuse,* in addition to including an article discussing ritual abuse in European countries, includes articles that deal with the concept of ritual abuse as it relates to other controversies involving false memory syndrome and recovered memories.

In case you are not familiar with the facts regarding our government's history of torturous mind control and medical experiments, which by my definition is certainly a type of ritual abuse, I submit the following information:

In the early 1950s when American POW's in Korean prison camps began making false confessions about such things as germ warfare, the United States military establishment took the clear inference of Chinese brainwashing techniques as a reality. In an address to Princeton alumni in 1953 (reported in *U.S. News & World Report*, May 8, 1953) CIA Director Allen Dulles stated that the Soviets possess the power to brainwash, which he described as

> . . . the perversion of the minds of selected individuals who are subjected to such treatment that they are deprived of the ability to state their own thoughts. Parrotlike the individuals so conditioned can merely repeat thoughts which have been implanted in their minds by suggestion from outside. In effect, the brain under these circumstances becomes a phonograph playing a disc put on its spindle by an outside genius over which it has no control.

Some time after this speech, Dulles, in an effort to win the "battle for men's minds" between the United States and the Soviet Union, set up a program called MKULTRA . He authorized mind control experiments testing such techniques as brain implants, sensory deprivation, ultrasonics, torture, amnesia-inducing drugs, biologicals, psychological stress, electroshock, and even hypnosis.

Further rationalization for conducting this type of venture was provided by a 1954 report for the White House by a secret group headed by Herbert Hoover which concluded: "It is now clear that we are facing an implacable enemy whose avowed objective is world domination. . . .. There are no rules in such a game. Hitherto accepted norms of human conduct do not apply." (Quoted in *The Secret Government* by Bill Moyers).

If many decades ago our own government recognized the potential of using these techniques in controlling people's minds, who could go on denying, in principle, that it wasn't happening?

The CIA, that's who.

On August 3, 1977, Senator Edward Kennedy confirmed the existence of MKULTRA in his opening remarks to a Senate investigation committee by stating:

> The intelligence community of this nation, which requires a shroud of secrecy in order to operate, has a very sacred trust from the American people. The CIA's program of human experimentation of the fifties and sixties violated that trust. It was violated again on the day the bulk of the agency's records were destroyed in 1973. It is violated each time a responsible official refuses to recollect the details of the program. The

best safeguard against abuses in the future is a complete public accounting of the abuses of the past.

Apparently no one listened to the Senator.

Under the Freedom of Information Act, law school professor, Alan W. Scheflin, read over 12,000 pages documenting that thousands and thousands of people including mental patients and children were subjects of CIA and U.S. Army mind control programs that extended over a period of twenty-five to thirty years. These were described in his book, *The Mind Manipulators*.

In *Psychiatry and the CIA: Victims of Mind Control,* psychiatrist Harvey Weinstein tells how, in 1979, while reading a review of an exposé by John Marks of MKULTRA titled, *The Search for the 'Manchurian Candidate': The CIA and Mind Control,* he realized that his father had been an experimental subject when he was hospitalized for anxiety at the Allan Memorial Institute in Montreal from 1957 through 1961.

By examining his father's records, Weinstein came to the conclusion that his father—in the name of medical science—had been endangered by heavy doses of LSD, electroshock, and sensory deprivation, purportedly to make his mind a clean slate. After these dehumanizing, debilitating acts, a prolonged drugged sleep was induced and for weeks, even months, through a procedure called "psychic driving," Mr. Weinstein was forced to listen to programmed, taped messages with the idea of creating a new personality. What it did for this man was to damage his brain, taking away the very essence of the high-functioning person he had been.

In 1980, with his son's encouragement, the elder Weinstein along with several other patients of Dr. Ewen Cameron, the psychiatrist who mistreated them, filed suit against the CIA. After many delays, the case was settled in 1988 just before trial without either the Canadian or the U.S. Government acknowledging responsibility for the crimes committed.

Proof that the CIA, Army, Navy, and Air Force have funded physicians and medical schools to conduct mind control experiments intentionally designed to create DID is provided by Colin Ross in his forthcoming book, *Bluebird: Deliberate Creation of Multiple Personality by Psychiatrists*.

On March 15, 1995, two courageous victims of mind control experiments stood before the President's Advisory Committee on Human Radiation Experiments to tell the world about the horrors they had endured in the name of National Security. Giving explanation and support for these young women was their therapist Valerie Wolfe, whom I quote:

I am here to talk about a possible link between radiation and mind control experimentation that began in the late 1940s. The main reason that mind control research is being mentioned is because people are alleging that they were exposed, as children, to mind control, radiation, drugs, and chemical experimentation which were administered by the same doctors who are known to have been involved in conducting both radiation and mind control research.

Written documentation has been provided revealing the names of people and the names of research projects in statements from people across the country. It is also important to understand mind control techniques and follow-ups into adulthood may have been used to intimidate particular research subjects in to not talking about their victimization in government research.

As a therapist for the past twenty-two years, I have specialized in treating victims and perpetrators of trauma and their families. When word got out that I was appearing at this hearing, nearly forty therapists across the country (and I had about a week and a half to prepare) contacted me to talk about clients who had reported being subjected to radiation and mind control experiments. The consistency of people's stories about the purpose of the mind control and pain induction techniques such as electric shock, use of hallucinogens, sensory deprivation, hypnosis, dislocation of limbs and sexual abuse is remarkable.

There is almost nothing published on this aspect of mind control abuse with children, and these clients come from all over the country having had no contact with each other. What was startling was that therapists reported many of these clients were also physically ill with autoimmune problems, thyroid problems, multiple sclerosis and other muscle and connective tissue diseases as well as mysterious ailments of which a diagnosis cannot be found. Plus somatization disorder is commonly found in these clients.

Many of the clients who have been involved in human experimentation with the government have multiple medically-documented physical ailments, and I was really shocked today to hear one of the speakers talk about cysts and about teeth breaking off because I have a client that is happening to.

Many people are afraid to tell their doctors their histories as mind control subjects for fear of being considered to be crazy. These clients have named some of the same people; particularly Dr. Greene, who was associated with client reports of childhood induction of pain. Clients who had seen him with a name tag identified him as Dr. L. Wilson Greene. A person with this same name was the Scientific Director of the Chemical and Radiological Laboratories at the Army Chemical Center, and he was engaged in doing research for the army and other intelligence agencies.. . .

[Another name that the speaker mentioned here was a Dr. Sidney Gottlieb.]

It needs to be made clear that people have remembered these names and events spontaneously, with free recall, and without the use of any extraordinary retrieval techniques such as hypnosis.

As much as possible, we have tried to verify the memories with family members, records, and experts in the field. Many attempts have been made through Freedom of Information filings to gain access to the mind control research documentation. Requests have generally been slowed down, or denied; although some information has been obtained which suggests that at least some of the information supplied by these clients is true.

It is important that we obtain all of the information contained in CIA and military files to verify or deny our clients' memories. Although many of the files for MKULTRA may have been destroyed, whatever is left, along with the files for other projects, such as BLUEBIRD and ARTICHOKE to name only two, contain valuable information.

Furthermore, if, as the evidence suggests, some of these people were used in radiation experiments, there might be information in the mind control experiment files on radiation experiments. We need this information to help in the rehabilitation and treatment of many people who have severe psychological and medical problems which interfere with their social, emotional, and financial well-being.

Finally, I urge you to recommend an investigation into these matters. Although there is a Commission on Mind Control, it did not include experiments on children because most of them were too young, or still involved in research in the late 1970s, to come forward. The only way to end the harassment and suffering of these people is to make public what has happened to them in the mind control experiments. Please recommend that there be an investigation on the mind control experiments as they related to children. Thank you.

Regarding one of the names that was mentioned in this testimony, I think it is interesting to know that Dr. Sidney Gottlieb, the man who directed MKULTRA was quoted in a 1994 article in *U.S. News and World Report,* "The Cold War Experiments: Radiation tests were only one small part of a vast research program that used thousands of Americans as guinea pigs," as saying that after retiring in 1973, he devoted the years "trying to get on the side of the angels instead of the devils."

In conclusion, I trust that this information is helpful and not too overwhelming for you. If, after reading this letter, you should choose to meet with me, I will also be happy to share not only what I have learned about the damaging effects of childhood trauma, but also what I have learned about the resiliency of an individual soul.

Dr. Kate Stewart who was at the luncheon in Boston will be sending you a letter stating that she is willing to talk with you off the record. She will be in my town the last week of October. If you want to interview us together, let me know and it can be arranged.

"That woman's a lunatic, albeit a creative one. Must be some kind of conspiracy nut."

Leslie turned around to face her boss who had come into the cubicle. "Good morning, sir. I think you're wrong about Dr. Klein. She's got a lot of data to support her statements."

"Does she really? From what I read this morning in her letter, it looks like she's been watching too much of the *X-Files.* Only a crazy person's mind is capable of thinking up that kind of fiction. It sounds as though this little woman straight out of the boondocks may be just the kind of therapist our investors were talking about."

"But don't you think parts of the letter are compelling? Such as the parody on the child's prayer. And if any of those declassified documents she mentioned have substance, then there's more hidden under this attack on therapists than hits the surface."

Leslie's boss closed the file and dropped it on the desk. Snatching the cigarette from his subordinate's hand and putting it in his own mouth, he leaned against the partition and took a deep drag. On the exhale, smoke curled from his mouth and recycled through his nose. "How can this Dr. Klein live with herself? Making a poor young woman believe all that bullshit about hidden people living in her body." He pointed to the file. "And that's not a letter. It's a damn treatise. Where the hell did she get all that nonsense?"

"With all due respect, I believe it's possible this old lady shrink," she glanced up at her boss's thinning white hair, immediately wishing she hadn't demeaned maturity, then went on—"can help us find out what's really happening in this recovered memory therapy which, incidentally, those psychologists at the luncheon last month said there's no such thing."

"No such thing!" He stepped past Leslie and stubbed out the ciga-rette in an African violet wilting on the windowsill. "Don't tell that to the thousands of fathers out there who've lost their children, their jobs, even their marriages because therapists made them believe those lies. Don't tell that to all the adults who thought they'd recovered memories of incest and, after they'd been therapized and hospitalized and groupized and taken to the brink of madness, in the end they realized nothing had happened after all."

"But she *was* convincing; almost zealous in her contention that the whole movement to discredit therapists is a diversion, a disinformation campaign to cover up some type of sinister government activity that took place a long time ago. And still may be going on for all we know. But I must say, the case of the porn star was touching—the poem, the prayer."

"The doctor could've made all that up too. Has anyone else agreed to go on camera?"

"Not a single person. But I did hear from that psychologist in Santa Fe. She'll be visiting Dr. Klein the last week of October and is willing to talk with me off the record."

"Well, we need to get on with this project and try to figure out how to visually portray this recovered memory movement and false memory syndrome and make some money in the process. As I see it, there are three interrelated questions which need to be investigated.

"First, what kind of person and what kind of motivation would it take for a therapist to cause all that trouble between parents and their offspring? Second, where do therapists come up with the satanic cult stuff? And third, what kind of hocus-pocus do they use to make their patients believe they have different personalities?

"Just so you'll know, Ms. Roberts, the investors have asked for a working proposal by the end of the year. Who knows? We just might have us a little cotton-patch of false memory planting down there to dig up." He snickered at his play on words. "Seriously, this Klein woman must have guts if she's willing to put her reputation on the line, so I'm authorizing you to go ahead and meet with her and try to find out what's really going on out there in therapy-land."

After her boss left, Leslie lit up a fresh cigarette. Through forbidden smoke, she glimpsed the world below . . .

I pray the Lord my soul to keep.

Chapter 36

Coupled with the raindrops blowing up the windshield, the rhythmic bump-bump-bump as they rode over the joints on the concrete interstate became hypnotic. Emily closed her eyes, drifting through a cloud of images: a dirt path winding to the top; people with torches coming around the mountain; a little girl hanging upside down on a cross.

When she opened her eyes, they were passing over the Eastern Continental Divide.

"Getting close," Jeff said. "The exit's coming up."

At first, the climb toward the once secluded church camp, now a plush conference and retreat center, was steep. Then the road became long and flat with peaks all around.

"This is what L'Amour called a hanging valley," Jeff said, "a small range within a big range of mountains." They were in a valley but at a higher level, another step up toward their destination.

On the other side of the entrance gate, the road became a dark narrow passageway under a canopy of draping spruce limbs framed by leathery mountain laurel.

"We've been up this road before," Emily said.

"We? What do you mean we? I never got to go to summer camp."

"No. I mean when we were real little. There was a big neon cross somewhere."

"I don't know what you're talking about," he said as they pulled into the parking area.

While Jeff was checking in, Emily looked over the hotel's brochure. She learned that it had been built in 1920 of copper-colored river rocks and that the inside had burned mysteriously near the end of the decade. Rebuilt in 1930, it burned down again. The present structure dated from 1946.

After they'd taken their bags to the room, she put on her hiking boots and set out to retrace her steps up the mountain to the outdoor altar, the sacred place where she'd promised God to always be good to little children.

"If you want me to, I'll go with you," Jeff said.

"No thanks. This is a walk I have to take alone."

Her memory was true. At least part of it.

There was a cross. It had fallen over and one of its arms was stuck in the ground.

Her memory was false. At least part of it.

She'd remembered it as a neon cross, but this structure had once been lit by ordinary light bulbs around the edges. Sixty, she counted. And it was made from metal; not the wood in her memory. White paint chips flecked the stone patio on which the symbol had stood. Opposite the cross was an altar.

Trying not to see the little girl hanging upside down in her mind's picture, Emily averted her eyes to the valley. Below was a large lake, a natural reservoir formed where several streams carrying water down the mountain had converged. In this beautiful place, opposing forces had existed since man had come through and desecrated nature: beauty with repugnance, tranquility with havoc, sanity with insanity, good with evil.

On a hunch, Jeff asked the clerk if the hotel kept old guestbooks.

"Yes we do. They're kept in the safe. Don't know why, though. You're the first person I know ever asked for them." She went into a back room and came out carrying three faded-green registries. "These begin in 1946. I suppose the earlier ones burned up."

He carried the oldest one into the lobby. Sitting at a walnut writing desk, he scanned the signatures of people from all over the South who had come to this place for inspiration. Looking over the guests for the summer of 1947, his eyes opened wide when he got to June 21.

With the book still opened, he took it back to the desk and asked the clerk to copy page number twenty-two.

When he got back to the room, Emily was waiting.

"You're not going to believe this." He handed her the guestbook list.

As if looking at a menu from the Village Diner, Emily read the words printed at the top of the page:

CHRISMONT INN
**Valuables must be deposited in the office safe,
otherwise Proprietor will not be responsible for any losses.**

Then, like a kid just learning to read, she slid her right index finger under each name, one at a time, saying it aloud:

Mr. Earl Elliott
Mr. and Mrs. Phil Owens
Dr. and Mrs. William Wilhelm
Mr. and Mrs. Casey Paxton
Rev. and Mrs. Wayne Miller
Mr. and Mrs. Jacob Lentz
Miss Amanda Jarrett
Mr. Cleat Klein.

She went back to the top of the list and counted each name: one, two, three, . . . twelve, thirteen.

Thirteen. The voice again. It had been quiet for a long time.

"They were here," she said softly. "Thirteen of them. Coming around and around the mountain . . . and I was here too. On that cross at the top of the mountain . . . maybe you were too."

"I don't know, Em. They could have all come up for a spiritual retreat or something."

"You *are* kidding, aren't you? What in heaven's name will it take for you to believe, for you to accept that our parents—that we—belonged to a cult of evil?"

"As I've said before, I just don't want to believe, that's all."

Obviously not wanting to talk any more about the possibility that Emily's mountaintop memory was true, he looked around at the elegant furnishings. "You know Hon, this place isn't quite rustic enough for me. What do you say we go find us a cabin somewhere?"

"I never thought you'd ask. From the moment I walked into that lobby, it felt eerie. Anyway, the place has already burned down twice. Wouldn't want to take a chance of it happening again."

They drove back down the mountain. In the hook of one of the hairpin curves was a chain-link fence with barbed wire on top. A small sign was tacked to the locked gate:

Private Property
U.S. Government
Keep Out

"Never noticed that before." He swerved the car back to the direction he'd just come from.

"Me either," Emily said. "Makes me wonder what all's going on in 'them thar hills.'"

Outside the open window, a cat was screeching.

Unexpectedly, Jeff felt hot all over. Springing from the twin bed in the '50s-style tourist cabin in the little village in the valley, he darted to the bathroom.

Suddenly feeling dirty, he stripped off his clothes and stepped into the mildew-encrusted shower, pushing back a curtain that was about to fall and shroud him with a personal history he'd never wanted to study.

"No . . . no . . . " Wearing coveralls made out of heavy material with tiny black and white stripes printed on it, the little boy is about five.

"Cut it open," the daddy demands. "For practice. If you get it right, you can do . . . a baby." The man puts the hand with the missing finger over the boy's hand. "Do it. Do it now."

Blinkers, his cat, is lying on its back with its belly shaved.

"I can't—don't make me. I can't. I can't."

The father shakes his son like he's a dirty dish rag and pushes his little freckled face down onto the makeshift altar. The child drops the knife and runs away into the woods.

A minute later, little Jeff, peeping around a tree, sees an older boy take his place beside his dad. It is Tommy Paxton.

In the corner of the shower, Jeff could still hear his father bellowing: "You ain't no son of mine, you sissy faggot! You little pussy."

Sobs of a terrified child drifted into his space.

The adult fell to his knees, pounding the gray ceramic floor, trying to demolish the humiliation of a little boy who couldn't please his father.

Emily opened the door. "Are you all right?"

"I'm okay. I just remembered something. That's all."

"Do you want to talk about it?"

"Later maybe. Right now I need to lie down for a few minutes."

His wife's arms were enfolding, comforting, as she led him through the door. For a long time they lay on the hard bed, engulfed by the damp mountain air coming through the window.

After several minutes of contemplation, Jeff described his memory in detail.

Emily listened intently, her only comment: "He can't hurt you anymore."

"But it was so real . . . it was like I was there. I felt little, ashamed, helpless. I felt Daddy's hand on my shaky little hand. And when I looked up, I saw those boiling eyes —"

"Me-ow. Me-ow." The cat outside the window was screeching again.

Fully back in the present, Jeff understood. "Strangely, as awful as it was to go though, I feel relieved. Now I know why he kicked me out. I was a wimp. A pussy. I couldn't pass the test. They called Tommy Paxton over to do what I couldn't. He took my rightful place in the group. A victim too. Like me."

In the bowels of the Great Smoky Mountains, Jefferson Winslow Campbell Klein had slammed against his truth.

Chapter 37

"Here's something I need to tell you."

A few days after their trip to the mountains, Jeff had stopped by his wife's office late one afternoon after spending the day at the State Archives doing some genealogy research on the Lentz family. "It appears that most of your ancestors on your daddy's side, for two or three generations in the early 1800s, were indentured servants."

"Nobody ever told me that. They must've been an angry bunch."

"No doubt. I thought you might be interested in hearing some of the things I've come across which would support the possibility that some of our German ancestors were participants in a transgenerational satanic cult."

"Of course. I want to know anything that would help me make sense out of everything that's been hurled at me by my clients . . . and my unconscious."

"Okay, here goes. From what we observed in the Black Forest and from what I've learned from studying Luther, our ancestors seemed to have germinated in a religiously superstitious culture where people honored witches and worshiped Jesus Christ. In one and the same breath, they wrestled with demons and talked with God. There's no way to prove any of this, but if I were writing a historical novel it could go like this: In the mid 1700s, two German families, the Kleins and Rheinharts—"

"Are you talking about the Rheinharts who're buried over there?" She pointed toward Olde Towne Cemetery.

"Just wait a minute. Let me finish what I have to say."

"Sorry. Go on."

"As I was saying, the Kleins and Rheinharts leave the Black Forest of Germany and migrate to America. In search of a future, they move to the area that became Campbell County carrying with them a chest brought from the homeland filled with black linen robes and other objects and implements needed to carry on their occultic traditions: knives, daggers, pewter chalices, and silver candlesticks.

"Joining a newly established Reformed church, they try to present the image of good Christian people. In 1835, they are accused of participating in 'frolics.' Thus, Frederick Rheinhart and George Klein, who are leaders of their respective clans, no longer have a cover for their perversions.

"They establish their own church on the Rheinhart plantation and name it Mt. Hermon—from the Book of Enoch—the forbidden place where the fallen angels took their secret oaths. Frederick and George elect themselves elders and call a preacher, a distant relative of George's, from the homeland. They erect a building of logs and paint it red."

"Where did you get all those details?"

"From different places. A little from my imagination, a lot from Mt. Hermon's records that were summarized in their 150th anniversary booklet. Back to the novel."

"Okay, I'll try not to interrupt again."

"The new church serves as a place of worship for sincere Christians who walk in the light and Satan worshipers who dance in the dark. In this case, they're not mutually exclusive. In 1850, Andrew Lentz, an orphan who has wandered from one home to another searching for food and shelter, winds up at the Rheinhart plantation as an indentured servant. Frederick likes Andrew and lets him keep his job, even after his contract is up. He introduces Andrew to his covert circle. In 1860, Andrew marries a neighbor named Mary Overcash. One of their children, Peter, marries Frederick's granddaughter, Hannah, who dies birthing her only child—"

"My daddy."

"You got it. So Frederick prepares Peter, your grandfather, for the secret religion. Meanwhile, George Klein also has similar aspirations for his oldest grandson, Martin, who was my grandfather. Martin and Peter fight over who should be the leader. Neither win. So Martin stays on to run things at Mt. Hermon and calls your mother's grandfather, one of the Keller preachers . . . maybe it's her great-grandfather . . . from Germany to serve as pastor. Are you with me now?"

"I think so, but it sure is complicated."

"Well anyway, Peter Lentz and his family and followers move to Chestnut Ridge. He helps establish First Lutheran Church and a cult of devil worshipers on the side. He also opens an ice plant and a slaughterhouse, thereby bringing convenience to both community and coven.

"Some thirty years later Peter's son—your daddy—follows his father's footsteps and gets involved in the Chestnut Ridge organization. The group meets formally to observe special occasions: Walpurgis Night, spring and fall equinoxes, summer and winter solstices—"

"Summer solstice. Like June 21? the day the cult checked in at Camp Chrismont." No matter how hard she tried not to interrupt when Jeff was into one of his long monologues, she just couldn't seem to help herself.

He was used to it by now and went on with the story. "They would have met on Allhallows' Eve or Halloween. And they would have met on Christmas for what they called the Grand Climax where they celebrate sacrifices, sexual orgies, bloodlettings, and other acts to pay homage to the forces of darkness."

"Wait just a minute. Let me get this straight. Would you diagram that family tree for me?" She pushed a piece of paper across her desk. He took a pen from his pocket protector and roughly sketched two family trees, bringing them together at the bottom of the page with the marriage of Peter Lentz and Hannah Rheinhart.

Emily took the pen away from him, turned the paper around, and printed "Hannah Rheinhart Lentz" in the top margin.

"Hannah *R.* Lentz," she said.

"That's what I wanted you to know, Em."

Showing no emotion, she softly acknowledged to Jeff and to herself: "Fred Crabtree was brutalized in an ancestor worship ritual . . . and murdered in the old Rheinhart family grave plot. . . . Fred was murdered over the decayed bones of my grandmother's ancestor—

And mine."

Chapter 38

What an opportunity!

Glancing at the entrance sign to Chestnut Ridge, Leslie Roberts could almost smell a Peabody brewing. Her first assignment; her first chance to win the most prestigious award in broadcasting. Following the hand-drawn map Dr. Klein had E-mailed, she crossed the city limits and passed a section of modest ranch houses decorated four days early for Halloween: a pumpkin on every porch, black and orange flags waving over front doors, and lots of straw men, women, and children lazing around brown corn shocks and green gourds. An announcer on the car radio drawled, "The county animal control officer has said there will be no . . . let me repeat . . . no adoptions of black cats any time this week. He's afraid they might be slaughtered by the devil worshipers."

Good God Almighty! What kind of place have they sent me to?

A rhetorical question to a mythical being. The documentary producer didn't believe in God . . . or Satan.

She parked the rental car in front of the Village Diner, a fifties-style building that looked like a house trailer wrapped in crinkled tinfoil. A little early for her luncheon appointment with Dr. Klein and Dr. Stewart, in dire need of a cigarette and trusting they'd have a smoking section, she went on in.

"Ms. Roberts, over here." A woman was waving from the end booth in the nonsmoking side of the long narrow dining area. Cramming the almost empty pack of cigarettes into the pocket of her navy blazer, Leslie walked over to the booth, not sure whether it was a Klein or a Stewart she'd be greeting.

Whoever it was, the brunette with long straight hair pulled behind her ears, wearing boots, a vest and printed skirt—about a size-five—looked as though she'd slipped right out of the '60s.

The woman stood up. "Hi, I'm Kate. Emily called early this morning to say she might be few minutes late. She's having some foot problems and was going to try to see a doctor. Did you have any trouble finding this place?"

"Not at all. Good to see you again Dr. Stewart." They shook hands. "I'm glad we'll get to talk."

"Me too, but not for very long. My plans have changed and I'll be leaving for the airport in a few hours." They slid into the booth facing each other. "Sorry I won't get to participate in your documentary, but the chairperson of our board decided it'd be too controversial. You're lucky to get Emily though. I've never known anyone more dedicated to her clients. Of course, there's no way for you to know it, but the Kleins probably own half the county and Emily wouldn't have to work a minute if she didn't so chose."

A waitress with a ponytail came over to the booth. She was wearing a yellow short-sleeved angora sweater and a flowing green felt skirt appliquéd with a white poodle on the front. "Are you ladies ready to order?"

"Not yet," Kate nodded, "We're waiting on someone."

"Can I bring you something to drink?"

"Iced tea for me," Kate answered.

"Water." Leslie's eyes were wandering around the room where pictures of the local high school's championship teams and old 45rpm records decorated the walls. "How do you and Dr. Klein know each other?"

"Well, let me see. We first met in graduate school in the mid-seventies when we were lab partners in Experimental Psychology. Then, I believe it was in 1988, we ran into each other again at an MPD conference in Chicago. It was during a break and we were standing at the message board when out of the blue she began to talk about a young man she'd been seeing for a long time who believed he'd been raised in a satanic cult."

"Satanic? That's really hard for me to believe, Dr. Stewart."

"For me too, at first. But then I began to see a few women reporting similar things. And began to think about cults in general. I suppose you could say I was in a cult of a kind."

"How so?"

"I'm an ex-nun, actually."

"Ex? Why did you get out?"

"You see, I was working as a psychologist in an inner city school in Charleston. One day, a fourth grader came into my office saying a priest had been molesting him. As required by law, I reported it to Social Services. Didn't get anywhere with them because when they confronted the good Father, he denied it. Then all hell broke loose. I was reprimanded for trying to destroy his reputation. Basically, how shall I put this nicely? . . . I was told I should've kept my mouth shut. But I couldn't do that, couldn't join that kind of conspiracy to cover for the . . . well, at any rate . . . I left. One step ahead of the order's invitation to do so, I suspect."

"That must've been an awfully difficult decision."

"Only one I had. Luckily, I had no trouble finding my current job in Santa Fe."

Momentarily, Leslie turned her attention to the jukebox selector attached to the wall. "Never seen one of these before."

"Really? Let me show you how it works." Kate put a quarter in the slot and punched a button.

"Oh -o oh yes, I'm the great preten-en-der," crooned a voice from the vintage jukebox across the way.

"Cool." Leslie smiled, then went back to the previous discussion. "What was it like becoming a nun?"

"Nobody's ever asked me that before. Let me think . . . how shall I describe it. Interesting . . . no, demoralizing—"

They both turned to see Dr. Klein come through the door and over to the booth. After greetings all around, Kate asked her friend, "How're your feet?"

"Not too bad during the day. But at night they feel like a pin cushion. The doctor said she didn't know what was causing it but would give me something for the pain if I needed it. 'No thanks,' I told her. You know how I detest pills of any kind. To change the subject, y'all won't believe what I just heard on the radio. The county animal control officer has decided that black cats can't be adopted this week because of Halloween."

"I heard that too," Leslie said. "Thought it was a joke. Do they really think that stuff's going on down here?"

"It would certainly seem so," the psychologists answered at the same time.

Emily laughed. "We're always doing that. My friend's pretty psychic, you know."

"Well, you are too," Kate said.

"Anyway," Emily continued, "the animal shelter guy must be talking about teen dabblers who're more likely to leave traces of their activity. From what I've learned, the intergenerational satanic cults don't leave any evidence."

"Oh yes, but they do," Kate disagreed. "What about the broken bodies and minds of their prey?"

"Granted. However, I don't believe people who participate in so-called Satan worship, especially the young folks whose parents aren't involved, are necessarily worshiping the Devil. Some do it because of peer pressure. To be macho. For power. Sexual gratification. But I suppose they get into a cult and get trained. Once they're made to perpetrate, it's hard to get out. A seed's been planted. Sometimes it germinates. Other times it lays dormant until the right time comes."

"But the training's not always successful," Kate added. "I believe a victim at some point, whether consciously or unconsciously, makes a decision to either follow the rules or get out. In my opinion, evil should be defined in terms of behavior—the behavior of one person or a group of persons assaulting human dignity. I'd like for people to quit blaming the Devil . . . take the whole thing out of the supernatural . . . and take responsibility for the choices they make."

The waitress came over and set a pitcher of tea, one of water, and three large styrofoam cups filled with ice on the table. She took an order pad out of her skirt pocket and reached for the short pencil that was resting on her ear.

"If you want some local flavor," Emily looked at Leslie, "I'd recommend the VD burger all the way. That means cole slaw, chili, onions—"

"A VD hamburger. Sounds gross." Forgetting for a second that she was supposed to be acting like a professional, Leslie brought two fingers toward her mouth then quickly put her hand back under the table. Afraid of offending a potential subject, the documentarian placed her order. "I'll have a VD burger all the way and French fries."

"Make that two," said Kate.

Emily held up three fingers. "I suppose I should get a salad— what the heck, there's always another Monday, another day to begin a diet—but hold the fries." Nostalgically looking around the diner, she said, "Ms. Roberts, you might be interested in knowing that this place was the local hangout in my high school days. I like to come here now because it reminds me of all the good times: Friday night football games, sock hops afterwards, and rock and roll shows at the Charlotte coliseum." She looked at Kate. "Did you ever go to one of those? . . . no, it would've been a few years before your time . . . in the days when Whites sat on one side and Blacks on the other."

"For real?" Leslie asked.

"Yes. At the time we didn't even think about questioning it."

The conversation turned to southern food, the weather, and other things older women talk about. Everything but false memory syndrome and the recovered memory movement.

"Excuse me," Leslie slid out of the booth, "I need to wash my hands."

In the ladies' room she lit a cigarette, wondering what she'd gotten herself into.

That Emily person, she's a talker all right and sounds intelligent but I don't know how she would come across on camera. Looks more like a farmer's wife than a Ph.D. And may really be a nut. Believes in satanic cults. Wouldn't surprise me if she believes in God, too.

When Leslie returned to the booth still pondering God, the psychologists were discussing hell. They didn't seem to notice her standing behind the waitress who was busy putting out burgers oozing all over red and white checked pasteboard trays, and greasy French fries piled high in plastic baskets.

After the '50s impersonator left, Leslie slid into the booth.

"Ms. Roberts, do you believe there's a hell?" Kate asked.

"Please call me Leslie. Well frankly, I don't believe there's a Devil; therefore, I assume there's no hell." When she picked up the sandwich, a glob of chili fell out, painting an oily stain on the collar of her white silk blouse. She took a bite of the conglomeration. It wasn't bad. Not bad at all. "What do you believe, Dr. Stewart?"

"I can't prove there's a Devil but I do know there's Evil . . . with a capital E. And please call me Kate."

"I still call her Sister Kate. She's nobody's sister anymore, but if I had a sister I'd want her to be just like Kate. And I'd prefer that you call me Emily. Now that we have all that out of the way, Ms. Roberts—"

"Leslie."

"Okay, Leslie. Exactly what do you want from us?"

"As I said at the luncheon in August, my goal is to present an objective view of recovered memory therapy."

"I certainly hope you can show that suing therapists or going after their licenses is not the way to do it. Aren't all memories recovered? Thinking about anything that happened before this second is a memory —a recovered memory."

Dr. Klein sure was getting defensive. And a little offensive, too.

"Well, I suppose I'm talking about recovering repressed memories," Leslie clarified. "Does that make more sense?"

Kate answered. "Depends on what you mean by repressed. I think of repression as keeping something locked out of consciousness. Like putting a self-imposed padlock on the gate to your own awareness."

Emily added, "More like putting a dead weight on the things you never want to see again and dropping them to the bottom of the ocean." She picked up the whole burger and took a big bite. Leslie and Kate waited patiently as she chewed and swallowed. "But before going on, you should know, we have a person with multiple personalities sitting right here in this booth."

Leslie didn't know what to say.

"Yes we do." Emily put her arm around Kate's shoulder. "My dear sister here is Good, Gooder, and Goodest."

"I don't know about that," Kate laughed, "but you could probably say I was forced to dissociate during my years preparing for and becoming a nun."

"What do you mean?" Something else leaked out of Leslie's hamburger bun. This time she caught it with a napkin.

"To tell you the truth, when I'd—willingly, mind you—first gone beyond the double doors of the convent parlor with my teased hair and wearing Weejuns and a Villager dress, I didn't realize the church's goal was to create a whole new personality out of me: a new person with a new name; an entirely different identity. Their methodology, it turned out, was to break down my will and destroy my own sense of self: to cut off outside loyalties, even friendships inside the cloister; and to make me a blank slate. They broke me down 'so God could build me up'— that's the way they saw it: coercing me to do 'God's will' . . . or, I should say, what my superiors concluded was his will."

"Brainwashing," Emily summarized.

"You could call it that. It was like going to Parris Island for basic training except the authority was God rather than the U.S. Government. You've got to know that I joined the order in the days before the reforms of Vatican II. They squelched my emotions. In retrospect, I overlooked the '60s and the troubles in the world. Much too busy being 'good for God.' They even censored the letters I wrote to my parents, preventing me from sharing my thoughts and feelings with anyone. You can guess what happened. My body converted those repressed feelings into physiological symptoms making me miserable and depressed. During the day, they required me to be stoic, making me eat whatever they set before me. At night I threw up, literally and figuratively, everything they'd made me swallow."

"I've heard nuns were taught to flagellate themselves. Is that true?" Leslie asked.

"Absolutely. It happened to me in the early years. They gave me a whip and I tried it."

"Why, for God's sake?" Suddenly realizing she shouldn't be cursing in front of a nun . . . an ex-nun, Leslie put her hand over her mouth.

"Supposedly the purpose was to whip myself with that knotted rope so I could identify with the suffering Jesus. They also gave me a chain with spikes to wear around my upper arm. Hurt like the blazes. But somehow I learned not to feel it."

"That's probably because it set off the endorphins, the body's natural pain killers," Emily explained.

"Yes and I'm ashamed to admit it, but I believe that for a while I became addicted to the high produced by the self-injurious behavior. It's only recently that I've wondered if they taught it as some kind of perverted means of sexual sublimation . . . their own."

"So why did you stay as long as you did?" Leslie asked.

"It was a calling. My vows were to God, not the institutional church. In the early '70s, when I came out from behind the closed doors and found out what the real world was like, I began to question why the church shuts out women, why the church ignores and trivializes the experiences of women. My graduate school professors allowed me to think for myself and I began to doubt some of the church's teachings. When I went back to the convent at night, my superiors stripped this newly found freedom—didn't permit any dissent. I was split again."

Kate paused to take a paper napkin from the metal holder and wipe her mouth. "To become more spiritual, to be free to express God as I understood him or her, I had to get out of the ungodly restraints of religious life. But there's a part of me who's always a Sister, the part on a spiritual quest. And I miss that sense of closeness to God found in the liturgy and formal worship."

"Makes me think of one of my clients." Emily stole a fry from Kate's tray. "She wants to be a Christian but doesn't like Christ; wants to get back to the God she remembered as a child in a mainstream church but says she can't honor some of their teachings on such things as abortion and homosexuality; wants to go to potluck suppers. Right now she's studying angels. Not because she believes in them but because the stories are wholesome, as she put it."

"I understand her longing." Kate squeezed a little more ketchup on her fries. "When I got caught up in the feminist movement there was too much inner conflict. I got tired of having to obey people who were making mistakes. And I could never compromise with the church's teachings on the ordination of women."

"It's easy to see why Kate ran from that male power enclave," Emily said. "She was a feminist nun—a real-live oxymoron."

"Don't get me wrong, Leslie. Although the life-style was not for me, I know many Sisters who are doing honorable and noble work for their church and community. Organizations are not bad in themselves. And not all people in closed societies are evil."

"Before Emily got here, you mentioned that you were in a cult of a kind. So are you calling the convent, or even the church in general, a cult?"

"I don't know that I'd go that far. But come to think of it, the priests do dress in black and white robes and perform lots of rituals."

Everybody laughed.

"There are good cults and bad cults," Emily said. "And I'd say the ones who inflict pain on children—ritually abuse them—are the bad ones."

"Exactly how many ritual abuse survivors have you guys seen?" Leslie asked.

Emily spoke first. "Before I answer, let me clarify something. I do much more than work with trauma victims. Probably 90 percent of my time is spent working with clients with everyday problems of living: situational depression and anxiety, marriage and relationship problems. Recently, I've seen several teenagers who're trying to come to terms with their homosexuality. And I've seen a lot of executive-types who just want to learn more adaptive ways to cope with pressures of job responsibilities or perhaps learn hypnotic techniques to help lower their golf handicaps."

Leslie wondered if Emily was trying to evade the question but didn't interrupt.

"Personally, I prefer to call persons who've been creatively abused in ritualistic or ceremonial ways, 'unwitting initiates into organized evil.' Of course, there's no way to know how many children survived such atrocities or how many didn't; to what degree and how long."

"So, how many survivors have you seen?"

"Let me think," Emily said. "In over twenty years of practice, I've seen five clients who reported clear and convincing memories of severe torture by multiple perpetrators. And a few dozen more whose dissociative behaviors, along a continuum from mild to extreme, were suggestive of early trauma and/or an inability or lack of opportunity to develop a strong-tie or attachment to a mother-figure."

"Where are those clients now?"

Rubbing her forehead with both hands, Emily looked down at the table. "Three are dead. One killed herself—that was the woman I described in the letter I sent you with all the documentation about ritual abuse and mind control."

"You wrote a very touching vignette . . . yes it was. And I really do appreciate your sending me that material because it gave me another perspective on the whole FMS issue."

"I'm glad it was helpful. About my clients, another was murdered and the third died of physical complications." Placing her hands back on the table, Emily raised her head, looking eye to eye at the documentarian. "The woman you'll be meeting on Friday made a conscious decision to learn to control the dissociation by not allowing traumatic memories to interfere with her life any longer. This was apparently successful. From all appearances, she's a highly functioning individual— personally and professionally."

"Can't wait to meet her."

"Excuse me." Emily slid out of the booth. As if trying to keep her feet from touching the floor, she walked toward the rest room on her tiptoes.

While she was gone, Kate told Leslie about the safe-house in Santa Fe which, in its fifteen-year existence, had sheltered more than a hundred defectors from destructive organizations.

When Emily returned to the table, Leslie reminded, "You didn't say anything about your fifth client."

"I really can't. The woman's still in therapy and doesn't want to be interviewed for your documentary. But while Kate's with us, I would like to talk a little more about cults in general."

"Sure." That woman is obsessed with this cult topic, Leslie thought.

"Secret cults and secret oaths," Emily sighed, "they've always been and always will be. Secret organizations are no respecters of class or culture. One of my former clients talked about a root doctor somewhere down in Black Bottom—"

"Black Bottom. What's that?" Leslie asked.

"It's the section down by the river where Blacks were once forced to live. Whites have always called it Black Bottom; the residents call it

Happy Holler. As I was saying, the root doctor both healed people and put evil spells on them. It comes from their African heritage. Probably a little voodoo mixed in, too."

"Speaking of secret societies, what about college fraternities and sororities?" Kate asked. "Yale's 'Skull and Crossbones' comes to mind. And the Masons? Or those special loyalty oaths the government required during the height of the McCarthy-era and the Cold War?"

"I suppose if you look at it that way, the Pledge of Allegiance serves the same purpose." Leslie was trying to follow their reasoning. "When you get down to it, people have always created ways to express their agreed-upon bond to an idea, haven't they?"

"Exactly." Emily motioned for the waitress to bring the check. "But what I'm concerned about are destructive cults. They could include anything from subsets of religious and fraternal organizations, to secret branches of our government, to families who've handed down the black arts from generation to generation, and even to the group of good ol' boys who pass around somebody's kid for fun and games after the neighborhood block party ... or perhaps, in these parts, after the monthly Ku Klux Klan rally."

"Now the Klan," Leslie said, "I could believe they were capable of committing ritualistic crimes against children. But in my opinion as a documentarian just beginning to delve into this material, it's the word satanic that gets everybody upset. Nobody wants to believe that satanic cults exist; that people actually worship the Devil and sacrifice children in the process."

The waitress brought the check to the table. Emily picked it up but Leslie took it from her hand.

Kate put a handful of change on the table. "It all comes back to good and evil. If evil doesn't exist, why do we have so many religions organized to fight it?"

"Good point," Leslie conceded.

Emily added a dollar to the tip. "Everyone wants to deny the reality of ritual trauma so these 'crazy' people—with their awful, unthinkable, unbearable memories—will just go away."

"Speaking of going away," Kate looked at the round Coca Cola clock hanging on the wall behind the cash register, "it's about time for me to leave. Leslie, if you're ever out Santa Fe way, give me a call and I'll find you a bunk for the night."

"Thanks. I may take you up on that sometime."

The psychologists slid out of the booth and hugged each other.

"Have a safe trip, Dr. Stewart," Leslie said, also leaving the booth.

Emily addressed Leslie. "I'm busy this afternoon but tomorrow I've blocked out the whole day. If you can come over to my office about nine, we can get down to business. Then Friday morning, I've arranged for you to interview the high functioning person I mentioned earlier."

"Sounds great. I have one more question though . . . for you both. Why did you guys go into the helping profession?"

Kate answered first. "It was my calling. I've always seen it as my mission to serve God and help others."

Then Emily. "To tell you the truth, I used to think it was to help people, but about ten years ago some things happened that made me wonder if, unconsciously, I really became a psychologist to help myself."

"I'd like to hear about that sometime," Leslie said.

"It's very personal." Emily looked upward at the faded football jerseys and heavy wool high-school letter sweaters hanging from the rafters. "And I don't really know if it has anything to do with . . . with your project."

———————

Leslie Roberts' professional problem was much worse than the one she was facing at the moment.

"Hi, I'm Cricket." As the friendly young woman greeted her at the door, Leslie held up her right index finger. "Ooh. How'd you do it?"

"Last night I was trying to get the dresser drawer in the motel unstuck and—"

"Visitor in town? Ya shore don't talk like you're from around here."

Thinking fast to explain her reason for being in Chestnut Ridge, Leslie introduced herself. "I'm a reporter from New York. I came down here to research mental health treatment in the South."

"Well then, I bet you'd like to meet my roommate. She's a reporter with the paper and could probably help ya get connected with the locals around here, if ya want to. How in the world did ya find out about me?"

"Dr. Emily Klein. I met her yesterday and when this happened, I called to ask her for a recommendation for a salon."

"Down here we called it a beauty shop."

"Shop, then." Leslie glanced to her right. A collage of heads covering the length of the wall—men, women, and children with various cuts and styles—stared at her.

"C'mon back." As Cricket led her to a manicure table, Leslie felt the eyes of the other stylists and their clients following her like she was some kind of creature from another world. "Have a seat and we'll get ya fixed right up."

"If you have time, why don't you just do a complete manicure?" Leslie asked, getting comfortably seated across from Cricket.

"Shore thing. Same shade?"

"Yes, that'd be fine."

Bubbling with energy, Cricket began working and talking at the same time. "I know Dr. Klein real good. In fact, she wuz one of my first customers when I came to town and rented a booth about ten years ago. Last year the owner died and would ya believe, left the whole business to me. Fine woman she is, that Emily. She's the only customer I have where I can do the talking and she just listens. And nothing I've ever told her, I'm shore, has left this building. Most of my customers just dump everything on me. To tell ya the truth, I'm like Emily: I don't tell nobody what I'm told neither."

"So you didn't grow up around here?"

"Law no. I'm from the mountains. But this shore has been a good place to live. Everybody's friendly. Leave ya alone if ya wanna to be left alone. Help ya if ya need help. Only person I've ever had any words with was Emily's father-in-law. He was my landlord when I first came to town. A drunk and about as obnoxious as any one you'd ever meet. And cluttery, lord-a-mercy, ya shoulda seen his basement."

Leslie was about to ask her what she was doing in the man's basement when one of the other beauticians called Cricket to the telephone.

"That was about our booth at the fall festival on Saturday," Cricket explained when she got back to the table. "They always have it around Halloween. This year it's out at the new Civic Center. Used to be a military school, I've heard. But the city built a big modern building out there and now they have all sorts of things going on."

"You'll be manicuring at the fall festival?"

"Not exactly," Cricket giggled. "We'll be painting faces for charity. If you really wanna get a taste of what us Southerners are like, ya should come on over if you're still in town. There's always something special and this year I've heard it's an exhibit of old railway cars. Hope that's not as boring as it sounds."

"I may do that. Talk about Halloween, have you ever heard of any real witches or devil worshipers practicing around here?"

"Nothing specific. There's so many churches in this town, I can't see how the Devil could make any headway at all. Maybe our police chief could help you out. Right after I came to town there was a murder and one of the rumors was that he was mixed up in the stuff."

"The police chief?"

"No, the victim."

"Thanks for the tip. I probably won't have time this week but maybe I can talk with him if I get back down here again."

The conversation seemed to have ended as Cricket began concentrating more on her art and Leslie began contemplating how to be unobtrusive in her mission.

After reading several articles and books suggested by the investors and watching tapes of two 1995 PBS documentaries, *Divided Memories* and *The Search for Satan*—supposedly balanced examinations of the FMS controversy—Leslie was becoming more and more curious about the therapist's side of the matter.

Having sat across from Drs. Klein and Stewart the previous day, she couldn't imagine that those two intelligent, extremely kind women were guilty of the types of things the therapists in these films had purportedly done. *Divided Memories* had documented a few examples of what most people would agree is bad therapy such as searching for memories in the birth canal. This program left the viewer with the impression that bad therapy is widespread. *The Search for Satan* had attempted to leave the viewer with the impression that multiple personality is a fad and that there is no evidence at all of widespread Satan worship. It painted doctors who treat such cases as charlatans and criminals engaging in insurance fraud.

Leslie wondered why another documentary was needed unless it was to offer one that was more balanced. However, she doubted if the investors for her project would sponsor such an approach. They seemed to have only one goal: to save the world from evil therapists.

If anybody else asked, how was she supposed to explain her presence in this town? That she was an investigative reporter looking for truth about false memories when she'd already been told what the truth was, what the story should be. How could she write a proposal for an unbiased documentary when the investors were definitely biased but apparently sincere in thinking theirs was the only truth?

"How's that look?" Cricket interrupted Leslie's consternation.

"Very nice. Thanks for working me in on such a short notice."

"Glad to help," Cricket said as they walked up to the cash register to complete the transaction. "Nice meeting ya. Hope ya enjoy your stay in our town. Come on out to the festival on Saturday and I'll paint your face."

Ten minutes later, Leslie was sitting in the waiting room of a building that looked more like a cozy cottage than a psychological clinic. She was contemplating her first formal interview with a person whom the investors would likely call a fringe therapist. Dr. Klein was with a client, leaving the documentarian more time to ponder her dilemma.

When they'd met on Wednesday, Emily had mentioned only one client who had agreed to be interviewed and wasn't certain if that person would allow her true identity to be disclosed on camera. How could Leslie show both sides in this controversy when alleged victims wouldn't surrender their privacy? Even if they did, or even if it were possible to find tearful parents to go on camera crucifying therapists, what did that show? One thing was certain: the impossibility of proving that something didn't happen.

It all came down to evidence.

In her dual roles as producer/director of this proposed documentary, how could she depict her findings without violating the confidentiality of her sources? Where would she find visual evidence that therapists are making clients remember things that didn't happen? Conversely, where would she find evidence that ritual abuse happens? Go to a cult meeting incognito? Not hardly. Leslie was smart enough to know that if you got caught in some nefarious activity, you'd be guilty by association. It's like the case of the journalist who was caught downloading child pornography onto his hard drive. His defense was that he was doing research, but it didn't work. And there was not much chance of his continuing the project in prison.

Some documentaries use re-creations but this technique wouldn't work either. To show people acting out the things many DID patients have alleged happened to them wouldn't pass the censors. Imagine the trailer: "Tonight on PBS we will take you into the world of occult crime where you will see fathers raping their children, babies being stabbed to death, children hurting other children, bestiality . . .."

Leslie was beginning to wonder why Dr. Klein had even agreed to be interviewed when the psychologist came through the waiting room door. "Good morning. Did you get to see Cricket?"

"Yes and she got me all fixed up. That young woman seems to be the epitome of southern friendliness. Even invited me to the festival on Saturday and promised to paint my face."

"So who do you want to be for Halloween?"

"Right now, I'm beginning to think I'd prefer to be anything but a documentarian. Since our meeting yesterday, I've been wondering how I can make something that is so . . . so cerebral and at the same time ambiguous, how I can make it visual. But that's not the only problem. As I told you in Boston, the investors are a group of parents who want to show how therapists are tearing up families—"

"Leslie, I volunteered for your project to give you a different side. Although I personally don't like to stand in front of a camera—I'd rather help behind the scenes—if that's what it takes to present another viewpoint, I've made up my mind that I can do it."

"Interesting. Most people I've met would do or say almost anything to get on TV. How do you think Springer, Montel, even Oprah survive? Would it be okay if I go ahead and set up my camera in order to get all your comments on tape?"

"That's fine. Had I known you were going to film today, I might have put on some makeup and worn a skirt."

"Don't worry. This is just for information gathering. For the real thing, if the project's approved, we'll fix you up to look like a news anchor."

"Whatever. But it wouldn't be me."

"Oh, I just about forgot." Leslie reached into her briefcase and pulled out a piece of paper. "Before we start, I need you to sign this informed consent form. Basically, it tells you all the risks of being a participant in a documentary."

"I understand. That's required in my profession, too. Didn't used to be, but today I've heard that's one of the main reasons therapists lose their licenses. Not telling clients the risks of therapy before they begin."

"Risks?"

"Yes. I'll give you a copy of my form, but honestly I don't see any real risks as long as a therapist upholds the ethical guidelines of the profession. In twenty years, nobody's ever made a board complaint against me. I can't imagine how I'd react if I got one of those letters. Any time I even see an envelope with the Psychology Board's return address on it, I get nervous. Like I've done something really bad. Thankfully, so far it's always turned out to be my renewal notice."

As Emily was reading over the form, Leslie recalled what one of her professors in graduate school had harped on: "Do no unintentional harm. Now there'll be times when the purpose of a documentary is to expose the wicked ways of some person or organization, but most of the time the purpose of behavioral-type documentaries is to show people just the way they are."

The psychologist signed the form. "There's not a lot of difference in this and the one I require my clients to sign. I explain what therapy's about and its possible positive and negative effects and make sure the person is competent to give consent." She handed it back to Leslie. "I suppose I could deal with the public ridicule that might occur if I speak out about this topic, but I certainly wouldn't want any harm to come to my clients or family members."

"I can't conceive of that happening," Leslie said, taking the form and placing it back into her briefcase. She took out a small video camera and attached it to the tripod Emily had set up in the corner. "Are you ready to begin?"

Emily nodded affirmatively and was talking before Leslie could get the camera locked and focused on her subject. "Do you realize that because of biased media presentations, most people in America believe that MPD/DID is just Hollywood stuff? Or that they caught MPD from watching the movie *Sybil*? What about reports from clinicians around the world—Turkey, Japan, England, Germany, Belgium, The Netherlands, Australia, Sweden, New Zealand, South Africa—who're treating MPD and ritual abuse and mind control victims? How do you let the general public know there's scientific support for such a diagnosis? The latest figure I've seen says that in the last ten years, approximately 1700 peer-reviewed articles about DID have been published in scientific journals. In my opinion, if a person has pathological dissociative symptoms and a therapist doesn't recognize them or call them what they are, that's malpractice."

This Dr. Klein person seemed capable of doing a one-man show on the topic.

"Do you believe it's possible to make someone think they're multiple if they aren't when they first come to therapy?" Leslie asked.

"No. Not using standard therapy techniques. In some of the mind control experiments, multiples were supposedly created by psychiatrists using mind-altering drugs and electroshock—"

"Like bona fide Manchurian Candidates?"

"That's what I'm talking about. It's also possible some clients may act multiple to please the therapist. But those factitious cases, I believe, wouldn't hold up very long in front of well-trained therapists."

"Okay, Dr. Klein, let's pretend that I'm on your side of this controversy now and am looking for a way to prove to the FMS proponents that memories can't be implanted—"

"I'm not saying that some false memories can't be suggested and a person begins to believe they're truth. In fact, some of the early hypnosis researchers have shown it's possible. But that's another story. I've got to tell you, though, no one has ever transformed someone's happy childhood to an abusive one using hypnosis. Nor has anyone implanted a traumatic memory with the accompanying symptoms . . . the panic attacks, depression, headaches, hypervigilance, and other posttraumatic phenomena. And another thing, no ethical therapists would do such things even if they knew how. By the way, since you're trying to see things from the other side now, I've collected several articles and books that you might want to browse through." Emily pointed to the boxes under the window.

"What do you have to say about the study that's frequently used in courts—it's called 'Lost in a Shopping Mall' if I remember correctly—to show that memories can be implanted?"

"Have you actually read it?"

"No I haven't."

"Well I'd recommend that you do and that you also read a recent article by Crook and Dean which examines the study. The authors conclude that the mall results are so unclear that they couldn't tell how many subjects, if any, completely—and completely is the key word here—believed the false memory.

"If I remember correctly, the way the shopping mall study went, a researcher found 24 pairs of relatives and had the older relative in each pair provide three true incidents and a believable false one involving the younger relative. The false incident was about a time when the trusted older relative supposedly remembered visiting a mall with the younger relative and the younger relative wandered off and became lost, cried, and was helped by an elderly woman. That's not exactly the same as suggesting that a child had been raped by her father when it was obviously not true. When the study ended, five of the twenty-four subjects thought that they possibly could have been lost in a mall when they were five years old."

"That's all there was to it?"

"Basically. However the study has been embellished over and over and not only cited in court cases, but also used in magazines, newspapers, and even scholarly journals to try to prove that therapists implant false memories."

"What about—"

For the second time that morning, Leslie was pre-empted by a ringing telephone.

"I'll be right back," Emily said.

While the psychologist was gone, Leslie looked through the books, pulling them out one by one, wondering how the mind can create images that never were? She was beginning to see some parallels between a documentarian's and a multiple's job. The task of both is to take all the visuals—flashbacks for the multiple and film clips for the documentarian—and put them together into a narrative: a structured, ordered, true story that makes sense.

Emily came back into the room. "Sorry, Leslie. That was the school calling. My granddaughter is sick and they can't get in touch with her mother. I'm going to have to close the office and go pick her up now. The woman who has agreed to talk with you called last night and said she can come here in the morning around nine o'clock. When I'm finished seeing clients I'll meet with you both, if that's okay."

"That'll be fine."

"You can take the books or anything else back to the motel if you want to."

"I'll do that, thanks."

"Oh yeah. As I was saying before the phone rang, sometimes we do find evidence: tangible, palpable evidence. As a matter of fact, I just happen to have some of it stored in a closet at my house."

"Now that sounds intriguing. What is it?"

"It'd be better if you see it first. If I don't forget, I'll bring it in tomorrow to show you."

———————

Unlocking her office door on Friday morning, Emily turned around to greet Leslie. "Good morning. Sorry about having to cut yesterday's meeting short."

"That's quite all right. I hope your granddaughter's okay."

"Thanks. She is. When her mommy came home, she got better in a hurry. Come on in."

"How many grandchildren do you have?"

"Two. My daughter and son-in-law have two girls. Winslow is almost nine and Alison just turned two. If you come out to the festival on Saturday, you'll probably get to meet them."

A young man came in the front door. Emily motioned him back to the therapy room, then turned to Leslie. "You can use the playroom for your interview. The tripod's already set up if you want to use it. The judge should be here in a few minutes."

"Judge?"

"Yes. The woman you'll be meeting. In my opinion, she's as credible a subject as you could find. I can tell you that she's a native of Chestnut Ridge, now serving as a district court judge in another state."

Leslie went back to the kid-friendly room and closed the door. After adjusting the camera, she plopped down on a big yellow beanbag and began to look through her notes. The door opened and Emily stepped into the room. "Excuse me. Thought you might want to read this. The judge has given permission to show it to you." She handed Leslie a copy of a letter addressed to the President of the United States dated May 26, 1997. "See you after while." Emily closed the door behind her.

Curiously, Leslie put her pad aside and read the letter:

Dear President Clinton:

In April of this year, you issued a formal apology to five remaining survivors of the 400 African-Americans whose syphilis was deliberately left untreated as part of a secret government study now known as the Tuskegee experiments. You stated: "What was done cannot be undone, but we can end the silence. We can stop turning our heads away, we can look at you in the eye and finally say, on behalf of the American people, what the United States government did was shameful, and I am sorry."

With this letter, I am requesting that you look into another matter in which my rights as an American citizen, as a human being, were horrendously violated. In 1995, I began to recover memories of having been subjected to unethical and torturous medical and mind control experiments during the 1950s which, I believe, were conducted and/or sponsored by various agencies of our government, possibly as part of its effort to win the Cold War. If there were any records kept on me, I'm sure you would agree that it is my right to have them. My medical condition is very complex and such information could be beneficial to both my current and my future health.

I am requesting that you take appropriate action to do the following:

1. Declassify all government files, documents, and tapes of any nature related to programs of mind control research and operations, and take steps to prosecute anyone who has engaged in criminal conduct related to such research or operations.

2. Determine the federal government's responsibilities for wrongs and harms done to human subjects since it's origination, both inside and outside the United States.

3. Determine appropriate remedies for those subjects who have been found to be physically or psychologically wronged or harmed.

4. Stop any current abuses immediately.

What was done to me was inhumane. I pray in God's name that someone really does care enough to listen and do what is right. I trust my government will be accountable and responsible and would like to believe that my amazing survival from such atrocities will not have been in vain.

Sincerely,

Margaret Rucker-Volz

Whoa! Leslie thought, if there's any truth to this, I doubt the investors will want me to deal with it at all.

Hearing a knock, the documentarian dug her way out of the beanbag. Opening the door, she was greeted by a woman carrying a large cloth-covered scrapbook. "Hello. I'm Margaret Rucker-Volz and I've come to talk with Ms. Roberts."

"That's me." Leslie offered her hand. "Dr. Klein said we could use this room. Nice to meet you, Judge Volz. I was just reading your letter to the President. I have a lot of questions, but first I need you to sign a consent form."

They sat across from each other at the child-sized table. After reading over the form, Maggie said, "I understand that for you to have a credible documentary you need to know my true identity; however, at this time I'm not sure if I'm ready for the general public to know who I am. For now, I'm requesting the option of having my identity disguised in your final production. Would that be possible?"

"Yes, Your Honor. Just write that stipulation on the form."

The judge jotted down a short addendum and signed the informed consent agreement. Pushing the paper across the table, she said, "Please call me Maggie."

For several minutes, the two women from very different cultures made small talk about the lovely fall weather, current Broadway plays, and even Halloween. The judge appeared to be a warm caring person, obviously intelligent, articulate, photogenic. There was something oddly familiar about the woman but the documentarian couldn't put her finger on it.

"You don't look like a multiple," Leslie blurted out.

"How's a multiple supposed to look?"

"Actually I've never met a multiple. Not that I know of. And you don't act like a multiple. Not like the ones I've seen on TV talk shows."

"How's a multiple supposed to act?" Maggie smiled, acting neither catty nor defensive.

"I'm sorry if I appear ignorant. There's a lot I need to learn." Having already determined that the woman should be able to conduct herself well on camera, Leslie asked, "Is it okay if I videotape our conversation?"

"Fine with me. As long as you honor our agreement. I'd like to do everything I *safely* can to tell the world about the secret Cold War 'multiplicity experiments.'"

Leslie got up and clicked on the camera. "I'm really intrigued with the letter you wrote to President Clinton. Can you tell me how you got to that point?"

"It's a long story. How much time do we have?"

"As much as you need." Leslie sat back down.

"Where do you want me to start?"

"How about when you began recovering memories of abuse?"

"To be perfectly honest, I'd have to say I have two sets of memories: those I never forgot and those that started with the snakes."

"Snakes?"

"I'll get to that later but first let me tell you about the ones I never forgot." Maggie stood up, stretching her arms. "Before we go on, I could use some caffeine. Can I bring you something to drink? Emily always has a fresh pot of coffee brewing and soft drinks in the fridge."

"No thanks." Leslie got up and turned the camera off. "But I think I'll go outside for a quick smoke."

When they both returned, Maggie asked, "Where was I? Oh yes. The memories. Of course, I never forgot the memories of being sick as a child."

"Wait a minute," Leslie said. She got up and turned the camera back on. "Now what were you saying?"

"I was getting ready to say, you may not believe this, but once when I was in the local hospital—I'm talking about in pre civil-rights days when Blacks were put in basement rooms with the boilers and pipes and I was waiting for them to take me to the ward or the dungeon as we called it—they left me out in the hallway in one of those beds with tall rails. The white folk would come by gawking at me like I was a monkey in a cage; like I was some kind of carnival attraction."

"How horrible." What else could Leslie say? Actually she didn't have to say much because Maggie was carrying the conversation.

"At first Emily thought that's why I was dissociative. You know, because of all those painful treatments."

"What does it feel like to dissociate?"

"Let me think a minute . . . the image that comes to mind is that of a little child being ravaged by a hurricane who suddenly finds herself trapped in its eye . . . everything's quiet . . . all communication lost to the outside world. No longer seeing or hearing what's going on in the outer world. It's as if her human inner core is somehow being protected in the midst of the storm."

"Great image."

The subject's eyes glazed over as she looked right past Leslie, saying softly, "But the damage stays with her a long time. Maybe forever."

The person across from Leslie Roberts didn't appear damaged in any way at all.

Maggie blinked. Looking directly at the interviewer, her demeanor changed to an excellent stage presence. "From my observation, dissociation is common in my culture, accepted. Perhaps it's related to the residuals of severe maltreatment blacks received during slavery. And later the blatant discrimination during the Jim Crow days, or the harassment we suffered during the civil-rights movement. Today, for Blacks to live successfully in an integrated society, we have to act one way in the white world and another in the African-American community."

"That's an interesting perspective. One I'd like to follow up on sometime but for now I'd like to hear about your different personalities. Were they created in therapy?"

"Surely you don't believe that's possible, do you? And even if it were, there's no way Dr. Klein could have, or would have, done that. She's always tried to help, not hurt me."

Leslie turned her eyes back to the letter. "In this letter to the President, you talked about medical and mind control experiments. Where did those memories come from?"

"From my mind . . . where else? . . . and they all came to me after I left therapy. Over the years when I've been in town, I've stopped by to talk with Emily about them. Fortunately, I've been able to manage the associated feelings—anger, rage, shame—on my own and by talking with people I've met at survivor conferences and over the Internet who remember having been put through similar atrocities."

Maggie's face became flushed and her previously warm gentle eyes seemed to change to cold transparent obsidian. She spoke as if she were a prosecuting attorney giving closing arguments in a court proceeding: "It has been established through declassified documents that in a program called MKULTRA, our government conducted inhumane mind control experiments testing such techniques as brain implants, sensory deprivation, ultrasonics, torture, amnesia-inducing drugs, biologicals, psychological stress, and electroshock. I don't know if you've heard about it or not."

"Yes I have. As a matter of fact, Dr. Klein described that program in a letter she sent me. I can't help but wonder why the general public hasn't heard more about it." Leslie was also beginning to wonder why the investors in her project hadn't mentioned government-sanctioned mind control experiments, when she noticed that the woman's eyes had changed back to warm and gentle.

"To answer your earlier question about integration, I believe I was split all to pieces in some of the government experiments." Maggie turned her eyes from the camera lens and digressed: "Just the other night I had an image . . . I guess you'd say a flashback. I was a little girl being ushered through some type of hospital setting and there were babies lined up in incubators against the walls. And knowing what I know now, I'm beginning to wonder if it was some type of eugenics experiment like I read about a few months ago in *The Wall Street Journal*."

"Could you tell me more about that article?"

"I don't remember all the details, but apparently in the early forties, the military funded psychologists to do research aimed at improving the human race." As if Leslie and the camera weren't in the room, Maggie went on analyzing her thoughts. "No . . . that couldn't have been it. I wouldn't have been born yet. And they certainly wouldn't have used a half-black kid—or half-white kid—which ever way you want to look at it. Back to what I was saying, I don't think they were successful in making separate parts with lives of their own. Granted, I have some of those, but I believe they resulted because of traumas right here in Chestnut Ridge where I was supposed to have been protected by my family. I believe the experiments only succeeded in making me dissociate the memories of the torture."

"I want to hear about that process, but first can you tell about the parts of yourself who, as you say, have lives of their own? What made them come out?"

"I'm pretty sure I know but let's talk about the MPD or DID diagnosis first. To tell you the truth, I'd always known my life was lived intermittently. For example, the person you see in front of you has little musical ability. When I sit down to play the organ or piano, I can't play a thing. So I take a deep breath and suddenly see my hands begin to work the keys."

"You're not musical, but there's a part who is?"

"That's correct."

"So are you . . . I believe the term is integrated?"

"I'm not sure if that's the appropriate term for the way I've resolved things. Let me put it this way: Before therapy, it was as though I'd been living in a boarded-up house. When I was in one room, I didn't always know what was going on in other rooms. In therapy with Dr. Klein by my side, I began to understand what was happening and the top of the house blew off allowing me to see what was going on anytime in any room. The shades came up, the doors swung open, and the walls became transparent. To use Dr. Klein's metaphor, I believe most of the closets are now empty."

Maggie went on talking as if unaware of the camera and potentially the world. "I became co-conscious with all the different aspects of myself. Although my life is still compartmentalized to a degree, today I can go in and out of the rooms freely. I guess you'd say the key word is control. Now I feel in control of my life. When the musician is needed on Sunday mornings, she comes out. When the judge is needed he . . . she comes out. There's even a party girl who shows up when I need to chill out. But thank the good Lord, she's not nearly as wild as she used to be. And there're always the child parts. But I believe everyone has at least one of those."

"Tell me about recovering repressed memories. Did your therapist use formal hypnosis?"

"No. I wouldn't let her. Now I know why. It was one of the techniques the experimenters used to control me and I suppose some part of me was not going to let that happen again."

"Do you think if you'd never gone to therapy, the memories would've come out? A lot of people are blaming therapists for implanting memories."

"Ms. Roberts, I can say without reservation that Dr. Klein did not implant memories in my brain. She was from a different world, literally. How would a white woman have been able to make me remember things like voodoo rituals? Or some of the so-called discipline techniques my grandmother used?"

"So why, after such a long a time, did you remember?"

"I'm sure some of it had to do with the stress of going public with what the town's favorite doctor did . . . and that's another story. But what I really think did it was the snakes."

"You mentioned them earlier. What was that about?"

"Before I tell you about them, let me show you my "Book of Memories." For the second time the judge had hedged on the snake question. Maggie laid the scrapbook upside down on the table so Leslie could see the detailed drawings. "Often at night just before I go to sleep, scenes flash into my mind, sort of like the panoramic slide shows at many of our nation's tourist attractions. In the morning, I'll sketch as many as I can remember. When I look at them in retrospect, all together, and when I talk to others on Internet chat lists who're remembering the same types of things, I'm often able to put them into a narrative, if you will, that seems to—."

"That's similar to my job," Leslie interrupted. "To get all the raw footage I can, then choose and organize it in a way that makes sense to the viewer."

"Good analogy." Opening the book to the first sketch, the judge offered, "You're welcome to flip through it and if you have questions, I'll try to answer them."

"I'd like to do that but if it's okay with you I need to adjust the camera to get close-ups." Leslie went over to the camera. Zeroing in on the scrapbook, she began to think of a way to produce her documentary. Possibly by showing the sketches, giving viewers ample time to see the memories of one person, they could decide for themselves if the client's memories could have been implanted by a therapist.

As the judge slowly turned the large pages, Leslie studied the images that had come from the woman's mind: a child on a gurney, wires leading to a black box, a laboratory lined with tiny babies in incubators, a room that looked like the set of Star Trek, men in white coats, men in black robes, helicopters, a dolphin, movie cameras and screens, a speaker hanging on a wall, a metal helmet, goggles painted with an array of colors, double doors opening into an underground chamber, needles, daggers, pills, snakes.

Leslie was about to ask about the snakes for the third time when Emily cracked the door open. "Can I come in?"

"Please do." Leslie got up again and turned the camera off. "I'm really going to have to ask my boss to get me a remote," she said.

Emily was carrying a white cardboard suit box. She laid it on the table, opened it, and pulled out some sort of age-worn costume.

"Where in tarnation did you get that?" An obviously surprised judge flipped to the last picture in her memory book. "Look! Here's one just like that. Right here."

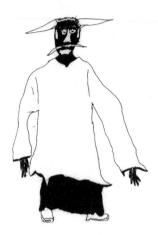

"It's a long story. Quite personal." Emily paused for several seconds as if trying to avoid an impulsive response; finally shaking her head: "If you really want to hear it, I don't mind telling you both. But what I'm going to tell you now is off the record; doesn't leave the room. Agreed?"

"Yes, I understand," Leslie said. "If you'd like, we could add that to your consent form."

"That won't be necessary. I trust you. Now with that out of the way, let's all go back to the therapy room where it'll be more comfortable."

The Honorable Margaret Rucker-Volz closed her memory book and the three women from three very different frames of the universe crossed the hall together.

Before they even got seated, Maggie looked at her watch. "Holy Moly! I didn't realize it was this late. I'm supposed to be somewhere else right this minute. When they found out I was going to be in town, the local bar association invited me to speak at their monthly luncheon. Ms. Roberts, it's been nice talking with you."

"My pleasure. If the documentary proposal gets the go-ahead, I'll be contacting you again if that's okay."

"Fine. Who knows? By then, I may be ready to go public."

"That'd be great . . . but one quick question before you leave: What was it you were going to tell me about the snakes?"

"Really, Ms. Roberts, I do have to be going, but maybe Emily can help you with that. She has my permission to tell you anything she wants to say about me. Bye now." As Maggie was walking out the door, she turned and looked at Emily. "Let's get together in January when I come back to speak at the King memorial service."

"Sure thing," Emily said. "Take care."

With that weird-looking figure wearing horns on his head standing in her mind, Leslie settled down in the recliner. Emily sat on the sofa. Taking off her loafers and arranging her body into a lotus position, the therapist began, "In the year of Hugo, I almost went to pieces . . . . "

———————

First in line waiting for the gate to open at 9:00 o'clock on Saturday morning, Leslie Roberts sat in the rental car, chuckling at the motto on the brochure that had come with her ticket to the fall festival:

WELCOME TO CHESTNUT RIDGE
AMERICA'S BEST KEPT SECRET

Although she'd seen it three days earlier on the billboard at the edge of town, today its meaning was deeper, more sinister, downright eerie.

How could such evil be lurking in this quiet little southern town? If those women I've talked with this week are telling the truth, I'd have to acknowledge that the world is full of pedophiles and child pornographers who hide behind costumes, clerical robes, white doctor coats and military uniforms. I'd have to believe that children had been—or are still being—traumatized in day-care centers, slaughterhouses, barns, Masonic temples, church basements, cemeteries, warehouses, suburban bedrooms and living rooms, hospitals, research labs, military bases, campgrounds, and caverns—just about everywhere.

Leslie had been sent south to expose the recovered memory practices of a lone therapist or two but was beginning to wonder if there was something more important that needed to be exposed.

What if twenty, thirty, forty, even fifty years ago there was a cadre of unethical scientists and high-level people in government who had no compunc-

tion about using evil for the greater good; whether it was for national security or for the gratification of their own bane needs for power, sex, and control?

And what if these people were also sadists and pedophiles willing to pay money to parents or institutional caregivers for the right to use dependent children in their diabolical activities?

And what if their failures, the ones who forgot not to remember, began showing up in therapy offices around the world?

And what if the survivors and their advocates began to compare histories, and to research declassified government documents, and to learn that through MKULTRA, mind control experiments were sanctioned by the CIA and that most of the records were destroyed in 1973?

Perhaps it would have been time for someone—maybe someone who had been involved in MKULTRA, or others who had been accused of physically, sexually, and/or spiritually abusing children —to begin a campaign to create a false disease; to brainwash an uninformed public into thinking that there's no such thing as repressed memory and that without external corroboration, there's no way to prove that traumatic memories obtained in therapy have any basis in truth.

As the journalist was considering the ethical choice she'd soon be required to make, the gate to the grounds of the rambling pink granite Civic Center building opened. A parking attendant directed her to the area on a section of pavement that had once been an airstrip.

On the greenway, dozens of tents had been set up to display historical pictures and artifacts; to sell food; and to peddle various arts and crafts. Only in South Carolina, she thought, walking past a booth where a purveyor of Confederate memorabilia was sharing space with a vender of traditional African clothing. An older white man sporting a military-style haircut and wearing a black suit and a clerical collar was looking at the latter. Why in the world would he dress like that to come to a place like this? Leslie wondered. Must have some type of insecure authority-figure complex . . . hmm . . . this psychological stuff is wearing off on me.

"Ms. Roberts." It was Cricket Cassidy calling from her face-painting booth. "Come on over. I'd like ya to meet my partner Danny Evans, the reporter I told you about."

They shook hands and Danny said, "Cricket told me you were doing a documentary. I'd love to give you an outsider's view of this town sometime."

"I'm sure that would be interesting but for now I'm focusing more on mental health treatment."

"If you ask my opinion," Danny went on, "all in all, Chestnut Ridge is a pretty good place to live. Like many small towns in the South, it's changed a lot since I came here ten years ago." For a reporter, the woman didn't seem to be listening very well and went on touting her community. "The population's almost doubled. The town is no longer run by a certain group of people; the names that used to be so prominent, you don't hear much anymore."

"It's a beautiful town," Leslie said.

"Yes it is. Especially since Syn-Tec, our chief industry, was bought out by a German Company. They pumped a lot of money into the community. I hear they're planning an outdoor pavilion for concerts over there on the other side of the railroad tracks."

Leslie heard a jingling sound and turned around to see an old woman wearing a tattered wool coat and brogans skipping across the lawn rattling a tambourine.

"China Doll." Cricket answered the question in Leslie's mind. "She's a town fixture. Sometimes comes into the shop preaching about the Devil. One thing about her, she ain't phony."

"She's psychotic, that's what. I'm sure she could tell you a lot about mental health around here." Leslie was waiting for Danny to say more when Emily came over. A little girl was clinging to each hand.

"Hi, Leslie. Glad you made it. Danny, good to see you again. Cricket, I brought you some business."

Cricket got down on her knees at eye level with the younger child. "Hey there, honey bunch. Who do you want to be today?"

"A pwincess."

"I think we can do that. And Winslow, what about you?"

"Nobody, thank you. I'm too old for that stuff."

"Leslie, these are my granddaughters." Emily touched one head, "Winslow," then the other, "Alison."

"They're beautiful." Hearing the unfamiliar tone of her own voice, Leslie was beginning to believe that southern charm was contagious.

"Thank heavens they took after their mother and not me," Emily said.

"But Gammy, you're pretty, too."

"Thank you, Winslow. Now would you do me a favor, please? Would you stay here till Miss Cricket gets your sister's face painted?"

"Uh-huh," answered Winslow.

"I'll be waiting at the table with Pop and your mother . . . see them over there. Looks like they're already eating breakfast."

Emily handed Cricket a ten dollar bill then turned toward Leslie. "Come on over with me. I'd like you to meet my husband and daughter."

Leslie followed, amazed that Dr. Klein had another life far removed from the cloistered therapy setting where, apparently by choice, she'd set herself up as a container for endless stories of unspeakable crimes.

The tall slender man and the attractive young woman who looked a lot like him stood up to greet them. Introductions were being made when an elderly man wearing khaki's, a gold knit shirt, and a baseball cap with "Winslow Manor" monogrammed on the front, stopped by. "Mornin' folks," he greeted.

Emily made another introduction. "Leslie, this is Henry Kiser. Henry, Leslie Roberts from New York City. She's been down here this week interviewing me, collecting material for a documentary she's putting together about mental health treatment."

"I could use some of that, Miss Emily." The man's laughter seemed to carry a German accent. "Well, not really. But I sure could've used some the first time I laid eyes on this place." He pointed to one of the old white clapboard barracks. "Over there. That was my home for a year."

"Mr. Kiser was a German POW housed here during World War II," Mr. Klein explained.

"To be honest," Henry said, "that was one of the best times of my life. Jefferson's grandparents—I worked for them in their timber business—were gracious people. As were all the townspeople I encountered."

"Really?" An idea for another documentary was developing in her mind. "I'd like to hear more about that sometime." Before she had time to say anything else, an elderly couple came over and sat down.

Emily introduced Sue and Dick Weaver.

"We were just talking about old times," Henry said.

"Mr. Weaver, were you also a POW?" Leslie asked.

"Not hardly. I was a Royal Air Force pilot sent over from England to train in 1941. The locals were very hospitable, often inviting us to Sunday dinners. We dated their daughters and after the war I came back to marry my favorite one . . . my bride here."

Mrs. Weaver blushed. "The Brits had something our boys were missing. Can't exactly say what it was . . . I'll never forget . . . he proposed to me over a two-dollar steak at Watt's Steakhouse."

"Yep. That restaurant's still functioning and so are we." The man winked at his wife. "Aren't we, Sweetheart?"

"Now Dick, let's not get too personal," Henry said. "Don't want to embarrass these young'uns."

"My food's getting cold," said Dr. Klein's husband. "Can I get anyone something to eat? Leslie, if you want to taste the local cuisine—"

Oh no, she thought, looking at his cholesterol-laden breakfast of thick homemade buttered biscuits, a big slab of salty-looking ham, a pile of scrambled eggs and grits—she assumed that's what the white gooey grains were—smothered with some kind of dark greasy broth.

"It won't kill you. It's just grits and what we call country ham and red-eye gravy." Mr. Klein must've been listening to her thoughts. "My grandmother ate something like this every morning of her life and she lived to be ninety-five."

"Thanks for the offer." Smelling a delicious cinnamon aroma coming from a nearby concession stand, Leslie thought about ordering one of those 5,000 calorie plate-sized apple fritters but refrained by saying, "I'm not really hungry. The motel provided a continental breakfast."

Emily broke into the conversation. "Well then Leslie, while everyone else is eating, would you like to walk around a little with me? We could check out the train car display."

"Fine with me," Leslie said. "But first I need to find a rest room."

———

The sophisticated New Yorker stood in the confined space of the Porta-Jon savoring the relaxing relief of the molecules of nicotine coursing through her veins. Oddly, she thought about the magnified picture of a bed mite she'd seen in a magazine on her flight from New York. With its saw-toothed claws attached to a big taut belly, it looked like a blood-sucking monster straight from hell. Interestingly, during her brief stay in Chestnut Ridge, she'd had trouble getting to sleep at night. Wonder if it was because she'd just learned that her mattress—any mattress—was home to a million mites waiting to munch on her dead skin? Or was it because of the things she'd learned this week from Emily Klein, Kate Stewart, and Maggie Rucker-Volz?

Leslie extinguished her cigarette in the open toilet and walked outside where a woman with long straight gray hair, wearing baggy jeans and a plaid flannel shirt, had come up to Emily. "Dr. Klein. Do you remember me?"

"Sure I do. You're Crystal's mother. I've really been worried about her. Have you heard anything?"

"Not a word. It's been over two months now and I'm beginning to fear the worst."

"I'm so sorry, Mrs. Griffin. If there's anything I can do to help, please let me know."

"Just pray for her. That's all I know to ask."

"I'll do that for sure," Emily said.

Since Emily hadn't acknowledged Leslie's presence or made any mention of the encounter as they walked toward the train cars, Leslie assumed that Mrs. Griffin's daughter had been a client.

Painted army green, the first car they came to was labeled in white letters on both sides:

United States Army
Medical Department
Hospital Unit Car

A Red Cross emblem guarded the sliding doors at the front.

At the base of the steps, a marker noted that the rail car had been used during War World II to transport injured servicemen to their homes across the United States.

"Do you smell coal smoke?" Emily asked.

"I wouldn't know what coal smoke smells like," Leslie answered, "but I don't smell anything unusual."

Leslie followed Emily as they carefully climbed three steep wide steps and entered the miniature hospital. A shower, bath, and two room-ettes for the staff were at the front of the car.

A tiny kitchen was next to a pharmacy. Thirty-six bunks, three tiers on each side, lined the outside walls. A long row of individual lights hung from the center of the ceiling. At the far end was a secured space, a cage actually—for the mental patients, she'd read.

"Night train . . . night train."

Leslie turned around to see the psychologist rubbing her hand across the cold metal operating table in the center of the car.

"What did you say, Emily?"

"Oh nothing. I was just talking to myself."

Chapter 39

All revved up!

Ever since stepping out of that hospital unit car on display at the fall festival, Emily had felt as if she were stuck on a treadmill going five miles per hour with no way to slow down or jump off. Ironically, she had awakened on Thanksgiving Day with the bottoms of her feet tingling with pain. Feeling compelled to write, she went downstairs to the rolltop desk and typed on her laptop.

> Chu-ca-lacka, chu-ca-lacka. Metal wheels over metal rails. The lonesome mourn of a train whistle coming close. You smell coal smoke.
>
> The train. It came to take you away. A nurse takes you inside and puts you on a table in the middle of the car. People all around. A doctor stands over you. Bright lights overhead. Somebody's sticking needles in your toes and the bottoms of your feet. It hurts. You scream. Shut up, he says. You kick. Hold still, he says. You spit on the nurse. Wet your pants.
>
> A mask comes toward your face. You sleep.
>
> Voices. The child will never make it. Not our type. Can't even talk plain. Not pretty enough.

The words ignited a vision:

A chubby little girl dressed up in a navy-blue double-breasted wool coat and a matching hat that ties around her neck is walking with her daddy across the cemetery toward a train car parked in the woods. A bunch of white letters that she can't read and a big red cross are painted on its side. Her daddy carries her up the wide metal steps and hands her over to a woman dressed like a nurse.

"Bye-bye Twisty Tail, I'll be back to get ya in the morning," her daddy is calling as he turns and walks away.

"I want Mommy," she whimpers as a nurse takes her over to the table in the middle of the car. Behind her the sliding doors clash closed.

When Jeff came downstairs at daybreak, she showed him the printout. "You remember what I told you about the Nazi doctors who came over after the war and got involved in the mind control business. Well, there's something I don't believe I've ever told you. As a little girl I used to lie in bed at night fantasizing that I was a brave and willing subject of torture. Now I'm beginning to believe that it wasn't a fantasy; that it really happened and I wasn't so brave after all. Apparently, I wasn't very good at dissociating and when they tested me by sticking the needles in my feet, I screamed and spit and they had to subdue me with drugs, probably ether or chloroform. Perhaps that's why I get cold chills . . . such a frightening, primitive stress response . . . every time I hear a train whistle."

Not giving her husband a chance to comment, Emily went outside and stood on the deck. She looked past the empty space where the mighty chestnut oak had once stood, contemplating the omnipresent morning mist simmering on the lake. Jeff came up behind her and she felt his arms reaching around her waist. "So I didn't pass the test" she said. "Thank God I failed. Things could've been a lot worse if they'd put me to work for Uncle Sam rather than just keeping me in civil service." Pulling away from his clutch, she turned around to face his eyes. "Laugh, Jeff. That's supposed to be a joke."

"It's really not funny, Em."

Glad he was serious, she finished what she wanted to say. "To tell you the truth, I feel so much better now that this piece of the puzzle is in place. But I *would* like to figure out where he put me on that train."

––––––––––––

"It's down here. I know it is." Emily was saying as they walked through the gate at the lower end of Mt. Hermon's cemetery late on Thanksgiving afternoon. After a decade on her spiritual journey, she'd learned to trust what her unconscious was saying, whether it spoke through words, images, sounds, or just pure gut-feeling. Maybe it was God who was egging on the unconscious. During a Communion Service a long time ago, she'd asked God what was happening in her life and God—he, she, or it—had seemingly answered. Surely it wasn't coincidence that Linda Lou Lackey had walked into her office that day.

"Well I'll be dammed," Jeff exclaimed when he saw the old rusty rail siding that was angling a couple hundred feet off the old track.

"You're right. It would've been a good place to park the car so it couldn't be seen. You can tell it hasn't been used in a long time. They must've closed it down when the tracks were rerouted around town."

Broken beer bottles and glass, rusty spikes, plates, and stabilizing bars were strewn all over the place. Poplar trees that were twenty to thirty feet high and cherry trees and cedars sprouted between and beside what was left of the tracks.

"Nature has reclaimed the evil's lair," Jeff said pensively, gratefully.

"I'm feeling dizzy. Drugged." Emily clutched her husband's arm, holding on with all her might. Again her feet felt as if they were being pricked with pins and needles.

"Okay, you've made your point," she shouted to her unconscious. Or perhaps it was God she was really addressing.

Chapter 40

W ired to a world without walls,

Emily sat in front of the monitor of her office computer waiting for the messages to download.

7 new message(s) . . .

From	Subject	Received	
Leslie Roberts	Documentary	12/30/1999	9:00 AM
Judge Rucker-Volz	MLK Day	12/30/1999	5:24 PM
Matthew Klein	Good News	12/30/1999	8:00 PM
Winslow Amato	Authors' Party	12/31/1999	7:30 AM
Carol Amato	New Website	12/31/1999	7:40 AM
S. Witherspoon	Cancellation	12/31/1999	7:53 AM
Jim Lentz	Happy New Year	12/31/1999	8:02 AM

She saved Leslie's to read last and opened Winslow's first.

****

Hi Gammy and Pop,
My class is having an authors' party on Wednesday at one o'clock. Can you come to hear me read from the book I made?
I love you.

Winslow
****

Mom, Dad

Just wanted to let you know the URL for our new website:
www.winslowhouse.com
Check it out!

Love ya,
Carol
****
Mornin' Mom, Mornin' Dad

At least I think it's morning. I've been on call for 36 hours and am too excited to think about sleeping. I got a call yesterday, I think it was yesterday, from the Human Resource Director at the hospital . . . I'm so tired now I can't think of its new name . . . Southeast Medical or is it Southwest . . .doesn't make sense, does it? What's it south of? Wish they could have kept the Campbell name in there somewhere. Anyway, they want me to come to work in July as an in-house cardiologist. I'm so excited and now I might even have time to date and get married and make myself a normal family.
Thanks for all your love and support
Give Winslow and Alison kisses for me.

Love, Matt
****
Dear Emily,

It was so nice to talk with you and the documentarian in October. I've talked it over with Wayne and have decided to tell Ms. Roberts that I will allow her to use my name if she wants to tell my story and describe the narrative I've drawn from my Book of Memories.
THE PUBLIC NEEDS TO KNOW!
Looking forward to seeing you in January when I come to speak at the MLK celebration.
Take care,

Maggie
****
Dr. Klein,

Please cancel my Tuesday appointment. I have to make a trip to Seattle but I should be back the following week.
Thanks! See you then.

Sandy

****

Hi Sis,

I finally learned how to do this E-mail stuff and remembered you'd given me your address last year when I called you on your birthday and decided to write. I'm in individual therapy now with a psychologist who was in Vietnam too and understands me and he has given me this new diagnosis called dissociative identity disorder and I hope it works this time because I guess an old man like me's not gonna have many more chances. I really am using Mama's money to help me find some peace. If I never did thank you for taking care of all that business and making sure I got my share of the estate, I'm thanking you now.

I never fit too good in the VA program. Not that it didn't help some people. It just didn't help me because I couldn't stand the groups they put me in. And nothing was really different in the hospital except I didn't get to drink. But all the legal dope they had me on made up for it. And another reason things are better is because I'm now in a stable relationship with a woman who was a nurse in Vietnam. I met her in one of those groups I hated. So I guess being there wasn't so bad after all. She has four grown children and a bunch of grandchildren so I'm getting to taste some of the pleasures of family life. I really do like playing grandpa. None of her children know about the money so I know they like me for who I am.

What I'm finally realizing is that my problems go back much further than Vietnam. To my childhood. I don't remember much about it except feeling resentful all the time. You know . . . or maybe you don't know, I was a mess before I left home. Come to think of it, I was probably already an alcoholic before I hit high school. Daddy sneaked around to get his liquor and I did too. As much as there was hidden around the house, he never missed it. And you may not know, I got picked up for drunken driving once just after I turned 14 and got my license, but Uncle Phil or Daddy, one of them took care of it, if you know what I mean. Can you believe that they used to let you get your license at 14 in S. C.?

Now that I'm totally sober because my girlfriend won't sleep with me if I'm drinking, I'm beginning to feel my feelings. Normal says my shrink. I think I've finally gotten over the anger at what my government had me do in Vietnam. I'm not alone in that and there are plenty others who are angry too. Now I mostly feel sad at the living I missed when I was drunk all the time.

Sadness that I've missed life. Sadness that neither Mama or Daddy saw me hurting as a child. There were some things that happened between them that I'm sure you're too little to remember. Things that happened in town too that I hope you never have to learn about. I'd like to see you and your family sometime before I die but I doubt that I'll ever set foot in Campbell County again.

I guess the real reason I'm writing is to let you know that I am truly sorry for the way I treated you when you were a little girl. I remember tying you up one time in the big magnolia tree in the front yard and leaving you there all afternoon and telling you not to tell and you didn't. I could've done anything and you never would have told. And there was the time Jeff was there when his grandmother had come over to play bridge and I hope you don't remember what me and Tommy Paxton and Dave Jr. did when we took y'all back to the car shed. I'm sorry about that too. I don't understand at all why it happened. And I'm really sorry about anything else I ever did to hurt you.

I trust you have some understanding now why I never came back home. I would've died living around our goody-goody mother and I would've been the world's biggest hypocrite to come home to mourn her death. Isn't it funny, she's helped me more as a dead person than when she was living?

I am so proud of my little sister, the doctor. And ashamed that I didn't turn out like you. Now that I've come to understand that I wasn't completely responsible for what went on in Vietnam, some of the nightmares are going away. It's weird but the flashbacks have taken on a different tone. The babies, the children I see bleeding and hear screaming don't have slanted eyes anymore.

Love, Jimmy

****

Dear Dr. Klein,

I want to thank you again for your good southern hospitality when I visited with you in October. It was nice talking with you and your friends Kate Stewart and Judge Volz, although I still shudder when I think about some of the things that we discussed. I now realize there is another side to this 'war of the memories' which somebody is not wanting the general public to understand. Unfortunately, my proposal which included examining both sides of the controversy was rejected by the investors. The Board of Directors will not consider seeking another source of funding to continue the project; therefore, I am faced with an ethical dilemma concerning whether or not I want my future to be with this company.

Please do not take this rejection personally. I believe that you and other therapists who deal with the aftereffects of organized evil on a daily basis will live to see the truth about this hidden holocaust exposed to the world.

All best,
Leslie Roberts

Chapter 41

"Have you got it all figured out?"

Jeff asked. He was fiddling with the fire that his son-in-law had built earlier in the evening. The grandparents were baby-sitting while Carol and Brad were out with friends bringing in the new millennium. The little girls had gone to bed at nine.

"Almost," Emily answered, "but I could use your help."

"Okay." Jeff set the poker down on the hearth and walked over to the card table where Emily was mulling over a thousand piece jigsaw puzzle, a high-difficulty level one that Brad had received as a Christmas present from Carol.

"There's a section here of dark ocean where the pieces all look alike. Very confusing," Emily said.

Jeff went to work. "This one goes here . . . this one goes there . . . this one—" In a matter of minutes it was completed.

They sat together on the sofa. Jeff clicked on the TV and started flipping through celebrations taking place all over the world. "Seventeen minutes till two thousand. I just thought of a good way to celebrate." He reached for her hand.

"But the kids might come down and walk in on us." As if her response were final, she picked up the afternoon paper from the coffee table. "Well whatta you know? Uncle Phil made the front page." Without asking Jeff if he wanted to hear it, she began to read aloud the article about Chestnut Ridge's most recent gala, an affair they'd deliberately forgotten to attend. It sounded more like an obituary:

At least a thousand people stopped by the Chamber of Commerce's reception at the Civic Center to pay respect to Chestnut Ridge's mayor emeritus, Philip Owens. He is well known throughout the region for his philanthropy, his involvement in church and civic activities, and his leadership in business and professional organizations. Instrumental in bringing investors together to establish the private Chestnut Ridge Military Academy on the grounds of the former flying school, he served as Chairman of the Board of Directors until it closed.

Later Mr. Owens led the drive to build a new Civic Center on those grounds. He has held various leadership positions in the local, state, and American bar associations, and is a member of the Board of Directors of Syn-Tec as well as the First Bank of Campbell and the Campbell Country Club. He is also a member of the Rotary Club, the Masons, the Scottish Rite Bodies, and the First Methodist Church, having served as lay leader for several years. His wife, the former Luella Keller, died in 1984. They had no children.

Emily put the article down and glowered at the fire. "Honey, I know you don't like to talk about this stuff anymore, but I'm beginning to believe that little runt was—and still may be—the man behind the scenes in all the organized child abuse activities in Chestnut Ridge."

"How in the world did you come up with that?"

"It just makes sense. Somehow when Phil came to town, I believe he may have managed to take the leadership position from the old-time generational powers-that-be—like possibly our grandfathers, if your little scenario about our legacy has any truth in it at all."

As if he were in for a long winter's night, Jeff went over and stoked the embers one more time. He sat down in his arm chair. "Why pray tell? And how did he break into such a close-knit society?"

"What I suspect is that he was working for the government in some sort of secret mission. Remember, during the war he was stationed at the flying school. He could've become friends with our daddies who told him about things going on in the underground and connected him with the other secret organizations in town: Satanic or Klan or both or neither . . . whatever was happening, it was evil. With his military connections, maybe Phil worked for the OSS . . . later the CIA or another agency, putting him in a position to deliver to them a pool of subjects— guinea pigs from transgenerational cult families—already trained to be obedient. After all, there was a ready-made laboratory at the school and he could've coordinated experiments conducted in the '50s and '60s. Lest we forget, your own daddy controlled access to those grounds for a long time and—"

Jeff interrupted, "And was tied to your father through his wife, Luella."

"Now you're playing, Jeff. This is a game isn't it?" She had not deliberately chosen to become a conspiracy theorist. "From the article, it looks like he had his hands in everything. I'm even beginning to believe there might be some connections to Syn-Tech. Crystal's father, Franklin Griffin, is still working out there as far as I know. Hope to God his love for filming little children—I'm almost positive that's what he was doing with his daughter—I hope it catches up with him some day. I've seen a few clients who've described a warehouse where they were taken to be filmed in pornographic movies. Could've been out there."

"Makes it look like there was a lot o' sinnin' out there at Syn-Tec," Jeff quipped.

Emily pulled her knees to her chest. "And don't forget, he was my mother's attorney and 'friend.' Whether it was for his personal gratification or for what he rationalized was for the good of the United States of America, Philip Owens had the resources for getting the job done: a group of citizens with unbridled dark sides, born and bred dissociators who apparently had no qualms about dedicating their children to evil; and plenty of secure places to conduct rituals and experiments, including cemeteries, church basements, the air school that had been made secure for the POW camp, and later the military academy with its stable of boys to gratify the needs of androgynous pedophiles. Maybe even Uncle Dave's funeral home. I've heard funeral homes come in pretty handy for some of their rituals."

"But Em, it's still hard for me to imagine a major conspiracy. We'll never know whether the local perps were working for the government or just having a good ol' time."

She placed the newspaper back on the coffee table and finished the rest of the conspiracy story in her mind.

Maggie had said that her mother worked for the Owens family and that they had lived in the servants' quarters after she was born. What if Phil had taken the two of them to live there so he could have ready access to the child to use for whatever purposes the community and government required?

Chapter 42

She had it all figured out except the hardest part: How was she going to tell Emily? Wearing a navy business suit, the Honorable Margaret Rucker-Volz had just finished her speech for Campbell County's Martin Luther King, Jr. celebration. As the clock on top of the courthouse struck twelve dignified chimes she looked upward, noting that the oyster-gray cloud which had been hovering directly over Chestnut Ridge had begun to float toward the coast, leaving behind a brilliantly bright sun and a clear turquoise sky.

A sign, she thought. Everything's gonna be okay. Rubbing her fingers over the Tuareg cross hanging on a gold chain around her neck, she glanced over the audience: a small crowd of Blacks, a smattering of Whites. Although it had been six years since she'd married and moved away, she recognized a lot of people: mostly distant relatives, church folks, and a few charter members of the Happy Holler Chorus. The majority of Whites, many of whom she didn't recognize, had probably come to the event because it was part of their job as civil servants. Philip Owens was sitting down front next to Chief Paxton. Throughout the speech Maggie had deliberately avoided making contact with either of those two pathetic hypocrites.

Where's Emily? she wondered as the president of the local NAACP was directing everyone to hold hands and join in singing the Negro National Anthem, "Lift Every Voice and Sing."

Near the end of the first verse, Maggie looked up to see Emily walking briskly down Main Street toward the assembled group.

"Sorry I didn't make it in time to hear your speech but the phone rang as I was going out the door and you won't believe who it was." Seated on stools at a tall round table for two in the back corner of Main Street's newest coffee shop tritely named, "On Common Grounds," Maggie and Emily were waiting for their *quiche de jour* to heat up in the microwave. "It was that documentarian, Leslie Roberts."

"Really? I was just going to ask you how to get in touch with her since I've decided that I am ready to go public with my story. A libel attorney told me that as long as I don't mention the names of alleged perpetrators who're still living, it's well within my first amendment rights to discuss what I believe happened to me. If Ms. Roberts wants more survivors to interview, several of my Internet friends who also remember having been used in Cold War experiments have agreed to go on camera, too. We're even thinking about getting together some sort of class action suit like the radiation victims did. Somebody in our government needs to take responsibility for atrocities that were committed in the name of National Security and if we don't get any results there, we're planning to take our case to the United Nations and—"

"Wow!" Emily broke in. "Before you go on, I should tell you what Leslie said. A couple of weeks ago she E-mailed that the investors had rejected her proposal. Today she attempted to explain—"

"So it's over, Dr. Klein. Don't you worry about that. Somebody else will do it sometime. The story *will* get out and I believe it will happen soon. That Roberts woman and the backers who tried to patsy her may not know it, but there's a groundswell of rage from hundreds, maybe thousands of us survivors that's growing up like a giant mushroom. One day it's going to explode and the world will have to take notice. We're looking at all sorts of tactics: civil suits against the junk scientists who testify in court that there's no such thing as repressed memory; suits against junk doctors who've diagnosed their patients or somebody else's patients with false memory syndrome and prevented them from getting the help they need; suits against the insurance companies who aren't granting coverage for appropriate treatment—"

"Whoa, Your Honor! I didn't know you'd become such an activist, but be assured that you have my utmost respect and support. There are therapists from across the country, around the world even, who are meeting underground for mutual support, trying to come up with ways to expose past atrocities and stop any that might still be going on."

"That's good to hear. Just as Blacks and Whites finally came together to help solve the civil-rights problems, perhaps therapists and survivors will one day be able to sit down and reason together about ways to combat ritualistic crimes against children. As I quoted from Martin this morning, 'We cannot walk alone.'"

Their number was called.

"I'll get it," Maggie said. Emily watched as this woman, who'd once been bound to a wheelchair and to the shackles of unresolved trauma, gingerly hopped down from the stool. She walked over to the counter, picked up their lunch, and brought it back to the table.

Slowly, as if weighing every word carefully, Maggie said, "I'm not sure where to start but there's another matter I wanted to talk with you about. It has to do with something my aunt told me a long time ago and when I saw Philip Owens sitting in in front of me this morning—"

"Excuse me Maggie. Before you go on, I need to go wash my hands." What Emily really needed to do was get by herself and decide whether or not to tell the woman what she'd figured out on New Year's Eve about her Uncle Phil.

Emily came back to the table and perched on the stool.

"To make a long story short," Maggie said, "the reason I quit therapy when I did was because I'd just learned who my daddy was—"

"And you knew he was my uncle," Emily impulsively interrupted. Maggie had a puzzled look on her face. "No-o. It *wasn't* Phil Owens."

Now Emily had the puzzled look. "Then who was it?"

Their eyes met head on, as though coming from opposite directions they'd slammed into each other right in the middle of a one-lane bridge.

Maggie spoke first. "He was . . . he was your daddy, too."

"Oh . . . my . . . God!"

"Honest, Emily. Until just now, I never knew how to tell you." Maggie reached across the table and placed her hands on top of Emily's.

Emily stared at the hands.

Her sister's hands.

Chapter 43

Perhaps if he had never spoken to the local ministerial association, they would have left her alone.

Asked to speak on a topic of his own choosing—and because he was beginning to look at historical figures as Emily looked at clients: to analyze them; sympathize with them; identify with them; to recognize the positive outcomes of their experiences—he'd decided to speak about a Protestant reformer. The presentation was titled: "The Dark Side: What You Didn't Learn in Seminary about Martin Luther."

At their first meeting of the new year, Jeff began his speech: "Today I will talk about the influence of evil on one person: Martin Luther. The man from Germany has been called many things: a leader, a heretic, a savior, and a crude hypocrite who spread racial injustices with his anti-Semitic views. Regardless of your perspective of the ideological and religious convictions of this religious icon, one thing stands out: evil was a concrete part of his reality. His opponents called his mother a whore and charged that he was a product of his mother's intercourse with the Devil. In their minds he was a child of Satan."

Looking around the long table in the private dining room of Watt's Steak House, Jeff tried to gauge the audience's reaction to his opening. He recognized everyone in the all-white audience of about a dozen Protestant preachers except the man with a military haircut wearing a dark suit and white clerical collar who, like a few of the others, had pushed his chair comfortably away from the table.

And who might you be? Jeff wondered, as he gathered his thoughts.

"Luther's early childhood religion was a collection of paganism's remnants blended with the Christian mythology of an unlearned peasantry. For these people, everything was inhabited by mythical beings such as elves, gnomes, sprites, fairies, or witches. The worst of these evil spirits were evidenced in floods, diseases, and storms, especially electrical storms. They believed demons afflicted people with sadness and depression because of their sins. It is well known that Hanna, Luther's mother, believed in evil spirits and passed this belief on to Martin.

"Bainton, in his biography of Luther, *Here I Stand*, wrote: 'Luther himself was never emancipated from such beliefs. Many regions are inhabited, said he, by devils. Prussia is full of them and Lapland of witches. In my native country on the top of a high mountain called the Pbelsberg is a lake into which if a stone be thrown a tempest will arise over the whole region because the waters are the abode of captive demons.'"

"If a stone be thrown," the stranger, nervously tapping his toes on the floor, broke in, "there have always been consequences for rocking the boat in one's community."

Nodding in agreement, Jeff went on. "As a young adult, Luther exhibited odd behaviors. In one episode which happened after he'd become upset reading an account of a man possessed by a dumb spirit, he fell to the floor in the choir loft of the monastery, raving and roaring with the voice of a bull, 'It is not me!' In his later writings, he referred to this as a 'fit in the choir.'

"In today's psychological terms, he might well have been labeled mentally ill. Even in those days, the chroniclers clearly considered young Luther to be possessed by demons; however, his 'fit in the choir' could've been what psychologists today call a dissociative episode with symptoms that included a partial loss of consciousness, loss of motor coordination, and automatic exclamations which he didn't know he'd uttered. It's my belief that Luther may have been a man with multiple personalities."

"How can you say a man who lived 500 years ago had different personalities?" Again it was the stranger. "I thought you were a history professor, not a shrink. Aren't you talking out of your field?"

"Maybe I should explain," Jeff digressed. "As some of you know, my wife is a clinical psychologist. Over the years she's worked with several horribly abused clients who somehow protectively constructed in their minds different personalities to some way portion out the trauma. Some of these people allege they have been tormented in ceremonies that appear to have been related to the worship of Satan."

"In this community?"

"Possibly." Getting tired of this man butting in, Jeff tried to stay calm.

"Satanic ritual abuse is a hot topic in some of the counseling workshops I've attended." A female Methodist minister had come to his defense. "Men and women from across the country . . . and the world are telling similar stories."

"What kinds of stories?"

"Stories about babies being sacrificed, 'marriages' to Satan—"

"That's incredible," said a Presbyterian minister.

"Why so?" The questioner was Jeff's own Lutheran minister. "History is full of accounts of ritual sacrifice." Pastor John picked up a Bible he'd brought along and read from Psalm 106: "'Yea, they sacrificed their sons and their daughters unto devils. And shed innocent blood, even the blood of their sons and of their daughters—'"

"Who did?—Surely not the children of God!" someone asked sarcastically.

"Oh yes they did," answered a minister from the Pentecostal Holiness Church. "Contrary to what their prophets taught, after making it to the promised land, the Hebrews intermarried with the heathen. They didn't forsake Yahweh but to be accepted they practiced the religion of their in-laws. It wasn't unusual for pagan cults to sacrifice children to the gods."

"Therefore they were able to rationalize that their god would appreciate the offerings of little children," said Pastor John. Several ministers nodded in agreement. "There're other accounts of child sacrifice in the Old Testament. For example, God asked Abraham to take his son, Isaac, to the top of a mountain in Moriah and present him as a burnt offering."

"Read without any context, that could've been a model for future Satanists who were required to murder children as a test of obedience," the Methodist minister added. "As it's written, God didn't intend for Abraham to murder Isaac. He was only testing his faith. When Abraham pulled out his knife to slay his son, God called it off . . . still I wonder how anyone who worships a good God could even think about murdering babies."

Clearing his throat, Jeff took back his platform. "I'm not saying that Luther personally knew anything about child sacrifices, but we know for sure that he was physically mistreated as a child. Once, his mother beat the blood out of him for stealing a nut. And from Luther's own words, 'My father once whipped me so hard that I ran away from him;

I was so upset till he was able to overcome the distance. I would not want to hit my Hans so hard, otherwise he would become timorous and estranged from me; I cannot imagine a grief worse than that.'

"Early childhood trauma is often associated with the development of multiple personality disorder which is now called dissociative identity disorder. There is no way to know for sure if Luther had been subjected to even more severe abuse such as satanic ritual trauma, but he definitely exhibited behaviors and symptoms similar to those who have reported phenomena such as having been brought up in two distinctly different worlds."

The man in the clerical collar had stopped tapping his feet and was looking at the floor.

Jeff realized the need to give his rationale for making what he knew had likely been received as a controversial statement: "First, Martin Luther was a man of conflictions. Afraid of both God and Devil. Some of his adversaries accused him of being possessed. He loved his God, but never enough. He hated the Devil, yet seemed to look for him everywhere.

"Secondly, he held contradictory beliefs in Christianity and witchcraft.

"As a third point, he was depressed. Some scholars have written that the Reformation was Luther's reaction to a father who tyrannized him—a manner of protest against all fathers whether they were called Papa, Your Holiness, the Pope . . . or God.

"Fourth, he suffered panic attacks—in one instance at least—triggered by satanic symbols. For example, upon looking at a woodcut titled, "Christ the Judge Sitting Upon the Rainbow," he became terrified over its images of horned demons dragging naked women into hell . . . of fire and smoke issuing from the ground . . . and a sword in Christ's ear.

"And fifth, but not least, there were reported encounters with, or hallucinations of, Satan. Luther fought his personal demons, real or imagined, from his early years until his death. Only two days before he died, he had spoken of seeing the Devil outside his window sitting on a drainpipe exposing his rear end."

"So the Devil mooned him!" someone called out.

Over the laughter, Jeff managed to ask, "Are there any questions?"

"Let me make sure I have this clear. Are you saying that Martin Luther, founder of the Protestant faith, was mentally ill?" The stranger wearing a 'halo' around his neck sounded hostile. "And are you saying that he was persecuted by Satanists?"

"Actually, I don't believe I said either. Luther was called demon-possessed in those days and would likely have been called dissociative today."

The Presbyterian minister raised his hand. "You said something about childhood abuse causing his problems—"

"Of course we have no way of knowing that for sure. We do know that he spent his life battling his dark side but, quite apparently, using his dissociative abilities adaptively—he taught, he wrote, he preached, he composed music . . . and he challenged the authority figures of his day." Well, I said it, Jeff thought, waiting for the expected backlash.

"And it got him in trouble. He was condemned by the Pope as a heretic for criticizing the Roman Catholic Church," said the stranger who by now was becoming a familiar voice.

"Yes he was," Jeff agreed, "but he hadn't wanted any of that controversy. To look on the positive side, he showed by his actions how a person can overcome the past, change himself, and even change the world."

"Amen . . . Amen . . . Amen," came the reaction from around the room.

"In conclusion, Luther had come out of the Dark Ages a reluctant hero, not even dreaming about a new church. But in 1521, after he'd been condemned by the Pope as a heretic—as the gentleman to my right has noted—he stood in the Bishops' Palace at Worms before the Holy Roman Emperor Charles V and strongly defended his criticisms of the Roman Catholic Church. When required to disclaim all he had said and written, he declared boldly, 'I cannot and will not retract anything, for it is neither safe nor right to act against one's conscience. Here I stand.'" Jeff paused, looking around the table in a moment of silence, then completed Luther's words in a clear firm voice: "'I cannot do otherwise.' Thus, when Martin Luther stood before his accusers to defend his faith and was ordered to recant and did not . . . some people say that was the dawning of the modern age."

Glancing at his watch, the speaker said, "I see that it's time for me to sit down. Thank you for your attention. If you have any further questions, I'll be glad to answer them after the meeting is adjourned."

As everyone was leaving, a few ministers came up to comment on the presentation. The stranger introduced himself: "I'm Cyrus Fisher.

"Nice to meet you." Jeff held out his hand.

The Reverend responded with a firm grasp. "My pleasure. In case you were thinking I was Catholic," he pointed to his collar, "I'm Episcopalian. Retired from the Air Force chaplaincy last year and I recently moved here to be with my daughter. If you really want to know my opinion, I believe that all those reports of satanic cults in this day and time are just somebody's imagination. Christians have always used the Devil to scare little children . . . don't you know that?"

"So how did it go? How did the clergy community accept your attack on their demagogue—or is it demigod?" Emily, standing at the kitchen counter pealing potatoes, asked as Jeff walked through the back door.

"Both. Neither. Depends on whose judging the man. Can't say I'd call it an attack. You should've been there. We even got into Satanism and child sacrifice. And I told them a little about your work in that area."

"That's not something I want the world to know. So why did you talk to—"

"It just came up, that's all. Most of them accepted it matter-of-factly, except there was this new guy there—an ex-military chaplain, the only one wearing a clerical collar—who was rather adamant about the non-existence of satanic cults."

"That must've been Cyrus Fisher," Emily blurted.

"How did you know?" Jeff looked surprised.

Thinking fast to avoid violating the confidentiality of one of her long-term clients, Emily answered, "Oh, I remember seeing a story about him in the paper when he first moved to town."

Chapter 44

Embarrassed for her family, her clients, her colleagues, and herself, Emily struggled not to see the sad-eyed child, dressed in a frilly pink dress, stomping her white-patent Mary Janes on the pavement doing what the grownups directed.

"Voodoo doc . . . voodoo doc," chanted a green-haired teenaged boy flaunting a pierced tongue decorated with rhinestones sparkling in the hot summer sun.

A man wearing shorts and a tank top stalked the therapist with a video recorder.

Suddenly Emily felt naked. Ashamed. Fat. Saturated by that weirdly erotic feeling, so out of place, that routinely hit when she felt threatened. Even though she now thought it might have come from some of those early experimental experiences on the train from hell, it was still a physiological reaction over which she had no control.

"Get off this property." She shoved the photographer down the steps. With camera running, he backed onto the sidewalk.

Unlocking the clinic door, she shrieked, "Y'all go away," as if trying to scare off a pack of wild dogs. No one listened.

Once inside, she called the police department and asked to speak to the chief. "Tom. This is Emily Klein.

"Well, do tell dahlin. It's been forever since I've heard from ya. How can I help ya?"

"I want you to send me somebody down here quick. Picketers are all over the place. They've got a camera and I don't want them filming my clients as they come and go."

"Perfectly within their rights as long as they stay on the sidewalk. It's public property, you know," he drawled in a taunting voice that gave her the creeps.

"But what if they bomb me or something? Like the anti-abortionists."

"Oh, dahlin. You always over react. Why would anyone want to hurt you?"

"Forget it." Trying not to visualize his sickening smirk, Emily hung up the phone, knowing that surely he'd be delighted if she weren't around to remind him of things he'd probably rather forget.

Beyond the protestors, two men were watching from a black Mercedes. An adolescent with baggy pants hanging off his buttocks walked up to the driver's side and talked for a few minutes. After reaching into the window and picking up a small package, the boy turned and trotted toward the building, not stopping until he got about three feet from the porch. Drawing his right arm over his head—

A missile sailed through the glass, thudding onto the darkly-aged hardwood floor. Frantically, Emily stooped down and culled through the rubble. She picked up a package shaped like a large potato wrapped in brown paper. Quick as a camera clicks, she read the note written in bold block-printed red ink, glancing up just in time to see the courier hustle across the street and fade through the open gates of the cemetery.

No. No. Not the girls.

Knowing Jeff would be in class, she called him anyway. His secretary answered.

"This is not an emergency," Emily lied. "But would you please tell my husband to come over to my office as soon as possible?"

"Certainly . . . oh, here he comes now."

"Hello Hon. What's up?"

"They're here, Jeff."

"Who's here?"

"Must be a dozen or more . . . I don't know who they are . . . some of them look like recruits from Acadia . . . calling me all sorts of names. And one of them just threw a rock . . . this place is a mess . . . with a note . . . some guy is taking pictures . . . and a little girl . . . . they're using a little girl—"

"Have you called the police?"

"Yes, for all the good it did. Tom said they weren't doing anything illegal."

"But they broke the window, didn't they?"

"That was after I called. And the little devil who did it ran off. Tom won't do anything. Why call again?"

"What did the note say? . . . forget it . . . I'll read it later. I'm leaving now."

"You don't have to come but if you want to that's okay." Emily put the receiver on the rotary phone—still, after twenty-one years, a functional conversation piece—and walked over to the window. Like a mannequin waiting for a caretaker, she peered out through the shattered glass. Listening to the sound of their obscenities. Wishing she were somewhere else. Anywhere else.

"I hate him! I hate them!" She screamed as Jeff came through the back door.

"Me too." He looked around at the debris. "Somebody's just trying to scare you."

"But why?" She handed him the note.

"IF YOU TELL, THE LITTLE GIRL DIES," Jeff read aloud. He crushed the ultimatum in his left fist and dropped it on the floor. Clasping his arms around his wife, he embraced her terror saying, "Jesus Christ! Somebody means business this time."

"Oh, Jeff. No way would I ever do anything to hurt either of our precious granddaughters. Perhaps I should just lock my doors and go home . . . forever."

"Settle down, Em." Like a sympathetic father soothing a fretful child, he patted her back. "We don't know for certain they're referring to Winslow or Alison." Releasing his clutch and stepping back from his wife, he pointed out the window. "Could even be that child on exhibit out there."

"They'd better not hurt her either, whoever she is." Emily put her hands over her face. "I'm really scared. I'd so wanted to be past that hysterical and paranoid stage therapists go through when they first realize the criminals in their clients' nightmares are living breathing citizens of the daytime world."

He came closer, bending slightly, offering his chest as a drain for the rare tears beginning to trickle down her cheeks like water from a leaky faucet.

"It makes me so mad, Jeff. The accused perps or their accomplices are harassing therapists all across the country, filing malpractice suits, trying to scare us into silence."

"It'll never work. Not if everyone is as dedicated as you." He pulled a handkerchief from his back pocket and wiped away her last tear.

She stooped to pick up a piece of glass.

"Don't do that, Em. You'll cut yourself. Let me call somebody to come over and board up this window till we get it replaced."

"It can't be replaced. It's a hundred years old."

"Well then, we'll just have to do the best we can."

Jeff made the call. Then picking up the smooth river rock and rolling it around in his hands, he said, "If a stone be thrown a tempest will arise over the whole region because the waters are the abode of captive demons."

"What in the world are you talking about?"

"Oh, it's just a quote from Martin Luther." Winding his arm like a fast-pitch softball player, Jeff hurled the present-day stone through the jagged pieces of original glass hanging precariously on the window sash, not seeming to care if it hit any of the protestors or not. "Do you want me to hang around?"

"That won't be necessary, but thanks for coming. As soon as I get in touch with all my clients and cancel their appointments for today—they don't need this kind of trauma—I'll wait till your window man gets here, then go on home."

They hugged again and he left through the front door.

Emily carefully stepped across the glass. Stationing herself at the window, she watched the love of her life silently walk past the teenager with green hair and the little girl in the frilly pink dress wearing white Mary Janes who was proudly carrying a sign that she was too young to read:

WITCH DOCTOR KLEIN DESTROYS FAMILIES

Chapter 45

"**I** want to keep myself from betraying myself," Sandy Witherspoon said, soon after her father had moved in with her. "I've learned a lot during therapy, made a lot of changes in my life, but unless I can get physically away from him I will never heal. Wouldn't be surprised if he's the one who set up the picketers."

Emily believed that her client might be correct. But she also suspected that Cleat was at least partly responsible, although she wasn't sure if he had enough brain cells left to instigate something like that.

"Where do you plan to go?"

"A couple of friends from college have asked me to move to Seattle. I might start there . . . regretfully find another therapist . . . I don't want to leave you but I have to get on with my life."

"What does your father say about that?"

"He's furious. Tells me I'm crazy and he wants to talk with you. Has for quite a while, but I don't want him in this room; don't want him to spoil my safe place. He thinks you put memories in my head so you could keep treating me and get some of the money I inherited from my mother's mother. . . some of the money he thinks he deserves."

"He came to Chestnut Ridge to live because you were here. What if he follows you out there?"

"I don't plan to tell him where I am; may even try to change my name."

"So he knows you're remembering things?"

"Yes. I've given him details of what, when, and where, but he denies any of it ever happened."

"Do you think he's still able to bring out personalities without your knowledge?"

"It's possible . . . he or somebody else can. There are times when I answer the phone, several minutes pass, and I forget talking with anyone. Thank God, it's been a long time, a few years since I've found myself somewhere not knowing how I got there. What I was wondering is, could you help me get deprogrammed all the way so those bastards can't ever mess with me anymore?"

"I'll try to help in any way possible, although I prefer the term relearning rather than deprogramming. Learning is based on classical and operant conditioning. If behaviors are not reinforced, they will extinguish. If we can figure out what they did to train you and you don't put yourself in a position for access by any of your perpetrators, it's possible you could reach your goal."

Sandy switched to an alter who called itself Cyberna. "I understand the programs. And I'll help you do it. Sandy needs to find some peace in her life, some continuity."

Feeling herself getting overwhelmed with the request, Emily remembered her philosophy of therapy: let the client lead the way.

From late July to early December, Sandy had come to therapy twice a week, sometimes for extended sessions. Like Nora who had committed suicide, Sandy appeared to have two distinct sets of alters: those she had created spontaneously to survive the horrendous things done by her father and his friends, and those who were structured and conditioned by the military experimenters to serve specific functions. In Sandy's case, in addition to the pornography which must've helped to keep the coffers of the organization (whatever it was) replenished, her ultimate purpose had apparently been to blackmail men in high places by getting them in compromising positions.

Steps were laid out to erase the artificial personalities. Self-parts created by Sandy's own mind were not to be affected. The procedure went like this: Emily helped Sandy go into a deep trance, a state similar to the one she had likely been in during various experiments. Next, the therapist followed the commands Cyberna had written, using numbers and letters in code form that meant nothing to Emily but apparently had meaning to Sandy's internal personality system.

When the 'deprogramming' which took hours and hours was supposedly complete, Sandy was hopeful she could no longer be contacted by her handlers without her conscious knowledge—but she wasn't sure.

Emily had two main questions for Cyberna: "How did you know what to do? Where did you get your knowledge of programming techniques?"

"I listened when the men—and women—discussed what worked, how it worked, and what problems they faced." Cyberna's speech sounded like a telephone computer voice. "It took them years to get the right configuration for Sandy, the white rat for their experiments. At various times they used drugs, hypnosis, electroshock, sleep deprivation, and starvation to get her in a state of low resistance to their commands. They developed alters to be used as sexual toys. Now that she knows what they did to her, she can resist their cue, their control. And maybe her physical self will get healthier. I'm sure they used radiation on her for whatever reason. That's why I believe her bones are so brittle; why's she's always getting sick in ways her doctors can't explain. They used to give her lots of drugs and shots. From what I can tell, she . . . we . . . I—"

The shift in pronouns suggested that Sandy was talking for herself; that she was becoming more and more co-conscious with the artificially-created personalities.

"Dr. Klein, I believe they may have used me in some biological experiments which could explain my chronically high blood count . . . that or . . . and this is the hardest thing—the most shameful thing—I've ever had to talk with you about. When I recently had some blood work done, it came back positive for some kind of canine virus. The doctor asked if I had any idea where I picked that up and I broke down and told her about the child pornography . . . about the bestiality."

"How did your doctor react?"

"Wonderful. She believed me. At least acted like she did."

In subsequent sessions, the programming began to break down even more and Sandy remembered other details about her past. She recalled being initiated when she was thirteen into a cult that used satanic trappings in its rituals. She was ordered to come back to that same group at thirty. That would've been almost nine years earlier in 1991, the year she had discovered her prostitute part and had first come to therapy.

In her images were nationally and internationally known figures. Even a movie star or two. Most embarrassing, even more than her adult memories, were her memories of having been used in child prostitution and pornography. "They put me in bed and photographed me with several pillars of the country—I wonder how many of those s.o.b.'s have made decisions throughout their lives based on those old pictures of black-mailable positions; I wonder how many humongous contributions have been made to political campaigns and university endowments to keep the sleaziness away from the media or some VIP's wife.

"I remember a nurse standing over me one time saying, 'At some point in your life, you will have a deep depression.' In another, I was given a shot that paralyzed me. Once after they'd attached electrodes to my head, I heard one of the doctors say, 'We're trying to locate the fear zone.' They were always giving me shots and pills. And I remember one time being left in a tank with a dolphin.

"A lot of the places they took me seemed high-tech before their time, reminding me of the set in the old Star Trek shows or a place that looked like NASA's Mission Control Center. There was a huge console with dials. I've had the sensation of being sucked through a metal tube and wonder if it was some kind of gravity experiment . . . they called it the acceleration chamber. It was so painful—being slung around in that thing; slapping my brain against my skull causing terrible headaches. And there were lots of times when I was strapped to a gurney in a stainless steel lab with people in surgical garb and masks standing around me."

No longer hiding under the guise of Cyberna, in her later writings Sandy used computer jargon: access codes, systems, exit, entry, programs, input, output, erase, sequences, loops. She remembered having heard words, letters, numbers, rhymes, and sometimes classical music played over speakers in a room where she had been isolated for long periods.

As TV had made the Cruise missiles an entertainment, Sandy's father, a man-of-the-cloth, had made his daughter an object of his pleasure. And as viewers had learned to dissociate from the Gulf War by literally switching channels when it became too horrid, Sandy had turned off her memories of being treacherously traumatized and exploited by her father and his friends, and other men and women who, she now believed without a doubt, were doctors working for the U.S. Government.

At her final session, Sandy expressed gratitude to her therapist. "Thanks for letting me be crazy in your office. For listening. But I have to move on."

"Keep in touch," Emily said.

"I will, Dr. Klein. But I want you to know that as long as my daddy is living here, it'll take an act of God to get me back to South Carolina."

Chapter 46

S o humiliating.

Head in the toilet bowl. Emily raised her head slowly, stood up, leaned against the bathroom vanity to catch her breath, and flushed the debris. Brushing the sour taste from her mouth, she turned away from the aging face in the mirror wondering why, even after understanding the dynamics, she couldn't prevent her perennial holiday nausea.

Nine days till Christmas.

This year, she'd hoped it would be different. Especially tonight with the kids around to "trim childhood's tree at the ol' homeplace," as Carol and Matt now wryly referred to their parents' annual family gathering. At this very minute, Winslow and Alison and their doting grandfather were probably tramping through a cold wet pasture looking for the perfect cedar tree to drag home. Emily was expected by everyone to be a put-together, able-to-handle-anything wife and mom, and a picture-book grandmother as well.

A bell in the evergreen wreath on the front door jingled. "Anybody home?" a voice called out tentatively,

Emily splashed water on her face, patted it dry, and walked out to greet the Saturday intruder who was dripping wet snow all over the waiting room floor. "Hi there, Jeannie."

"Mornin', Doctor Klein." The woman glanced down at her boots. "Sorry about that . . . I have a certified letter for ya."

"Well there's the proof," Emily said, looking at the floor to hide her own uneasiness, "so I guess I can tell it for the truth: neither rain nor wind nor sleet nor snow —"

Setting her bulging leather bag on the floor, the mail carrier grinned. "Had an aunt used to say days like this were 'cold enough to freeze the words coming outta your mouth, so don't open it'—your mouth, that is." Chuckling at her own story, Jeannie handed Emily the clipboard and pen. "Gonna cramp a lotta parties if this keeps up." And then, as if it were all somehow part of one seamless thought she was having, "Dead now, God rest her soul . . . but she was a funny one, my Aunt Maudie."

"I always hate this . . . signing for letters. Makes me wonder what I've done wrong," Emily said, and wished immediately she hadn't. Quickly she scribbled a signature and handed the clipboard back to Jeannie.

"Don't worry about it. Lots of things are certified nowadays. Probably a fancy invitation or something. Well, gotta run now." The young woman threw the mailbag over her shoulder. "Hope you and yours have a good holiday."

"You too." Emily was moving politely toward the door with the young woman as though she were a guest. "Drive carefully now. It's gonna get worse."

The psychologist walked a few feet across the room toward her office, stopped, turned the envelope over and studied it for a moment. Maybe you just forgot to pay your dues, she told herself.

Fighting a fresh wave of nausea, she ripped it open, shook it. Two pages fell into her hand. Her eyes raced over the first sheet. Ignoring the salutation and opening lines, she quickly reached the phrase:

> Be it known that if the allegations in the enclosed letter are found to be true, you will be guilty of—

Without finishing the first page, she went to the second. It was the copy of a letter obviously typed on an antique typewriter that hadn't been cleaned in a long time.

Hands trembling, Emily shuffled back to the first page:

> —practicing psychology in such a manner as to endanger the welfare of clients. You will be subject to disciplinary action by the Board, including revocation of your license to practice psychology in this state. Assuming that you will exercise your right for a hearing to defend yourself against these charges, we have scheduled a time for you to meet with the Board at 9:00 AM on April 13, 2001.

She scanned the letter from the complainant. Two words popped out from the page like objects in a 3-D movie.

morally incompetent

The phrase launched a frenzy. For a person who'd spent her life trying to abide by the Christian principles laid down at her mother's knee, no accusation could've cut deeper. She paced through the building—from the therapy room to the biofeedback lab and back to the waiting room—envisioning a lifetime dissolving in chaos while everyone watched.

And a career.

Stopping at the front window, Emily looked toward Olde Towne Cemetery, whispering a scream into the foggy windowpane: "Don't cry yet. Don't be afraid. Not now. Not ever again. You can cry when it's over."

She collapsed on the sofa behind her. "Why me?" she begged the God of her childhood. "I only wanted to help people. I certainly didn't ask for this bungee ride . . . up and down . . . titillated and terrified . . . never knowing when the cord might snap."

She picked up the phone from the end table and called home.

Jeff answered.

"Y'all find a tree yet?" Her voice was quivering.

"What's wrong, Em?"

She couldn't fool her husband.

"I just got an awful letter . . . from the Psychology Board. Oh, Honey, my worst nightmare has come true."

"What did it say? Wait a second, let me close the door . . . Matt just got here and he and Carol are already out there picking through the ornaments arguing like they used to about which one goes where. Part of the tradition I suppose."

Emily swallowed hard and began to read:

> I lost my daughter, Sandra Witherspoon, to the recovered memory movement. During her therapy with Dr. Emily Klein, she came to erroneously believe that she was abused in childhood by me and a group of my friends. Some of the things she claimed to recall would have had to happen before she was three years old.
>
> As a retired military chaplain, it is outrageous for anyone to think I was capable of molesting my own daughter. The doctor should have contacted me to determine if the allegations were true. I consulted a

psychiatrist who diagnosed her with false memory syndrome (FMS), a condition created by therapists. Dr. Klein also made my daughter believe she has dissociative identity disorder (DID) formally called multiple personality disorder (MPD) which I understand is a controversial diagnosis and that many psychiatrists do not believe in its existence.

By now Emily was having difficulty catching her breath.

I contend that this psychologist, using hypnosis, willfully and maliciously implanted false memories of abuse into my daughters mind, including the preposterous claims that I allowed her to be used in bizarre satanic rituals, as well as child pornography and prostitution and government-sponsored mind control experiments. My daughter's fabricated accusations and her ultimate reaction to them have caused me severe mental and emotional stress. I request that you discipline Dr. Klein, in the harshest possible terms, for her act of malpractice. In my opinion, she is morally incompetent to practice psychology.
Rev. Lt. Col. Cyrus Fisher (Ret.)

The letter was dated December 5, 2000, the day Sandy had closed out therapy in preparation for her move to Seattle.

"What in God's name is that all about?" Emily could've sworn she felt heat coming off the earpiece. "Some holier-than-thou Bible thumper accusing you of putting memories in his daughter's head? How absurd! Sounds like a smoke screen to cover his own inadequacies as a father. Contrary to more popular belief, in my opinion, preachers often make lousy parents. Too involved in others' problems—too little time to go around—and worst of all, too often beginning to believe what their cheerleaders tell them."

"Jeff, this is not about preachers."

"Why that egocentric Episcopalian asshole! No wonder he was so critical of my Luther speech. Wouldn't even know how it is to live in the real world. Em, you've done more to help people than he has even thought of helping. Malpractice? Bullshit!"

"But what if I *did* put memories in her head? Made her—"

"If they get your license it won't be the end of the world. You could retire."

"Don't say that. Sometimes I wonder if you ever really wanted me to get a career."

"Now you *are* getting crazy. Don't do this to me again. Come on home. We can talk about it later. Everybody's waiting for you."

In the background, she heard little Alison: "Me talk. Me talk."

"Not now. Gammy'll be home after while," Jeff said, calming down a little.

"Let me speak with her." Emily said, easily drifting over to the other role.

"Hey, whacha doin' Gammy?"

"Working. I've got a few more things to do but I promise I'll be home soon. Did you find a tree?"

"Yep. Guess what?"

"What?"

"Pop's gonna hold me up and wet me put a big angel on the tippy top."

"That's wonderful. Wait for me so I can help too. Bye now."

"Bye-bye. I wuv you."

Buoyed by her husband's indignation, Emily put the phone down, stood up, and as if the summons were merely a senseless piece of junk mail, carried it back to her office and tossed it on top of her already cluttered desk.

In a deliberate, determined, controlled manner, she grabbed her ski jacket, purse, and car keys and marched through the front door, locking it behind her.

Fixed on the immediate goal of getting home to her husband and children before the roads turned to icy glass, she carefully descended the steps, avoiding the swiftly spreading patches of ice—suddenly, oddly, remembering the first day Fred Crabtree had climbed those same few steps onto the porch of her office changing her life forever: taking her down to a totally alien worldview; bringing her back up to a place of mission and meaning.

So she'd believed. Until now—

There were people who didn't want this town's attic disturbed.

April 13. Four months, came the sound of words outside the attic of her own thoughts: You'll be ready. On time. You always are.

They weren't nearly done with Emily Lentz Klein.

And they meant for her to know it.

As she reached for the handle of her car door, she glanced back toward the building. Her eyes were drawn to a sign left by the picketers on Friday afternoon. Three vinyl letters—*T*, *H*, and *E*—had come unglued and were scattered on the grass leaving an eerie message intact:

TRUST GOD NOT _ _ _ RAPISTS

Perhaps years from now, the coincidentally unglued letters would be a story to laugh about. But right this very minute, nothing was the least bit funny.

———————

Stopping at the wall of windows in the sunroom, Jeff looked out over the back yard, his thoughts blocking out the crackling of limbs in the bitter wind and the 'making merry' noises in the other part of the house.

Where in the world is she?

He paced back to the family room.

"Dad, when are you going to get a store-bought tree?" Carol asked. "You could make it look so neat and pretty."

"'Tis purty, Mommy," said Winslow, all wrapped up for Christmas in a red velvet dress and sucking on one of her long auburn curls.

"Wouldn't want to do that," argued Matt who was unpacking the box of presents he'd just brought into the house. "You'd spoil the family ritual. I'll always remember the first year I first went to the woods by myself and got one. Chopped it down, put it in the bucket of dirt—"

"And cut the top out to make it fit under the ceiling. Ugliest tree we ever had." Carol looked at her husband. "But Mom made us keep it."

Little Alison came into the room carrying a Christmas present shaped a lot like fishing gear. "Open it Pop." She lifted it as high as she could.

Jeff rolled it around in his hands, jiggled it, felt it through the paper. "Must be a new pair of shoes."

"No sil'wee, it's a wod and weel."

"Thanks my little cherub." He patted the top of her head. "Let's wait till Christmas Eve to open it." Taking a cell phone from his belt clip, he dialed Emily's office. No answer. Tried her mobile phone. No connection. "Now that really ticks me off! She got that thing so we could keep in touch in times like this. Must've let the battery run down. Could be stuck in a ditch somewhere. Get your coat on Matt . . . Carol, you and Brad stay here in case she calls."

———————

Entering through the wide stone archway, Emily turned left at the huge magnolia tree and stopped at the third plot on the right. She got out of her car and walked over to the Lentz plot. From the spreading cedar tree in the corner, she peeled a dangling strip of bark from its trunk and shred it into tiny strips.

Suddenly she saw the familiar marker in a different light. About three feet high, two feet wide, and eight inches thick, it resembled a closed book. The cover was naturally gray with a cross embossed in the center. An engraved rose hung from the upper left corner; a lily from the right.

Emily knelt and slowly traced the inscription with her fingers:

Hannah R. Lentz
(1887-1912)
There where the wicked trouble not
She laid her head to rest.

A current of knowing pulsed through her blood. "It's yours, isn't it Hannah? Your voice that's always telling me that everything will be just fine."

But will it?

Her mind formed the words her mouth would not allow to escape: *They're gonna get me, Grandmother. I'm so afraid.*

Still on her knees, Emily began to pray like she had not prayed since she was thirteen and had made that strange vow on the mountaintop.

So when was it, God? Ten, twelve years ago? I gave you a puzzle: What's happening in my life? And you gave it right back. I opened myself up for the unthinkable, never dreaming it would call for a voyage to the depths of my unconscious, even to the dark side of my very core. But you took me there.

"What does it profit a man to gain the whole world and lose his soul?" Preacher Miller used to ask. Or was it Jesus? Or Mama?

Somewhere along the way, all those Bible verses got jumbled up with science and psychology and history and—

"For then I saw through a glass, darkly . . ."

Mama said: "You must forgive, you must forget . . . if he did anything."

But didn't your son, Jesus, say that if anybody put a stumbling block in front of any of your little ones, he should have a millstone tied around his neck and dropped into the sea? Doesn't sound too forgiving to me.

Anyway, what good does it do to forgive someone who admits no wrong? And God, do you really want me to forget? I think not. Why else would you have showed me the way to remember?

"Be a good little girl now. Daddy loves you. See you next week. Here's your present early." He handed me the silver dollar minted in 1887, his mother's birth year.

Good Lord! Emily looked upward for a second. *No disrespect to you.* Then back at the marker.

I was thirteen and didn't have to be his little girl anymore. But I didn't know it at the time.

So I grew up. Got married. Became a mommy. Then a therapist. To help the hurting, I'd believed. Not knowing that beneath the layers of self-protection, hiding way back in the closet, was a split soul waiting to heal itself. Asking—

Why God?

If you really are out there, why do you let little children suffer? I know, theologians will say that you suffered with us. Some therapists will say you gave us the gift of dissociation. Worked pretty well for me until those other suffering children of yours came parading into my office. To be absolutely honest, all those horrible things like cannibalism, bestiality, child sacrifice go way beyond my understanding of you and your rival—if either of you really and truly exist. Perhaps my theological and demonological understanding needs further development.

There're still some things, God, that I don't have straight in my mind.

Why would my daddy choose to turn me over to strangers? To take me to all those doctors like Mama said he did. Put me on that Red Cross train? I must've been a dummy, thank God—thank you—because I'm pretty sure I didn't meet the test for any of those special government programs like Bluebird and MKULTRA. But I was apparently good enough to be used by the good ol' local boys who got their kicks from little kids, doing only you and they know what.

Why would Mama choose to not know?

That my mother betrayed me is the most difficult thing I've had to accept.

And why would Cleat choose to despise his own son?

Where does Grandmother Hannah come into all this. Sometimes I feel that I'm her or she's me. Is she hanging around, a spirit waiting to find rest? Or an inside protector I made up in my head when I was little? You know what I'm beginning to believe, God? I'm beginning to believe that she died giving birth to my daddy because she had inadvertently walked into an intergenerational satanic cult family and couldn't endure knowing what lay ahead for her little baby.

And I've never really thought of it before. But now I wonder if that might be why Jeff's mother killed herself.

This prayer stuff brings out the crazy in me, doesn't it? Or perhaps it's not prayer at all; only free association and false memories.

How can good people do evil?

How can you let it all happen?

Choice. Free will. The theologians are answering again. But wonder how many of those academicians, as children, were ever laid on that altar and 'sac-

rificed' to the Evil One? How many were ever strapped on that gurney while a burgeoning life was ripped from their not-quite-grown-up bodies? How many had their souls shattered to shards?

Yes, God. I know all the right answers.

But sometimes they don't fit the questions.

If you're still alive and children are still being hurt . . .

And now the letter from the Board. It's like there's a leviathan—or school of leviathans—just floating around out there waiting to pull me under one final time, waiting to drown me in my own do-goodism.

But I'll hang on, God. I'll make it to the shore. Remember. I'm a strong swimmer . . . you do have a sense of humor, don't you?

Finally noticing the wet cold seeping into her knees, she heard a child praying:

"Now I lay me down to sleep
I pray the Lord my soul to keep
If 'ishudie' before I wake,
I pray the Lord my soul to take."

God, as a little girl I didn't know about death. And thought "ishudie" was one word. Although I never had a visual image of you, I'd learned from the simple prayer that my soul belongs to you and that you would take care of it—whatever it is.

"But then face to face: now I know in part."

Now I see it clearly. My soul is the facet of me that is spirit: a higher power within; my connection to you, the highest power in the universe . . . whatever, whoever you are.

She stood, celebrating her epiphany.

That's it God. That's why I survived the attempted murder of my soul. They couldn't penetrate the God-part within me.

And in that cold, cold cemetery, Emily Lentz Klein rose to her feet and shouted to the living and the dead, whoever may have been listening, and to Matt and Jeff who had come to take her home—

"They couldn't murder God!"

Chapter 47

"**L**ooks like you're bound and determined to ruin the family name!" On the day before Christmas, Cleat came stomping into his daughter-in-law's kitchen like a master ready to discipline an errant servant. The old man threw a shopping bag full of presents onto the table, griping as usual. "Damn, it's hot as hell in here." He took off his heavy jacket, laying bare a sweatshirt imprinted with the CK emblem over his heart. "They're for y'all's kids and my great grandbabies who I never get to see much—thanks to you, Mizrez Klein!"

"Merry Christmas." Trying to keep her revulsion at being physically close to this man and the strong odor of alcohol coming off his breath at bay, Emily continued placing miniature marshmallows on the scooped out orange cups already filled with mashed sweet potatoes.

"Merry Christmas," he mimicked. "Everybody who rides by your office is gonna think you're a nut. Breaking up families and all."

"It's none of your business what I do." She swallowed the acid gurgling up in her throat. "And I can't help what Carol does. She doesn't want you near her girls."

Carol had never liked her granddaddy and she didn't want him and his drunken behaviors to frighten her girls like he'd always frightened her.

Wanting to tell him what she'd remembered about his part in her own childhood, Emily bit her lip. To keep the peace, she tried to understand Jeff's point of view: that it wouldn't do any good to confront Cleat; that he would deny it all anyway, and make things worse. But she knew Cleat knew that she knew. And Cleat knew she knew he knew. Why couldn't they just get things out in the open?

"Where's that boy of mine?" he asked.

"At church. In case you don't know, it's Sunday."

"You don't have to get smart with me, woman." Cleat put his coat back on. "Will ya just tell him I stopped by to wish y'all a Merry Christmas?"

"I'll do that." In a lapse into pity, a thought about inviting him to the family's Christmas Eve supper sloshed around in her head, but she let it sink. As she watched him open and close the kitchen door, a faint tinge of icy sweat moistened her palms and forehead and she rushed to the bathroom. Determined to break the cycle of Christmas-triggered body memories, she bathed her face in a hot towel.

Looking past the aging face in the mirror, she could almost see the children marching up and down the street in front of her office, doing what the big people ordered them to do.

Out of the blue, she remembered Fred's voice on the tape: "Once't I asked Grandpaw why Mr. Casey hated kids and he said it was 'cause he was disappointed in his own boy."

It was *not* Ca-sey.

It was K-C; Klein-Cleat.

Of this she was almost sure.

"Bet you can't guess who dropped by this morning?" Emily said, walking into the family room where Jeff, who had just returned from church, was building a Christmas Eve fire.

"I give up. Who?"

"Your dear ol' Dad."

"No kidding. Did he come by to wish you a Merry Christmas?"

"Of course. And he left some presents for the kids."

"Still trying to play Santa Claus in his own way, I suppose. You have to admit he was a good Santa. Giving out gifts and movie tickets at the Empty Stocking bash. Who knows how many bicycles he fixed up and gave to needy kids?"

"Or what else he did for those children," Emily said under her breath. Then so Jeff could hear, "The real reason he came was to tell me to do something about the picketers."

"What does he want you to do? Shoot 'em? And why does it matter to him?"

"Don't pretend you don't know. He wants me out of practice; always has from the day he learned that I was working with cult-abused clients. He knew he'd be found out."

"Exactly what did he say?"

"Not much, except he implied that I'm an embarrassment to your family name. Like I'm ruining the good old Ku Klux Klein clan, huh?"

Jeff didn't laugh.

She wasn't sure what that look in his eyes meant, but knew this was not the time to go where she really wanted to go. "Just kidding, but I wouldn't be surprised if he's the one who's been paying the picketers to harass me. They look like a bunch of misfits and winos recruited from Acadia. I've tried to talk to them but they ignore me. Would you believe, the other day a girl with a pierced nose and rhinestones in her tongue had the audacity to ask if she could use my rest room? Maybe she's one of his puppets . . . or somebody's."

"Did he tell you what he's doing for Christmas?"

"Didn't ask. Don't care. But I don't want him ruining ours." Her stomach was getting queasy again. "Let's don't talk about him anymore."

"Suits me. What time's dinner?"

"Early. About five. Alison's bedtime is seven, eight at the latest. That'll give us time to eat and open presents. After both girls are in bed, we get to help play Santa Claus. Then I was hoping we could go to the midnight service. Just you and me."

"Sure. I'd like that."

After lunch, they went into the family room. Jeff stoked the fire one more time, then sat down on the sofa beside his wife and picked up the remote. "The *Messiah* should be coming on PBS in a few minutes."

Tired from all the Christmas cooking and cleaning and decorating and shopping, Emily drifted off to sleep during the "Hallelujah Chorus." When she awoke, Jeff was talking on the phone.

"Sure, Dad. I'll be right over."

The fury smoldering in her gut burst into a full flame.

He put the phone down. "I'm sorry. Dad's having chest pains again and is out of Nitro. I hope I can find a pharmacy that's open."

"Do what you have to do. I understand." But she really didn't. Cleat was always calling with some excuse to get Jeff to come by. She didn't understand why Jeff would risk alienating his own family by missing dinner; by not being around to open presents or help play Santa.

All to please his daddy.

Without Jeff, the dinner at Carol and Brad's was gloomy. Opening presents was no fun. After the little girls were in bed, Emily went home alone.

When Jeff had arrived at the apartment, his daddy was passed out on the floor. He called 911. The EMS people came and took the old man to the emergency room. Tests showed that Cleat had experienced a heart attack and he was admitted to the hospital.

By the light of a midnight moon, Jeff unlocked the front door as quietly as he could and walked stealthily into the dark house. Climbing the stairs, his hands touched the cedar garland on the railing and he smelled Christmas. On the landing, he glanced through the doorway of the guest room. Emily was sound asleep in the rocker.

What an ass I am, he thought. I'll make it up to her in the morning.

Tubes and drains were all over the place. Machines were beeping and bopping. A potted Norfolk pine decorated with tiny colored lights lit up a corner of the dim room. The old man with liver spots on his crusted face looked at his surroundings, trying to think himself into the right time and place. Christmas. It must be Christmas, he thought.

The tall man with a neatly trimmed white beard who was shoving a paper in his face looked familiar, but Cleat couldn't quite place him. He smelled gauze, urine, antiseptics, disinfectants. Needles pricked his arms and he felt a raw ache in his chest. Hell couldn't be any worse, his body seemed to say.

Maybe this is it! Maybe they have Christmas in hell, too.

Shoulders crunched into cold metal rails, he was suffocating in the narrow bed on wheels. Lungs, rattling with each breath, seemed full of salt water.

All his life Cleat Klein had been swimming in two parallel rivers that never touched each other, that rarely came in conflict. In one, he was violent and intolerant to his own son, hated snobby people like his mother-in-law; in the other, he loved animals and was generous to needy children. But right this minute, he was stuck in an estuary where the rivers' currents were meeting the sea's tide. His life, like sand in an inlet, was hanging in a volatile balance.

Had he been in this place a long time? Or only a few minutes? The little hand on the clock was at twelve, but he didn't know if it was morning or night. His mind ticked with the bright red second hand, finally pausing to give him a moment of lucidity.

"Do you know who I am?" asked the man looming over him.

"You damn right I do. What do you think I am, crazy or something? When they gonna let me out of this stinkin' place? Stupid. They wake you up to put you to sleep. What day is it?"

"December 25, 2000." The tall man pushed a paper in front of his face. "Dad, here's something I'd like you to sign. It's a power of attorney. Do you know what that is?"

"You damn right I do. It means I'm more dead than alive. Give it here." For a brief interlude, Cleat had come back to his limited vocabulary and his habitually obnoxious self.

"I'll hold it for you." Jeff handed his daddy a pen and held the clipboard above his face.

Clutching the side rails, Cleat tried to pull himself up but couldn't make his withering body rise. "Goddammit! They got me tied down. Get this fuckin' strap off."

"Now try to relax." Jeff loosened the restraints. "They just don't want you to roll out of bed and hurt yourself, that's all."

With a trembling left hand his damaged brain was trying to control, the elder Klein scratched his name as close as he could get it to the signature line.

"What difference would it make if I fell out?" The helpless man rustled under the sheet. He tried to sit up again but fell backwards, howling an obscenity two blocks long. Rolling over on his side, he curled up into a fetal position, squealing like a wild wounded creature. "Don't let 'em . . . help me," he moaned in a voice of long ago. "It hurts . . . I couldn't help it . . . they made me do it . . . I'm so scared . . . help me." Fumbling around with his fingers, Cleat managed to push the call button.

A woman dressed in white came into the room. She pulled a pair of latex gloves from the wall dispenser, stretched them over her hands, and began to prepare a concoction of drugs designed to quiet the man who was rambling out of his head.

"Don't do that!" Jeff grabbed the nurse's arm. "I want to hear what he has to say."

"Let go of me," she demanded, "or I'll call security." Jeff released his grip and she went about her business.

"To help you get some rest, sweetie," she said, infusing the IV with a clear liquid.

Not dead yet, another Cleat winked at the buxom redhead, then retracted in the face of still another man's lament: "Oh Katherine, my beautiful Katherine . . . you've come back . . . with the baby."

"That was my mother's name. He's hallucinating." Jeff explained.

"Wouldn't you be?" She pulled off her gloves and on the way to the door, dropped them into a wastebasket.

"There's an ugly woman in here," the patient yelled.

"Pardon me, sir." The nurse turned around. "Are you saying I'm—"

"Not you. Her . . . over there." Cleat was pointing to the metal locker in the corner. "Get her out of here . . . get that bitch out of here! I want my Katherine."

Shaking her head with resignation, the earthly woman left the room.

Cleat extended his cold blue bloodless hand to his son. "I'm leaving now," he said, and wandered off to a plane somewhere between now and forever. Moving . . . faster and faster . . . spinning . . . splitting. Eyes inside his head saw bits and pieces of a lifetime: table saws, likker cycles, pistols, naked women, Puffy Poo and Sarge. He heard chanting voices and babies crying. A little boy came to his side, reaching for his hand.

Jeff, the adult, walked into the midst of his hallucinations.

Before the father had spun all the way to the realm of the unconscious, he looked up at his son through hollow sunken eyes and, hedging his bets, pleaded, "Pray for me."

Jeff flopped back on the dark brown vinyl recliner to continue the deathwatch. Thinking about his daddy's age regression, he became furious at the nurse for tranquilizing the tormented tormentor, for not allowing the old man to finish his story.

He didn't want to be in this place, snared in the milieu of critical care hearing moans and groans sweeping through the halls, the slamming and clang of dishes as aides were getting meals on trays, and the rumble of an elevator transporting a body to the other side.

What was he to do? Leave the old man to die alone?

Hawking magazines, candy bars, and soft drinks, a Pink Lady parked a squeaky cart in the hall and stuck her head in the door. Seeing the old man with his mouth locked open and his glazed eyes ogling the ceiling, she moved on.

A man in hospital greens brought lunch and left it on the tray. Jeff was hungry, but not for bullion and ginger ale with Jell-O on the side. Did they expect him to pour this scrumptious meal down his daddy's throat? With any awareness at all, the steak and whisky man would've been mortified.

As if suddenly deducing his fate, Cleat let out a caterwaul of desperation. "Ah . . . oh . . . ah . . . oh—"

Emily came through the door carrying a briefcase. "Are you all right?"

"I will be." He wiped the sweat off his forehead. "But I gotta get outta here for a while."

"Yes. You need a break. I'll stay with your daddy. Why don't you go home and take a shower? Get a bite to eat."

"Thanks. But I'll be around somewhere. Just beep me if you need to."

Before leaving, the son took a last look at the father. "By the way Em, he remembered something. He was whimpering like a child being hurt . . . being made to do something he didn't want to do."

As always, when his wife didn't know what to say, she talked "It's all right, Hon. He can't ever hurt us . . . hurt anyone again. Who knows why he did what he did?" She answered the question herself. "Probably so he wouldn't have to face what maybe even happened to him as a child. Your daddy was just sick. Plain old soul-sick."

"He can't hurt us anymore." Jeff walked out of the room leaving Emily to sit with the dying man and her lonely thoughts.

In a straight-backed chair with a floral cushioned seat that looked like it belonged in a formal dining room, Emily sat in the future she'd often imagined: at the place of her birth on the third floor of Southeast Medical Center, formerly Campbell Memorial Hospital. In a room, once pea-green, now painted a neutral gray as if to tone down illness and death, she sat beside the most repulsive man she had ever known.

Opportunity was now.

She could tell him what she'd always wanted to tell him. Whether he heard or not, at least he couldn't talk back.

But not a word came from her mouth.

She felt the abominable nausea. Tired of letting her father-in-law control her autonomic nervous system, Emily was determined she wouldn't let him get her down this time. As if she were trying to rid herself of all the dirt the pervert had ever heaped on her, she went over to the vanity and squirted a glob of Kind-Kare hand soap from the wall dispenser into her palm then turned on the hot water faucet.

Behind her, Cleat was blathering like a mad dog. "Help me . . . help me . . ." She thought they may have been the most genuine words he'd ever uttered, but she went on washing her hands.

"If ya remember what we done ya have to kill yourself. And always keep the knife with ya in case ya have ta die."

Had the old man just spoken? Or was it her imagination?

"Hi Mom. How's he doing?" Matt—Dr. Matthew Klein—had come into the room on his short lunch break.

"He's out of his head." Emily turned around to acknowledge her son. "That's all I know. Glad you came by."

"Where's Dad?"

"Probably down in the cafeteria or lobby."

Matt picked up Cleat's chart from the foot of the bed. "We're losing him, Mom." He wiped his eyes with his fingers. "We're losing him." His pager beeped and he checked the return number. "Gotta run. I'll try to stop by later."

A different nurse came in to take Cleat's vital signs, no doubt observing Emily's coldness toward the patient. "His doctor says things are deteriorating fast. They want to do a cardiac catheterization to see if there's anything else we can do."

An orderly came in and rolled the patient out of the room. A few minutes later, a janitor wearing kneepads swished through the room as if cleaning up for imminent death.

Emily picked up her briefcase. She stepped across the hall to the visitors' quiet room.

To pass time, she looked through the pamphlets and magazines in the rack. An old copy of *Working Woman* had an article on hormone therapy and one extolling the benefits of short-term psychotherapy. Drive-through therapies. Where would she be if she'd depended on managed-care and had been told she could have only ten sessions with Julie. Or what would've happened to those clients of hers who'd spent years in therapy trying to cope with the aftereffects of human cruelty if their care had been managed—or as one of her colleagues called it, mangled—by some inexperienced mental health worker who had never sat with a ritually abused patient.

The bold black caption on a pink flyer advertising a nutrition workshop caught her attention.

YOUR MOTHER WAS RIGHT

It's subtitle was, "Eat vegetables and watch cholesterol."

Emily Lentz Klein could hardly remember what her mother looked like, but many of the old programs instituted by Gladys Keller Lentz had been indelibly cast throughout the folds of her brain.

She walked over to the vending machines, bought a Snickers and a Diet Pepsi and took them back to her chair. Fueled up to write, she took the computer from her briefcase and opened it on her lap. On the blank screen, her thoughts began to appear in words:

What should I feel? Contempt? Anger? Elation? Ashamed of my feelings toward him? Now that the old man is finally dying, all I can think about is pity. I can't stand to see anyone suffer. Not even Cleat.

What was it I learned about object relations?

A part of Cleat is still like an infant whose perception of the people and objects around it are an extension of itself and exist to meet its needs. Anything the baby does to subjugate others makes it feel better. As a child, Cleat must have lived in a split world. In a world where no one talked about sinning Saturday night, but on Sunday morning in Mt. Hermon Lutheran Church repented, "Not only for outward transgressions but also for secret thoughts and desires which I cannot fully understand but which are all known unto thee."

The promise of forgiveness. For some people, a license to kill.

Pushing a walker, an elderly woman came rushing across to the rest room. Emily continued her task, trying not to hear the tinkling sounds invading her privacy.

Cleat is asking for help. But it's too late. Too late to work through his own victimization and grieve his own losses including his son and his grandchildren. Too late to accept responsibility for his actions.

Here I am swimming in the sea of ambiguity again like a dolphin who's lost its radar. There's no way to prove he hurt me when I was little. My automatic writings and the graphic pictures in my mind are the only evidence. Perhaps graphic is a truth in itself.

Apparently, Cleat had never been able to forget that his son had brought dishonor to him in front of his peers. However, the child in Cleat had wanted to be like Jeff and couldn't. And he hated Jeff for that.

I'm almost certain that Fred's teacher in the cutting business had been Cleat Klein, C-K backwards. K-C. Not Casey Paxton. Maybe it was Cleat who killed Fred or had him killed.

The woman came out of the rest room and sat down. Emily closed the computer and her eyes so that she wouldn't have to carry on a meaningless conversation with a stranger. Rather, she talked to herself: "So, Dr. Klein. How do you feel?"

Hate? I'm not sure what hate feels like. Never been allowed to hate. It's kinda hard to hate a dying man. If Mama were here, she'd tell me to forgive him. How can you forgive someone if they don't even believe or even admit they've done anything wrong? . . . Uh-oh. I'm feeling something. I know it's anger toward Jeff for running off and leaving me alone with his disgusting daddy . . . if no demons had ever lived on this earth, Cleat came pretty close.

Under portraits of his grandparents and other dead benefactors of the hospital, Jeff was drawn into the design of the lobby's checkerboard floor. The marbled stone tiles, covered with a haze which kept them from being their original pure black or white, were at least two-feet square. As a child, he'd played here when his grandmother visited sick friends. And in later days, when fathers were not allowed to be with their wives during labor, he'd anxiously waited in this place when Emily gave birth, first to Carol, and two years later to Matt.

The community hospital, established in the late '30s through a trust set up by his Grandfather Campbell and nourished by various fund raisers like the one Jeff had hosted at Acadia over a decade earlier, was now a conglomerate-owned, state-of-the art medical complex offering both open-heart and brain surgery. Every new technology you could think of was upstairs and his daddy was wasting away and nobody could do a damn thing about it.

He looked up to see Emily coming toward him. "They're doing another catheterization," she said.

Jeff nodded. Sadly. Resignedly.

For a long time they sat in silence, together and alone.

"Know what?" she finally broke the quiet. "I do believe it's possible for people to have false memories. Your daddy and my mother did. Both of them would have said our childhoods were wonderful."

"Maybe Dad was just chronically drunk. They say alcoholics can't recall what happens during a blackout; may not even know they've been out."

"That's possible. However, when he was hurting little kids he could've been re-enacting his own trauma and, as he most likely did as a child himself, just blocked it out."

"Maybe he simply lied," Jeff said. "Sociopaths do lie, don't they?"

"Yes, it's their nature. In my opinion, anybody who could rape a child or murder a baby would hardly be beyond lying. And there's always the possibility of conscious, deliberate denial."

"What if Dad had admitted—"

"Do you mean, would he have been treatable? Who knows? Would he have been able to take responsibility for what he did?"

"If you really want to know what I believe, but can't prove, is that Dad never told about the cult because of some kind of oath. Probably very much like the Klan's oath, maybe even patterned on it. If he told, he'd have expected to die. That simple. In a twisted way, he was an honorable man, at least in regard to what he considered his purpose for being."

Cleat's cardiologist came wandering into the lobby, interrupting their discussion. With a recognizable trained neutrality, almost a nonchalance, he looked at Jeff. "Your father went into cardiac arrest during the procedure. I'm sorry. There was nothing else we could do."

There was no funeral, no memorial service, no nothing to celebrate the life of Cleatus Adolphus Klein (1922-2000).

Jeff stuffed himself into a jumpsuit and draped a white scarf around his neck. After picking up the baggage, he climbed into his pickup and headed toward the plantation. The day was warm, definitely out of character for the last week in December. Since he had called to tell the mechanic he was on his way, his gorgeous canary-yellow biplane was waiting on the airstrip.

First thing he did was put the baggage under the pilot's seat and unbuckle the belt which held the control stick in check. Before taking off, he walked around the plane and gave it a thorough ground inspection: examining every nut and bolt and screw; wiping his hand over the propeller to check for nicks; and looking at the control surface, the antenna, the lights, and instruments.

Once airborne, the son began talking to his daddy as if the man were right by his side. For the first time he could recall in his entire lifetime, Jeff spoke to Cleat without being criticized or interrupted:

What should I feel? Sadness? Remorse? Anger? Pity? At whom? Surely at you! But what? You lived your life as you wished. I hated you for the way you talked about and treated the people close to me. I hated you because you would never talk to me without attacking either me or my opinions. I hated you for your one-sided ugly narrow-mindedness.

And most of all I hate myself for not taking a baseball bat and making you sit quietly while I told you what I knew about your life in the cult.

I could never prove anything. But inside me I knew the truth.

I hate myself for knowing that to have had such a conversation would've been useless. You would've admitted nothing. You could not have done so. Not only would your desire for self-preservation have kept you from it, you were never a big enough man to do it.

You were nothing like I thought you were when I was a kid and I hate you for that . . . and I feel so guilty for hating you as I do.

A little over an hour after takeoff, Jeff dipped down as low as he safely could and picked up the baggage—a white biodegradable cardboard box— and, like a World War II pilot dropping a small bomb over a German city, tossed it out the hatch.

When his daddy—what was left of him—was out of sight somewhere in the dense pine forest surrounding Slicky Rock Mountain, Jeff finished his dialogue with the dead:

Now that you're gone, we can all have some peace . . . peace at last.

And turned toward home.

Chapter 48

"**D**o you think they'll survive?"

Standing at the front window, the Kleins watched the snow blowing like spun sugar as it coated individual twigs on the shrubbery. In the background, a TV weather reporter from the local cable channel was making a major story out of the surprise first-day-of-spring storm. "The temperature will be just above freezing all day so we expect no accumulation of snow in the Midlands. We're looking at three or four inches in the mountains and significant erosion on the coast. Wind gusts of 30 to 50 miles per hour are expected. If you have to travel, watch for falling trees and power lines."

"Who're you talking about now, Em?"

"The gardenias." They were her favorite flower. Extremely fragile. Lightly touching or breathing on them could turn the petals brown.

"I thought you were talking about your clients . . . with all the worrying you've been doing about the board hearing coming up."

"That wasn't even on my mind . . . not consciously."

"About the gardenias, then. Of course none of the buds are out of danger yet. We could still have a hard freeze. But even if there's a wipe-out, they'll come back. Always do."

The siren-like noise on the TV heralded a special news bulletin. A young woman bundled up in rain gear came on the screen. "Good morning. This is Sarah Smith broadcasting from Chestnut Ridge's Upper River Bridge. We're waiting to learn the identity of the body —"

The couple turned around to see what was happening.

Several empty cars were lined up on the bridge behind a late-model silver Cadillac. People were standing on the walkway looking down at the water, some with hands over their mouths, others muttering to those at their sides.

"What happened?" Sarah Smith asked a bushy-bearded biker dressed in black leather and wearing a skull rag under his helmet.

"I wuz followin' that car all the way out of town and it stopped dead on the bridge and the first thing I knowed, that man, he got out and went to the side and throwed hisself over the rail and just let go. Kinda flipping over head first. Didn't hear 'im holler or nuttin. And I can't swim and didn't know what the hell to do but pick up my cell phone and call 911."

The news person walked up to an elderly man hanging over the railing who was rambling to anybody who was listening. Looking down to see what he was seeing, she gasped at the sight and stuck her microphone in front of his face. "Why did they call in those fellers?" he asked, pointing toward two divers in wet suits climbing up the bank. "Whoever it wuz done dove into shallow water and rocks. Just look down there. His head's busted wide open."

Tom Paxton came into the picture, ordering the bystanders, "Get along now. Y'all are gettin' in the way." Turning toward the reporter, he got ready for the limelight. Wearing a double-breasted suit and a stiffly starched white shirt with a red, white, and blue tie, he assumed a military-style position: standing straight and tall, chest out, one hand behind his back.

The reporter spoke to the camera: "With me here is Police Chief Thomas Paxton." Then to Tom, "Good morning, Chief. Have you identified the body?"

"Yes ma'am, we have. It's that of one Franklin B. Griffin, a man well known in this community. He recently retired as CEO at Syn-Tec."

"Oh, my God!" the woman exclaimed, apparently forgetting for a moment that she was on camera. "The Mr. Griffin who was in court this morning? Who pled guilty to—"

"Yes, ma'am. That's the one."

Looking back at the camera, as if she'd just scooped the story of the year, Sarah Smith said, "We'll be back in a minute with more from Chief Paxton."

Without making any comments, the Kleins went over to the sofa and sat down.

"Lumber . . . lumber . . . lumber." A bald man in bib-overalls was hawking products from his family-owned home-supply store. Emily clutched the wheezy sensation in her stomach, waiting for Jeff to make some snide remark about Tom Paxton. He didn't let her down. "The sniveling bastard. To tell you what kind of man he is, as if you don't already know, when he first came home from college, he walked up to me at the Homecoming Dance and asked, 'Are you still dating that Lentz girl?' When I said I was, he said with that ratty supercilious voice of his, sticking his nose up in the air, 'Well, I think I'll just take her away from you again.'"

"What did you tell him?"

"As I remember, I just laughed, saying something like, 'Just try. She's not a piece of property. You don't know Emily Lentz like I know Emily Lentz.'"

Before Emily could react, the news show was back on. "This is Sarah Smith again. I'm out at the Upper River Bridge where we've just learned that the man who jumped off the bridge was the Franklin Griffin who earlier today pled guilty to sexual exploitation of minors, a story which incidentally was scheduled to air on our noon news. He had previously been charged with possessing and distributing child pornography on his home computer." She pointed to the side rail. "Less than an hour ago, this prominent man in the community plunged to his death, fatally escaping from all responsibility for the crimes he committed and for which he would have been sentenced on April 6, 2001 in the U.S. District Court." Again, placing the microphone near Tom's mouth, she asked, "Can you tell us more about those crimes?"

The once macho-man pushed back a thin chunk of gray hair blowing over his forehead and tried to talk with intelligence. "We believe Mr. Griffin was a member of the global child pornography operation known as 'Wonderland,' a computer club in which members had to have a minimum of 10,000 pictures of child pornography encrypted on their hard drives. Several weeks ago, our department was instructed by the U.S. Customs Service to seize the home and office computers of this man."

"What did you find?"

"It was amazing. Both shocking and disturbing. Even for us seasoned investigators. Images of children tied up, some having sex with animals or adults or other children. Made me sick on my stomach. Some of the kids looked like they were younger than two years old."

"There's the evidence!" Emily yelled, slapping her husband on the back. "But too late for Crystal," she sighed.

"Thank you, Chief Paxton." The reporter looked away from the camera. "I see that our former mayor has just arrived." She walked across the bridge where a feeble-looking Phil Owens was stepping out of his car. "Good morning, sir. Can you tell us anything about Mr. Griffin? It's my understanding that he worked with you for many years."

"I just can't imagine what happened." Phil wiped his cheek. "Franklin was a good Christian man as far as I knew. And a superb business man."

"I'm sure he was," Emily blurted.

Jeff nudged her with his elbow. "Keep quiet and listen."

"There're some of us around here who believe he may have been framed but had no way out but to plead guilty." Phil glanced down at the ground for a second or two. "It's a crying shame he never got a chance to tell his side of the story. We do know he was despondent after his daughter ran away from home about a year ago."

"One of my sources told me there's state-of-the art video equipment out there at Syn-Tec?" The astute journalist had made a simple statement into a leading question.

"Certainly we . . . they do. They use it all the time in their training films."

"And the satanic paraphernalia found in one of the warehouses?"

"Way to go Sarah Smith." As Phil paused to think about his answer, Emily beat on her thighs cheering the reporter on. "Keep him jumping."

"I-I-I have no idea where that came from," Phil answered.

"Thank you, Mr. Owens." The camera panned the river below just before a commercial for pre-owned cars glared on the screen.

Walking back over to the window, Emily said, "Now, thank God, Crystal . . . or Star will have her proof . . . if she's still alive."

The skies were clearing; the snow on the gardenia bush had melted away. But the wind was still coming in strong.

Chapter 49

*W*earing no robes,

the judges were cloaked with the power to drain her very lifeblood.

Seven pairs of probing eyes burned images into her brain.

Tell us about your soul, Dr. Klein, demanded the pipe-smoking man in a deep voice from hell.

Do you use hypnosis? challenged the man wearing a black armband lettered with HMO.

Are you an initiate? Have you ever been in therapy? chimed a chorus of women's voices.

"Yes . . . yes . . . yes!" the woman sitting at the head of the table lamented.

Snippets of memories glowed in the dark:

A neon cross on the mountaintop, the Red Cross, frosted windows, a stained glass, the baby's frozen face.

Hands. Big hands. Little hands. Hands that looked like witches' hands. A tiny hand on a huge penis. Grandmother Hannah's hands. Her mother's. Maggie's.

The alarm went off and the warning resounded:

When you stand before the judgment seat, the book of your life will be opened. Everything will be made known. Everything you've ever done, every thought you've ever had, every word you've ever uttered, every secret will be exposed. The final judgment will be public. There will be no way to hide your naked shame.

Three hours later, Emily Lentz Klein, Ph.D. would face her accuser. Alone. Entitled to counsel, she'd chosen to represent herself. It was her challenge. No one else's. The strategy was to show her integrity as a human being and as a therapist. Offering a defense, it would be difficult for her to separate the personal from the professional.

She wanted to know that everything would be okay but was not sure that it would.

She wanted to believe that she was a good wife, mother, grand-mother, and therapist but was not sure that she was.

Not sure. Not sure of anything.

Today, holding in her mind an incredible body of data without specific proof of anything, she would sit before a jury of her peers trying to guarantee that she was not . . . morally incompetent.

It was Good Friday. The day they crucified Jesus.

All eyes of the Psychology Board were upon the accused as the Secretary ushered her to the head of the table. Without an interrogation chamber of its own, the licensing body was holding the hearing in the psychology department of the university where twenty-two years earlier she'd defended her doctoral dissertation ironically titled, *Predictors of Memory Retrieval in Gifted Children*.

Decor in the musty basement conference room had changed little since the seventies. Commercial carpet, multicolored (not the old avo-cado green), covered the cold damp floor. There were a few more scratches on the table's veneer. The brown, cracked Naugahyde chairs were the same.

Of course the faces were different. And so was she: wearing a teal blue business suit; exuding self-confidence; holding her one-shade-of-gray head high; knowing she'd done nothing wrong; thirty pounds lighter than she was ten years before; and feeling younger than when she was a graduate student.

"Good morning." The chairperson, a retired professor wearing a tattered sports jacket with suede patches on the elbows and defying authority by smoking a pipe in the smoke-free building, opened the quasi-judicial proceeding. As he introduced the other six board members, all appointed by the governor, Emily matched faces with resumes and vitae. She was acquainted with Charles Williams, having served on the State Mental Health Board with him in the early '80s. Two female psychologists were in clinical practice. One worked in a Christian counseling center; the other was in private practice. There were two male psychologists: a researcher who'd probably never seen a patient/client professionally, and a reviewer for a health maintenance organization (HMO). Lay members on the board were a male accountant and a female kindergarten teacher.

"Shall we begin?" Looking directly at his peer seated at the opposite end of the long conference table, Dr. Williams stated, "You have requested this hearing to offer evidence that you are innocent of the complaints brought forth in the letter I will now read."

Numbly—thank God for normal dissociation in times like these—the accused listened, hearing only scattered words and phrases.

. . . recovered memory movement . . . discipline . . . harshest possible terms . . . malpractice . . . morally incompetent . . .

The chairperson summarized: "Dr. Klein, you have been accused of implanting false memories of abuse in the mind of this man's daughter. Furthermore, you have been uncooperative by not relinquishing your case notes; therefore, this board has been unable to evaluate how you carried out your responsibility of therapy with this woman."

"With all due respect sir, in light of the 1996 Supreme Court ruling guaranteeing absolute confidentiality between client and therapist, it would've been, without my client's permission, unethical for me to release those notes, even to this board."

"The board was unable to locate your client."

"I'm aware of that. Because of harassment by her father, Ms. Witherspoon chose to change her name and move from this area. In my opinion, it would've been better if he could've responded to his daughter's allegations before she left."

"Do you know where she is?"

"As a matter of fact, I do—"

He didn't give her a chance to finish answering the question. "The Reverend has filed a formal complaint and this distinguished board will respond to it. He is here in this room and you have the right to confront him as he does you."

"Dr. Williams," Emily spoke just as sternly, "it is my understanding that when a healthcare provider is accused of malpractice, any such accusations must come directly from the party who claims injury. In my opinion, Ms. Witherspoon's father is not my client; therefore, I do not owe him a duty of care."

"Uh . . . uh," Dr. Williams stammered, "that may have to be decided in a court of law. Right now, as I see it, the question before this board is, did you, in fact, implant false memories in your client, the Reverend Fisher's daughter, Sandra?"

"No sir, I did not. But with the board's permission, I've invited Ms. Witherspoon to speak today, to tell her side, and then the board will be in a better position to consider the man's charges against me. For your information, she's waiting outside in the hall right now."

Reverend Fisher let out a huff heard around the room.

"We will allow that," Dr. Williams said, "but first the board would like to ask you some questions."

The HMO reviewer began the grilling. "Are you trained to do recovered memory therapy?"

"I'm not sure what you mean by that term. I help people deal with the problems they bring to therapy. Sometimes memory retrieval is a crucial part of getting better. If clients come to me saying they want to remember their pasts so it can enable them to understand how it may be affecting their present functioning, I'll do what I can to help. Some people say they know they had a horrible childhood but don't want to remember it. I also respect that stance."

"Can a therapist literally put memories in someone's head?" the accountant asked.

The HMO reviewer didn't wait for Emily to respond. "Of course, they can." Walloping his fist on the table, he defended his position. "From reviewing hundreds of cases a year of patients who claim without a shred of evidence that they were sexually abused by their parents, I believe false memory syndrome is real."

Breathe deeply—and sit on your hands.

"To my knowledge," Emily rebutted, "even in the numerous and often frivolous lawsuits which have been thrown at therapists in the past several years—although some therapists have been accused and found guilty of misconduct and malpractice—no one has ever been convicted of implanting false memories or lost his or her license for that reason."

"Well, we see a lot of the same therapists reporting they are treating these cases using recovered memory therapy," the reviewer was grandstanding. "Patients come in with depression and relationship problems and things like that and because of techniques like hypnosis and visualization and art and drama and some silly trivia called sandtray therapy, they begin to recall all kinds of things like sexual abuse and even something being called SRA or satanic ritual abuse. It's my opinion that therapists are making big bucks off of these patients they make dependent on them and making them desert their families whom they've accused of abusing them. By making them imagine things that didn't happen like that so-called ritual abuse and mind control and programming and decompensating, so that they will need more and more care and pay them hundreds of dollars a week for therapy and putting them in hospitals that cost several thousand dollars a day and giving them sodium amytal to make them spurt out things that didn't happen."

This man seems as if he's about to decompensate himself.

"Those things may be true for your insureds," Emily countered, "but I have to tell you, the first MPD client I saw more than twenty years ago revealed those types of crimes very early in his therapy. At the time, I'd never even heard of satanic ritual abuse and had been taught in graduate school that MPD was extremely rare. I certainly did not suggest that he come up with memories of something I knew nothing about."

Both the private secular psychologist and the Christian psychologist nodded in agreement.

Emily continued her defense: "I've never urged severance from families or isolation from the outside world. I've never encouraged any of my clients to file lawsuits against their perpetrators, although I understand why that would be tempting for those persons who are trying to pay for therapy and other medical expenses related to the aftereffects of trauma. Many are too disabled to work and need money for living expenses. About the claim that therapists implant false memories for financial gain, I don't know about other therapists, but for many of my clients, I've more often than not provided treatment *pro bono* or on a sliding scale."

"But how can someone be so wounded and not remember it?" asked the accountant.

"That's not difficult to understand," the teacher answered. "What about the date-rape drugs that have been so much in the news lately? Victims could have unknowingly been given similar drugs that caused disorientation and confusion, even amnesia."

"That makes sense, but there's another issue," the accountant said. "From what I've seen in the media, there are a lot of unscrupulous therapists who mistreat patients. Even have affairs with them."

"There are some," Emily agreed. "And I wouldn't defend an unethical therapist any more than I would defend an unethical priest, politician, or educator . . . or accountant. I've even seen a couple of women who say they were sexually exploited by their former therapists. And I've heard of still other dual relationships. One of my clients was a receptionist for her former therapist. Another spoke of having lived with his therapist for a while. I try not to be judgmental, though, because I really do understand how someone can get overinvolved. Even so, that doesn't mean the person's memories are unfounded."

Emily paused to take a sip of bottled water. "Of some interest, in fact, I'd like to ask you this: why would you so readily believe someone's memories of having been molested by a therapist, but—and, for the moment, this is hypothetical, of course—deny outright a person's memories of having been sexually molested by, let's say, a family member? What makes one report so easily true to you and the other so patently false—so implanted?"

No one answered her questions.

"Why does anybody want to remember anything bad that's happened in the past?" the accountant asked. "Even if you lost a job or didn't get picked for the team or didn't go to the prom or whatever, isn't it best to just forget it and live in the present? And if people did hurt you, I think you should be forgiving and just get on with your life."

Funny, you don't look like mother. Another unthought-thought had bubbled up from Emily's always active well of humor.

Before the defendant could respond to the accountant, the experimental psychologist questioned, "Is it even possible to deliberately create these extra personalities as Father Fisher has charged?"

"Yes," Emily answered. "I believe it's possible to create multiple personalities in powerless subjects by inflicting severe pain combined with operant and classical conditioning techniques. During the Cold War, the CIA sponsored mind control experiments under a project called MKULTRA in which they tried to create alter personalities programmed to carry out undercover jobs such as spying, prostitution for blackmail purposes, and things like assassinations.

"Incredible!" exclaimed the kindergarten teacher. "Are you telling this panel that our government was involved in such atrocities?"

"Yes, that is a fact. Dr. Colin Ross has documented this quite nicely in his book, *Bluebird: Deliberate Creation of Multiple Personality by Psychiatrists*. And people are coming forward now saying they were subjects in those experiments. I should note that some of these researchers were working either directly or indirectly for the government. In one book that's just come out titled *Secret Weapons*, two sisters, in collaboration with a former police captain and a professional writer, tell how they were used in Cold War experiments similar to those that Ms. Witherspoon recalled. In another recently published book, *A Nation Betrayed*, a woman who remembers having been tortured as a child in government-sponsored behavior modification programs tells not only about her own experiences as a victim, but also provides pages and pages of documentation that such programs, including MKULTRA, existed."

Emily paused to take a another drink of water. "But I must point out to you, my fellow psychologists, that I believe we, as a profession, are also at fault."

"What do you mean?" asked the experimental psychologist.

"In many cases, it was apparently psychologists who conducted the experiments. Who else would have known as much about the power of positive and negative reinforcements in controlling human behavior? And we know that when the National Institute of Mental Health was created after World War II, it opened the 'money doors' for academic psychologists who could then get grants for research on human behavior. I'm not saying that everyone who did experimental work was involved in some kind of clandestine operation, although some of them could've been without even knowing it."

"Why did they use children?" The teacher appeared to be closely following Emily's concerns.

"First, let me clarify this issue by stating that, to my knowledge, because most of the MKULTRA documents were destroyed in 1973, there are few, if any, records to show exactly who was used. What we know is that the government conducted mind control experiments during the Cold War and that adults today are reporting childhood memories of having been used in such atrocities. It's interesting to note, however, that therapists across the country who have the courage to work with these—if you prefer to say alleged—subjects, and frequently the clients themselves, are being harassed and intimidated in what appears to be a very well-organized manner."

No one bothered to ask Emily about the false memory movement to which she had just alluded.

"Why do you think all this programming you talk about failed?" asked the experimental psychologist.

"I can only conjecture, but the programming could be time sensitive. Maybe even soul sensitive. Meaning there's an inherent rebellion toward being controlled. There's something I've wondered about recently: Could it be that when innate intelligence is tampered with, the mind is capable of taking on new and larger contexts; healing itself, if you will."

"Let's get back to our agenda," Dr. Williams directed the board.

Pointing to Reverend Fisher, the HMO reviewer asked the accused, "Did you create personalities in this man's daughter?"

"I definitely did not. Although it may be possible to structure a psyche to be multiple, this is certainly not something I know how to do, or would do, with any of the people I serve. Ms. Witherspoon's various personalities came out spontaneously during hypnosis to help her learn ways to cope with physical discomfort."

"So you did use hypnosis?" asked Dr. Williams.

"I did. As you know, the relaxed state produced by hypnosis can lower stress-levels in the body and—"

"Did you call for personalities to come out?" the HMO representative interrupted and took over the questioning.

"No. Because at that point, I didn't know she had any."

"Did you tell her she was multiple?"

"I only told her what I'd observed. Over the course of treatment, she came to accept the diagnosis of dissociative identity disorder, saying it explained so many things: the voices, lost time, the fugue states."

Dr. Williams addressed the board again: "Dr. Klein has said she didn't create personalities in Ms. Witherspoon. We know the research is not at all clear on the mechanisms involved in the recollection of traumatic memories."

Then he addressed the defendant: "Did you, in using hypnosis . . . did you implant false memories in your client?"

"No, I did not. When I used hypnosis, it was at her request with the intent to help her relax. In an altered state, probably similar to the dissociated state she entered when she was being abused, she had images of being tortured by her father and by other perpetrators. Knowing that the damage caused to clients and their families by mistaken accusation is usually irreparable, I neither encouraged nor discouraged her to believe what she claimed he and his friends did. Parenthetically, I also know that discounting the testimony of adults who were traumatized as children is also devastating: they weren't believed as children; they aren't believed as adults."

"Did you tell her that you believed she was deliberately traumatized?"

"I don't impose my beliefs on any person."

"You didn't answer the question."

"With all due respect Dr. Williams, as I see it, whether or not I believe is not the issue."

"And what about her claim of remembering things that happened before she was three years old?

"There's some good research showing that one to two-year-olds are able to remember specific events. For this reason, I believe we have to give up the assumption that adults can never recall things that happened in infancy."

Dr. Williams didn't give her a chance to give the citation before asking, "Or that Reverend Fisher dressed as Satan? Do you believe that?"

"That's not the issue."

"She's right." One of the clinicians came to her defense. "That's not the issue."

"Thank you," Emily nodded to the psychologist who appeared to be her second ally on the board.

Dr. Williams looked at his watch. "We should be able to hear from Ms. Witherspoon, or whatever her new name is, before lunch." He motioned for the Secretary to bring in the witness.

As her former client came into the room, the defendant stood. "May I introduce Sandy Witherspoon—at her request I am withholding her new legal name—one of the most courageous women I have ever known. She spent almost ten years in therapy with me trying to learn adaptive ways to cope with the sequelae of having been tortured. From what I could observe, the perpetrators of the heinous crimes against this person had tried to destroy her very identity." Emily glanced toward Sandy's father, suddenly having the impulse to run around the table and kick him in the groin but quickly recalled her professional self and sat down.

"Before I tell my story," a healthy-looking, normal-weight Sandy began, "I'd like to say that the more I tried to convince myself those things didn't happen, the more I knew they did. The more I wanted to change what is true . . . the clearer it became . . . my feelings come and go . . . my reactions to what happened come and go . . . but I cannot change what happened to me . . . I cannot change truth."

Glaring at his daughter with maniacal eyes, the Reverend pushed his chair back from the table.

"My abuse . . . no, as Dr. Klein just said, it was torture . . . was not only carried out by men and women in robes appearing to be paying homage to Satan, it was by my father and his friends doing things—I believe mostly for our government, perhaps the CIA—that they didn't want to get caught doing themselves. And the perpetrators enjoyed every minute of it . . . every disgusting sadistic minute. For some reason, they liked terrifying little kids. How much power could they have felt by scaring two-year-olds? They were playing God; creating robots who could service their bodies, even as toddlers; thinking of all the creative ways they could torment. I still feel sick when I think about it. Whether in the name of worshiping Satan or defending our country from the Commies . . . or whatever . . . the harm was done." For the first time, Sandy tried to make eye contact with her father but he was looking down at the floor. "And I'm not the only one it was done to," she said emphatically.

"Just what is the connection between Satanism and the CIA?" the experimental psychologist asked with obvious deriding disbelief.

"This is only my opinion, but I believe that both types of organizations could provide a venue to carry out the vilest forms of child exploitation. And when the government needed guinea pigs for their mind control and medical experiments, what better place to find them than multigenerational satanic cults where the children's training in dissociation was already underway? Now I'm not saying that everybody in the CIA is corrupt. Most, I trust, are looking out for the good of our country. But some, I'm sure, have used their top-secret positions as a cover for their own perversions."

Dr. Williams interrupted. "Notice she said that was her opinion."

"I was told I was doing all this for the President—to help stop Communism. I was taught to provide sexual favors to powerful people who were, in turn, secretly filmed and probably blackmailed and made, I suspect, to give large donations to charitable causes, universities, and politicians. In fact, I've met three women who like me were used in experiments in a secret military complex somewhere up in the mountains—Georgia, North Carolina, South Carolina—I'm not exactly sure where.

"Since I left Chestnut Ridge in December, I've met mothers whose children were ritually abused and used in child pornography in daycare centers. I've even talked with some of the children themselves. And I've met both women and men who're convinced they've had brain implants and some agency is monitoring or perhaps even trying to control their every move. Some who first thought they were UFO abductees got to deeper layers of memories and found the UFO equipment to be a ruse . . . like satanic paraphernalia may have been for others."

Emily broke in. "All this may sound inconceivable if you're hearing it for the first time; however, I'd like to remind you, so did the Holocaust. Persons from the United States, Canada, Europe, and Australia have reported being targets of electronic surveillance and/or experiments using nonlethal weapons for mental and physical attacks. Today's technology—using lasers, acoustic devices, and electromagnetic waves—was described in an article titled, "Wonder Weapons" in the *U.S. News and World Report* magazine in 1997, maybe it was 1998. Is it not possible that such government-developed weapons could've fallen into the hands of various individuals and destructive cults who've learned how to use them for their own purposes?"

Sandy continued. "I'm in a network of survivors from across the country who were tortured in mind control and radiation experiments. Our stories are similar. We recall many of the same places and perpetrators . . . and the hideous ways we were used. Some of us in child pornography—which, no matter how despicable the idea may seem to you, is a business venture of known international scope—often used even by terrorist groups to finance their activities. One of my friends was a black-op for the CIA. She was trained to kill and claimed that before realizing her mind was controlled, she'd been sent to Europe as an assassin. Other survivors, often independently citing the same places and MO's, talk about well-known people in medicine, politics, the entertainment field . . . and even religion who have been part of organized perpetrator groups."

The young woman looked directly at her father some six feet away. "I'll always love the part of you who took care of me after Mother died; who made sure I got dancing and piano lessons; who sent me to college and helped me get my first job. That part I protected all these years in my mind . . . and, in a way, still do. I haven't gone public with my memories. Not until today. And this is supposed to be confidential." She glanced at Dr. Williams. "And I don't want us to wind up in some tabloid or TV talk show." Then back at her father, "I can only assume you didn't choose to hurt me or my therapist . . . and have been coerced into attempting to do so by the people who are trying to keep all these crimes against children silent."

Reverend Fisher was looking at the floor.

"They tried to gain control of my mind by splitting it into many parts. I want to tell you people today that I'd much rather be able to stand here and recant all that I've said . . . I'd much rather believe my therapist made me remember things that were not true . . . than to believe they made me forget things that were."

After fixing each and every person on the board with a singular moment of individual eye contact, one by one, the young woman ended her testimony. "As God is my witness, I stand here today telling you unequivocally: Dr. Emily Klein did not implant false memories, or any memories, in my mind."

Dr. Williams asked, "Are there any questions for Ms. Witherspoon?"

The room was still—except for a whimper coming from the Reverend who had cupped his face in his hands, and the classroom clock Emily heard ticking on the wall at her back.

Or was it her heartbeat finally slowing down?

"Then we'll adjourn," the chairperson said, "and meet back here at two o'clock."

Jeff was waiting in the basement hallway. "How's it going?"

"It's almost over. That's all I can say."

"How about some lunch?"

"My stomach wouldn't take it. Could we just go down and sit by the lake?"

"Sure." Amongst college kids dashing to class, throwing frisbees, and consorting with their laptops or lovers, the Kleins walked across the university's quadrangle.

Sitting on a park bench, Emily picked up a pebble and tossed it into the water. Watching the concentric circles spread wider and wider, she asked, "Jeff, am I a bad person?"

"Don't be ridiculous. You're reacting the way anybody would under these circumstances."

"Do you believe me . . . believe what happened?" A frisbee whizzed past her head, landing in the lake. "Then and now?"

"You know I do. Don't forget, we're in this together. Always have been."

Years ago—before the Bull and the poltergeists and her practice and her own therapy and Jeff's few memories—he probably would've sluffed her off; told her to quit whining, to keep her feelings to herself. Not that he didn't seem to respect them but he'd said he couldn't bear to see her hurting. Or didn't want to admit that when she was vulnerable he felt vulnerable, too.

But today she knew he understood.

"Should I tell them about my memories? Perhaps then they'd believe I know what I'm doing, that I know how to treat others who've had the same types of experiences that I've had."

"If you tell your personal story it could ruin your professional credibility. They might conclude a trauma victim shouldn't be doing trauma work."

"But Jeff, I was never dysfunctional; never missed a day of work except for the surgery in all these years. Granted I was hurt, severely hurt, and for a brief time—before I discovered why my body and mind were reacting the way they did—I'll admit I acted a little crazy at first. But I was never in the bad shape my mother claimed I was, unless finally being able to feel—and show those feelings—is abnormal."

"You don't have to convince me, Em. I know you're stable. You're a fighter. And you can be pretty aggressive when you have a cause. But you know me, I believe it's sometimes best to just stand pat: not to run; but not to deliberately pick a fight either. Some of those jokers on the board, the uninformed ones, might really think it's madness for a person to go on trying to help at the constant risk of her own—"

"So you do think I'm nuts, huh?"

"Not I, madame. However I don't know what your less experienced colleagues would think. But then again, so what? If 99 percent of the world believed you were a virtual nutcase—as wife, mother, daughter, or therapist—what difference would it make to the truth?"

"Well, a lot . . . if they get my license. But I'd rather be nuts than believe the reality of such evil. I'd rather go back to the days of our innocence—maybe everyone's innocence—when we thought no evil of that extent could exist in a quiet little town like ours. I'd give up all the material blessings I have if I could change the way our personal family histories have turned out to be."

"Me too, Em."

Centered, as though balancing the burdens of all her clients on her shoulders, the psychologist—left hand on the rail, right hand under the arm of her childhood sweetheart—descended the stairs to judgment.

"I love you," he said.

"I love you." She left him in the hallway, restless on a straight-backed wooden chair. In the light beaming from a ground-level, bar-protected window, remnants of auburn glistened through his fluffy white hair.

When everyone in the conference room was seated, Dr. Williams looked at the defendant. "Dr. Klein. Is there anything else you would like to say to the board?"

"Thank you. Yes, I would." And there she was surprising herself, standing before her peers making a speech prepared by . . . perhaps one of those parts of herself whom it had taken so long for her to acknowledge and honor:

"For nearly two decades I have sat almost daily with adult clients who relive with terror the screams of their childhoods. They tell of secret groups who traumatize little children. Mr. Fisher"—she just couldn't call him Reverend . . . or Father—"has claimed that I implanted false memories in his daughter. He was not my client. His daughter was. And she told me of horrible things he and his friends did to her. You have heard her side of the story, so I ask each of you: Do you believe it's possible for me or any other therapist to convince you that you were molested as a child—if you were not? Therapy isn't about convincing people that horrible things happened to them. It's about empowering them to do what they need to do in order to recover and move on. I can't imagine, even if it were possible, why therapists would implant horrible memories. Don't you think if they had that much control over someone, it would be much better to imbue positive attitudes?

"There are other questions I ask you to consider before you pass judgment on my competence as a psychologist. How can you explain the accounts of adults who recover memories of sexual abuse before they enter therapy? How do you explain the behaviors of children now living in protected environments who can't stop the flood of memories, the nightmares, the excruciating body sensations; who can't understand why big people in masks made them, as they say, do yucky things?

"To my knowledge, no one has ever offered a satisfactory alternative explanation for why certain people report images and memories of torture by organized groups including those using the trappings of Satanism. If it's not real, how can we account for the sheer number and consistency of reports and symptom-patterns from all parts of the nation? And from other countries as well. How can I account for reports from people who have never met each other naming the same perpetrators?"

The defendant paused, toying with the idea of telling the board about Linda Lou Lackey and the Bull; telling them how Lou had fingered Jake Lentz; telling them about her own spiritual journey. But a voice in her head—this time it sounded like Jeff's—said, "No!"

She went on. "Horrific memories are imprinted—not implanted—in the minds of vulnerable children. Some store those memories in mental closets for decades until they can find a safe time and place to let them come out. I beg you, please don't take away my legal right to provide a place to listen to their stories, and if necessary, hear their screams, and help them find their own kind of peace."

The accused sat down.

"Thank you. Does the board have any further questions?" the chairperson asked with perfunctory courtesy.

The room was as quiet as Lentz Mill Pond on a windless night.

Looking at Dr. Klein for the last time, Dr. Williams announced: "This board has ninety days to render a decision on your case. We'll send you our verdict by certified mail. Thank you for coming."

On the way back to the parking lot, the levee which had stood to block her tears of relief, rage, sadness, joy, worry, hope—all the emotions she rarely allowed herself to feel—caved in.

Her husband said nothing to disrupt the catharsis.

Settled in the car at last, Emily sighed, "What can I say? What can I do? It's out of my hands. I wonder if anyone on the board heard what I was trying to say or if they'd already made up their minds."

Jeff turned on the ignition. Leaving the gear in park and his mind in neutral, he listened.

"From the questions they asked, I'd bet the two clinicians and the kindergarten teacher are supportive. The HMO reviewer clearly expressed his feelings about memories and private therapists. And if the experimental psychologist doesn't know the research showing how traumatic memories are processed differently from normal memories and that infants do remember and that patients have corroborated memories uncovered with the help of hypnosis, he'll probably be inclined to agree with the few studies showing that spurious, nontraumatic memories can be suggested in a laboratory situation. Now I'm sure Charles would go the way that would serve his own best interests."

When she finally paused for a breath, Jeff quipped, "Perhaps we should offer to endow a psychology chair in his name." He turned the car's motor back off and waited patiently for his wife to talk and talk and talk until she had nothing more to say.

"The accountant has no idea what the controversy is all about and will probably base his vote on whether or not he likes me. Even after all these years of working with clients and working through my own trauma, I still want to believe what the HMO guy was saying. Because

I want to believe that my childhood was unblemished. That my parents were loving and caring."

"We don't get to pick our parents, my dear wife. Nobody does. Neither did Cleat."

It was the first time she could ever remember hearing him use his father's given name.

"I've loved you all my waking life, Em . . . but never more than I do this very moment, right now. Right here and now."

Jeff started the engine and backed out of the parking space. They headed toward home through a world ablaze with fragrant colors. Pink dogwoods and azaleas, yellow buttercups and forsythia were dressing up southern yards for the coming Easter Day. Magenta Judas trees spattered the greening woods.

Turning into the driveway, he noticed a white blossom in a bush under the front window. "Look Hon, a gardenia. They don't usually open till June."

"That's odd," Emily said, suddenly feeling as if a wand had brushed her heart. In her head, she heard a clear polished feminine voice saying:

"Everything will be just fine."

Chapter 50

When Jeff opened the basement door, molecules of lingering cat pee, cigar smoke, mildew, and alcohol drifted up the stairwell. It was difficult to tell what was real and what was memory.

At first he had made up his mind that the demolition crew could just bury the junk in his daddy's basement; however, returning from the airport after taking Emily to catch a flight to Santa Fe, he'd changed his mind and decided to go through the apartment one last time. After Cleat died, he'd donated the property to the YMCA who'd been looking for a site to put a skateboard park. They didn't have money in the budget to demolish the duplex and the woodworking shop, so Jeff had volunteered to clean up the place.

He'd already hauled most of the furniture and clothes over to the Goodwill Store. The local Habitat for Humanity organization would be coming by to pick up any salvageable construction materials.

Jeff pulled out his billfold and flipped through an accumulation of credit cards, ID's, and a few snapshots of the children and grandchildren. He couldn't help but smile at a black and white studio proof of Emily's high school senior picture with SAMPLE stamped across it. The yellowed business card touting *CK Custom Furniture* was on the bottom of the stack. Could it really have been a dozen years he'd carried that combination around with him?

Standing under the stairs in front of the gun safe, Jefferson Klein was a little boy again about to mess around in forbidden territory.

Left to 99 four times . . . Right to 29 three times . . . Left to 54 two times . . . Full right until dial reaches positive stopping point.

The door opened to an interior covered with deep purple crushed velvet. There was not a single gun in the whole safe. Cigar boxes with duct tape holding them closed and army green ammo boxes were stacked about four feet high.

Five rusted cans of 16mm film sat on the top shelf. He picked up the one labeled, "The Wedding." Whose wedding? he wondered. Taking out all the cannisters and placing them on the old table, he was already making plans to check out a compatible projector from the college media center. Who knows? Maybe he would see his mother.

His eyes drew his hands to the ammo boxes. Each had a dime-store padlock protecting its contents. He looked around the room for something to force them open. Not seeing anything, he went upstairs and out to his truck where he found just what was needed.

Back in the basement, with urgency in his gut and a tire iron in his hand, he took the ammo boxes out of the safe and pounded on one of the locks until it popped open.

Perhaps he should've just closed the first box, but he didn't. Perhaps he shouldn't have cracked open the rest of the boxes, but he did. Sitting under a single dim light bulb, the son looked through the father's warped eyes at hundreds of pictures of naked children, infants even — seeing, feeling, and knowing the terror in their eyes as they were being posed for and pushed into unthinkable acts of degradation.

Why would Cleat have wanted Jeff to have the combination to that safe of iniquity? Were the contents supposed to be his inheritance? Or was it some kind of sick joke the old man had played on his way out?

Jeff didn't even bother to open the cigar boxes. Whatever was there, he didn't care. It could've been cash, government bonds, old deeds, anything. He didn't want to ever again have to harbor anything that had touched Cleat Klein's filthy hands.

Neither did he want anyone from Habitat for Humanity to come across the pornography. That would be embarrassing, to say the least.

He stacked the boxes in a couple of old wooden orange crates and put the films in a paper grocery bag he'd found on a shelf above the *Playboys.* It took him two or three trips to get everything out to the truck.

One man's treasure is another man's trash, Jeff was thinking as he tossed the boxes into the trash compactor at the county landfill. Feeling dirty, ashamed. Whatever his unconscious or conscious motivation had been, he was abhorred that he had succumbed to his base instinct, his almost compulsive need to 'taste the forbidden fruit.'

Evil lurks in Everyman.

He could've chalked up his behavior to research. How can moral people fight child pornography if they don't know what it's really all about? he rationalized.

As he picked up the last box, a cigar box which was much lighter than the others, a horrible thought crossed his mind: If a policeman, say, a Tom Paxton, had caught me with child pornography in my possession on the way to the dump, I could've been locked up for a long time.

His hand turned loose of the box. Just before the big crunch, he noticed a faded label stuck to the lid on which his daddy had written in his infamous backhand, "Letters from KC - 1942."

KC . . . CK. Cleat Klein. That's crazy. Why would the old man have saved his own letters? he wondered, walking back to the truck.

KC.

His heart seemed to tumble in his chest.

Katherine Campbell.

They had to have been his mother's words in that box.

All gone.

Crushed.

Chapter 51

*D*rive slowly to avoid potholes.

Turn right at first gravel road. Road narrows. Veer left then right, down steeply. Then up. Heading always toward mountains. Pass white dog in middle of road where it curves sharply. Turn right at top of hill. Follow narrow dirt lane to tall cedar tree. Go left.

"I made it!" Emily rejoiced when she finally spied the sign at the entrance to the *Center for Restoration*. The directions Kate had sent were perfect, down to the dog in the middle of the road which had undauntedly, taking its own good time, stood up and moved to the ditch to let her pass. When she had looked into the rearview mirror, it was already back in position, sitting sentry.

At the locked gate, she braked the rental car and punched the speaker button. "Emily Klein has arrived."

"Happy birthday," Kate answered. "Welcome to Santa Fe. You can drive on up to the main lodge—it's straight ahead—and I'll give you a key to your cabin. Actually, it's not exactly yours. You'll be sharing it with seven other men and women."

Emily parked in front of a century-old adobe farmhouse surrounded by piñon and juniper trees. She walked into a walled garden courtyard full of people who, until this moment, had been faceless names on their Internet list. They were from a dozen states and Canada, Germany, the UK, Israel, Sweden, the Netherlands, and South Africa; from clergy, law enforcement, social work, psychology, psychiatry, general medicine, journalism, law, and academia; both mainline and conservative Christians, Jews, Humanists, and Atheists; people of different ages trying to respect each other's political and spiritual beliefs, unifying for a common cause; professionals, many who were trauma survivors themselves, coming together to chart a course for exposing, for combating the personal, religious, political, and commercial exploitation of children.

In addition to her Internet group, she had heard about networks of therapists, clergy, and other professionals who meet in secret to discuss things they can do to help and/or protect victims of crimes against children, to get information out in a context to which the general population can relate. Why secret meetings? Because when the meetings were public, the presenters and participants had often been harassed; their offices toxed with pesticides, herbicides, and other chemicals; their lives and the lives of their children threatened. Like computer hackers, a few of these people have infiltrated destructive groups and are collecting anecdotal data via hidden cameras and tapes that will someday be made known. Therapists and clergy and untainted law enforcement officers, not as flummoxed as their detractors would probably like to believe, are collaboratively amassing large bodies of information about this hidden holocaust.

One day, hopefully soon, the world will know!

The conference was unlike any Emily had ever attended.

Kate and her staff provided a breakfast every morning of milk and coffee, seasonal fruits, yogurt, and various cereals and cheeses. Surrounded by a library of spiritual and psychological writings, the place was traditional Santa Fe with rough-sawn vigas and latillas overhead; a floor of wide planks worn smooth by years of use and polished to a shiny warm glow; a beehive fireplace in one corner; three walls decorated with artwork by Native American artists and former and present residents of the center. On the fourth wall was a sign printed with the same mocking words that were on the sign that had hung over Jonestown two decades earlier when Jim Jones, leader of the Peoples Temple cult, had ordered 913 followers, including 270 children, to drink cyanide-poisoned punch.

There were no leaders; no formal presentations. For three days and a greater part of the nights, a cadre of crusaders in pairs and small groups—frequently intermingling with residents who'd come to Santa Fe as part of their spiritual journeys—walked, talked, plotted, and sometimes prayed together.

On Sunday evening, exactly twelve hours before Timothy McVeigh —the thirty-three-year-old Desert Storm veteran who had rationalized the killing of children in the Oklahoma City bombing as "collateral damage"—was scheduled to be strapped to an execution gurney, an extemporaneous discussion was held in the common room.

Waiting at the open window for everyone to come into the room, Emily gazed out across the high desert wilderness and its multicolored rock formations, listening to the stillness of the sunset. She felt someone tapping her shoulder. "Hey girl. What did you think about the conference?" Kate asked.

"It was wonderful, terrific, inspiring, energy producing, but there's one thing I didn't like about it."

"What's that?"

"You and I didn't get to spend any time together."

"Then why don't you just stay a little longer?"

"I'd love to but Jeff and I are planning to spend the whole month of July at the beach celebrating our anniversary—"

"Which one?"

"Can you believe, our fortieth? He's been thinking about retiring at the end of the year, and who knows, I may have to retire too, depending on what the decision of the Psychology Board is."

"When do you think you'll hear from them?"

"By the middle of July anyway. Their ninety days will be up."

"They're not going to take your license," Kate said with assurance.

"I appreciate your optimism. But to tell you the truth, I just don't know how it will turn out."

When everyone was in the room and seated in a circle, Kate opened the meeting.

Throughout the evening Emily took a few notes, made a few comments, but mostly just listened:

—I don't know if it involved creating multiple personalities, but on a national radio show last year Gordon Cooper, one of the seven original astronauts, disclosed that in the '50s and '60s NASA involved gifted children in a mind control program designed to develop their psychic abilities.

—Amazing. Whatever for?

—He said that it was in case we ever needed some way to communicate with extraterrestrial beings. Who knows what terrible things the kids might have gone through under the guise of National Security?

—What about the claim that because the government did it, therapists can also make someone MPD?

—That's malarkey. Very few of us, if any, have access to or know how to use drugs, electroshock, or other aversive techniques to alter people's minds.

—Or have unlimited access to clients. You can't tell me that asking a person if they were abused in their daddy's bedroom or in a satanic cult or in a laboratory is going to make them remember being raped or ritually abused.

—Or make them have panic attacks or severe headaches or shake all over when remembering the traumas.

—There must've been some major flaws in the early experiments. Why else would ex-subjects have been marching into our offices?

—Yeah. I'm wondering if their experiments also produced some wild cannons, perhaps like those criminals out there bombing federal buildings and shooting up school houses. It was rumored that McVeigh had an implant somewhere in his body but since he requested no autopsy, we'll never know, will we?

—In my opinion, the greatest enemy to us is our own profession. Like all those hospitals who under fear of lawsuits quit treating DID's.

—No they didn't. They just give another diagnosis to avoid getting sued.

—Same with psychiatrists and therapists who've defected from the field; who've quit using hypnosis or other techniques to access dissociated parts; who've quit helping clients uncover memories they so desperately want.

—But I'd venture to bet there are still hundreds, probably thousands, like us around the world who continue to treat survivors, whether they've been ritually abused in destructive cults or robots of shadow governments.

—As we all know, there are no quick fixes. From my experience, a person's healing usually comes because of the relationship, not by any specific techniques. It comes through the therapist's ability to receive and work with what the client brings to the sanctity of the therapy room.

—That's it in a nutshell. I don't believe anyone, including so-called experts who don't see validity in a treatment unless its efficacy has been proven in scientific research, has all the answers. Just because we don't always know why it works is no reason to deride the successes of interventions using EMDR or the various energy therapies such as EFT, TFT, even theophostic prayer and process healing or other mind-body or spiritual healing techniques.

—Hey listen. I'm not a therapist. I'm a cop. Can someone please tell me what all those letters mean?

—Let me think: EMDR stands for Eye Movement Desensitization and Reprocessing; EFT, Emotional Freedom Techniques; and TFT is Thought Field Therapy. I'm sure if you go "googling" on the Internet, you'll find everything you need to know about them.

—So what do you guys think about the deliverance procedures used by some Christian counselors? The ones who believe in a literal devil.

—Well I've never been to an exorcism, but a colleague of mind said that if you've ever witnessed one by a team of caregivers like he did, you'd have no difficulty believing in demonic forces.

—That may be true for your colleague but since I don't believe in a God or a Devil, I'm sure there's another explanation. Those of us who work with clients who've remembered being brainwashed in satanic rites have no trouble believing in the power of evil. Somehow we need to stop the misconception that cult and ritual trauma is only inflicted by Satanists. Any secret or closed group or organization has the potential for shielding perps.

—Or that it happens only in this country.

—From what I've learned over the years, ritual abuse of children is a worldwide phenomenon. I know of a fairly recent study in Germany documenting 354 cases in treatment. And a special commission over there studying cults found what they call 'split data' because of the discrepancy between what therapists are hearing from survivors of cult crimes and the lack of evidence that police are finding. Even so, they recommended that police get special training about the phenomenon of ritual abuse.

—Wow! That's more than our U.S Government is doing.

—To make any headway in exposing these evil activities, we'll have to show what we've learned in a manner that has context to the general population. In my practice, I'm seeing what I believe to be a common denominator: child pornography.

—Me too. I believe what we're dealing with in many instances is the commercialization of child abuse. I read somewhere that the U.S. Customs Service estimates 100,000 websites are involved in some way with child pornography.

—That many? To stop it, there's got to be worldwide cooperation among law enforcement agencies like we had with the Russian authorities in Operation Blue Orchid. They were able to close a Russian website that was offering custom-made videos for 5,000 dollars a piece. Whatever the buyers wanted, they could get.

—An article came out in *Der Spiegel*, a German news-magazine, last September reporting that several persons were arrested in Rome and Moscow who were part of an international child pornography ring that distributed pictures of violence, torture, and murder via the Internet. It said some of the victims were younger than a year. The movies were sold in Germany, the States, Italy, and Russia for up to six-thousand dollars apiece.

—You folks may remember reading about the serial-killer Marc Dutroux in Belgium. About four years ago police found three hundred or more videotapes in his basement depicting sexual crimes against children. News stories circulating at the time suggested ties to organized crime, satanic ritual connections, and involvement of the upper crust of society in sex orgies and viewing of snuff movies.

—How can anyone deny that ritual abuse goes on when it's right there on film?

—Just watch Germany. They can deny it all the way. When that huge pedo-network based in Italy was busted and they found videos of killings that had gone over the Internet—parts were shown on Italian TV just to prove this exists, and of course people lost their jobs over it—the German police immediately pointed out that these scenes had not reached Germany . . . as if the Internet stopped at the borders.

—Did any of you see the special article in *Newsweek* in March called "The Web's Dark Secret"? It told about a Catholic priest and three colleagues in Sicily who found photos on the Internet of child rape involving toddlers and infants—

—They better watch out. One thing that makes child pornographers so difficult to prosecute is because people who are curious to see what it's all about run the risk of getting arrested themselves. From what I understand, just clicking on such a website renders one liable to prosecution.

—I'd say that the Internet, even with its risks, makes it easy for the pedophile. They can chat with friends of like mind—don't even have to belong to a local group—they make friends around the world, meet vulnerable children online, do the traditional grooming by E-mail, and setup a place to abduct victims . . . all in the click of a mouse.

—I just had a thought. Perhaps the computer which makes it so easy to partake of kiddie porn will be the pedophile's downfall. What with the way they like to keep detailed records of who and when and where and how many times they've sexually exploited a kid, it's possible those records will someday be found on their hard drives, giving us all the evidence we need to bring those criminals to justice.

—If we could stop the traffic, if they didn't make money, it could possibly kill much of the pornography-based ritual abuse.

—Maybe so. But sadly, in my opinion, most of the burden of proof is on the children who've grown up and are working the streets; those in prisons and mental hospitals; those in therapy offices; and those who, if they're lucky, have been helped by supportive community or church organizations.

—It's easy for us to see children in pornography as faceless names (as in Internet chat rooms) or nameless faces (as on porn sites). But what if one of those faces belongs to the little girl abducted from her bedroom with her parents sleeping down the hall? Or, heaven forbid, your own child or grandchild or niece or nephew who was entrusted to the care of a priest, a camp director, Social Services, a day-care teacher? Would you have the courage of the parents in Europe—whose children reported being filmed as they were ritually abused in day-care settings—to sift through a database of pornographic images looking for your child's picture? I know of at least one mother in Europe who identified her child in an Interpol lineup.

—The atrocity is global. And images of children tortured, shamed, humiliated, and silenced in pornography are its most visible and prosecutable evidence. However, unless there are admissions of guilt or criminal convictions, sexual predators wearing black robes, white coats, military uniforms, biker shorts, or nothing at all may forever be able to cry, "False!" to the claims their accusers make regarding previously dissociated memories of sexual trauma: whether it occurred in the child's bedroom with only two people present or in a ritually-abusing cult chanting the mantra, "If you tell you die," or in a university laboratory, or on a military base working for 'Uncle Sam.'

—One of my clients used to fantasize about surfing the Net and finding photographs of her 'marriage to Satan' when she was seven years old, or videos of her thirteenth birthday party when she was 'laid bare' to the elders in the local cult. Actually doing such a thing would be a no-no. Peaking on to porno sites to unmask criminals would be at the risk of my client herself going to prison.

—I wonder what would happen if pedophiles or groups of pedophiles continue to make slip-ups as they did in Wonderland and

Blue Orchid, and the pictorial records of their crimes against children show up in the hands of some law enforcement agent with integrity.

—Or if law enforcement agencies would use computer technology to cross match images found on porn sites with faces of missing children, or faces of children reporting recent exploitation, or childhood pictures of adults who remember having been filmed in sexual scenes as children.

—Or if a vigilante group whose mission is to track and take down child porn sites on the Internet was given the legal authority to view the sites and collect the faces of the children to post for anyone who is interested in trying to identify and rescue the victims.

—What if we could infiltrate the playground of pedophiles and snare them in their own Web?

It was almost midnight when Kate stood up to close the conference. "I just want to thank all of you who've helped make this retreat a success. There's one more thing I want to say, and I trust it doesn't get lost amidst all the horror we've talked about in the last few days. From my perspective as a psychologist, I know, as Coffey asserted in her book, *Unspeakable Truths and Happy Endings*, there can be positive outcomes for those who survived heinous crimes; for those who are willing and able to learn about their pasts in order to find peace in the present; and especially for those who are fortunate enough to find someone to listen compassionately and sensibly to their stories of having been intentionally traumatized."

A couple of the clergy in the group said, "Amen."

And Emily used the opportunity to tell the group a little about her sister, the Honorable Margaret Rucker-Volz: "With your indulgence, I'd like to quote from an unwitting initiate into organized evil whose battle cry was "Hopeless Optimism," who won the war in her mind, and is no longer dominated by the aftermath of human cruelty. When I was talking with this person recently, she commented with conviction 'The more I know, the more I tell, the better I feel.'"

After saying good-byes to her friends and colleagues, Emily headed toward the door. Crossing the threshold, she turned around to ponder, one last time, the sign hanging on the opposite wall:

**THOSE WHO DO NOT
REMEMBER THE PAST
ARE CONDEMNED TO REPEAT IT**

Chapter 52

I want him dead. I want him dead.

Whom did she want dead? Her unthought-thought didn't make sense.

Crystal's daddy, the old pervert, had been dead almost three months. Her daddy was long gone.

Cleat was gone.

Uncle Phil was too old to matter.

Jimmy. He might as well have been dead because she didn't expect to ever hear from him again.

For just a second, she wondered if there was an ego state who didn't understand Jeff's love for her; who was only remembering something that may have happened in the past.

I want him dead.

Emily really didn't want to delve into this. Afraid of what she might find. But the thought was keeping her awake at night.

1:30 . . . 2:30 . . . 3:30 . . .

Summer had begun.

Sometime before daylight Emily sat down at the computer to get in touch with whatever part of her wanted 'him' dead, whoever 'him' was. Lightly touching the keyboard, the internal dialogue seemed to appear automatically, brain to screen.

> Tell me. Who wants who dead? I've got to know. And why.
> Who's talking?
> Me.
> Who's me?
> Emma Wee.
> How old are you?
> About five.

Who are you afraid of?
Tommy?
Tommy. Why?
He's mean.
What did he do?

Her body was beginning to ache all over and she felt as if she'd been tied up and confined for a very long time.

It is hot summer around dusk and a bunch of neighborhood kids are in the Lentz yard playing hot-summer-around-dusk games like Kick-the-Can, Capture-the-Flag, and Snake-in-the-Gully. Jeff is there because his grandmother has come to play bridge. Tommy is also there. He lives way across town but sometimes his daddy drops him off to play with her brother Jimmy who is ten years old. Gladys had asked Jimmy to watch out after his little sister and their cousin, Dave Keller, Jr., who is Emily's age.

"Let's play war," Jimmy suggests after everybody but Emily, Tom, Jeff, and Dave have left. "Me and Tommy and Dave, we'll be the Krauts. Jeff, you and my little sister can be the Yanks."

"I want to be Hitler," Tommy yells, rubbing some black dirt under his nose for a mustache. "Emily and Jeff can be our prisoners. And Jimmy, you can be my general. Dave, you're the guard."

Seven-year-old Tommy Paxton has taken over control of the play group.

Neither Jeff nor Emily seem to realize they have a choice in the matter and simply obey orders as Hitler and the general and the guard march them around to the back of the white house on Main Street, forcing them to climb the outside steps to the storage area above the car shed.

Someone pulls a chain to turn on the single light bulb that is hanging from a rafter.

At Hitler's command the general puts some type of blindfold over Emily's eyes and ties her to a bench. Somebody takes her shorts and panties off—

The frightened little girl goes away in her mind . . .

She comes back to hear Jeff screaming, "No! No! Don't." The general rips off her blindfold.

"Hitler says watch," the general tells Emily, turning her head toward a table where Jeff is lying with his arms tied behind his back, his legs held apart by the guard, as Hitler, holding a Boy Scout knife in his hand is—

"Please don't! It hurts!" Jeff screams again. Hitler looks around the place until he finds an old oily rag to stuff in his prisoner's mouth. "That'll keep you quiet, Mr. Klein."

All the time Hitler is carving on Jeff, Jimmy is stimulating his sister's, sweet spot with his finger; all the time making sure Emily's eyes are on her sweetheart.

Watching blood gush over the splintered floor, Emily hears the little Hitler speaking to Jeff in a deep false voice. "See that cute little girl over there with the big brown eyes, your little friend . . . well I think I'll just take her away from you."

Emily stared at the words on the screen. It couldn't have happened like that, she argued with the part of her unconscious that had released the story.

It had to be a metaphor.

But it wasn't, her body had already begun to say when she first remembered the knife in Tommy's hand headed toward Jeff's groin and Jimmy's finger in her vagina.

Pain paired with pleasure.

Could it be that the out-of-place sexual surge that often came over her when she believed she had done something wrong, or felt threatened, was a body memory of this horrible war game from long ago?

———————

A little after dawn, Emily was sitting in front of the Little Country Market on the outskirts of town. At seven o'clock the longtime proprietor opened up the window boards.

"Good mornin', Miz Klein. Come on in. How can I help you today?"

"Well, Mr. Buck, I woke up this morning thinking I'd like to fix a good country supper tonight for my kids and grandkids. You know, like my mama used to do."

"Ah yeah. I remember your mama. Fine Christian woman she was. Used to bring you in here with her when you weren't no bigger than a June bug." He pointed to several baskets filled with peaches. "Those are freestone. Picked this mornin' fresh out o' my own orchard."

"They sure look good." Emily picked one up and rolled it around in her hand. Bringing it to her nose she said, "Smells good too. Give me about a peck, would you please?" she asked, already knowing how she was going to use them.

"Yes ma'am. What else?"

"Let me just look around a little." She picked up a hand-basket and stepped over to a crate of corn still in its husks. "This white or yellow?"

"White Silver Queen. It's kinda out of style now. Most folks around here have gone back to yellow but I still like the white."

"Me too. I'll take two dozen ears. My grandkids love it on the cob and I'll use the rest to stew with some of that good-looking okra and tomatoes over there. Add a little onion and that's my favorite summer dish. Mama used to fix it all the time."

As Mr. Buck was picking out the corn, Emily walked up and down the aisles filling small plastic bags with okra, tomatoes, a couple of Vidalia onions, a mess of green beans, and a handful of cucumbers.

There was something wonderful about going down to the little produce stand and loading up with fresh vegetables and fruit right off the local Carolina farms.

Almost spiritual.

Cleansing.

———————

Making ice cream. Homemade ice cream. You peel the peaches and mash them up good. You mix a cup of sugar, a little bit of flour, add a dash of salt and about two cups of milk and cook it in a double boiler till it gets thick. You add a small amount of this hot mixture into two beaten eggs and put it all back in the pan together, cooking and stirring over low heat for a minute. You add a pint of whipping cream and a tablespoon of vanilla. Then you cool it off, stir in the peaches, and pour it all into the freezer can.

That's how you did it in the days when nobody worried about cholesterol and fat grams or too many calories.

That's how Gladys did it. When the mixture was ready, she'd tell Emily to call her daddy and ask him to bring home a block of ice and some ice cream salt. Emily would pick up the black phone receiver off its base and speak to the operator: "7-6-W, please." Her daddy would answer the phone at the slaughterhouse and say, "Jake Lentz speaking. How can I help you?" And Emily would answer, "Mama said—"

———————

The modern Klein clan—Jeff, Emily, Matt, Carol, Brad, Winslow and Alison—had just finished eating a good country dinner cooked up by Gammy on her day off and were still sitting around the dining room table.

"Imagine," Emily said, "my mother used to cook a dinner like this everyday. That was back in the days when the largest meal was served at noon. Except she'd always have some type of scrumptious home-baked dessert: fruit pies in season, a variety of cakes and custards, or maybe even brownies or different kinds of cookies."

"Just so happens," Jeff had stood up to take his plate to the kitchen, "we've got a big surprise dessert for this evening."

"What is it, Pop?" Winslow asked.

"Wait a minute." He went into the kitchen and came back carrying an old green bucket with rusty metal bands barely holding the pieces of wood together. Opening the lid of the freezer can sitting in it, he motioned for his granddaughters to come over and look. "Do you know what that is?"

They both looked puzzled.

"It's ice cream," he said.

"No it's not," Alison giggled. "It's too wunny."

"Yes it is," said Pop. "But there's some work you kids have to do first. And we have to go outside to do it."

"From what I remember," Matt said, "it's compulsory to make ice cream under a big shade tree. Too bad the old oak's gone. I'll take some lawn chairs out and we can sit under the pines."

Jeff said, "Sounds like a good idea, son. Brad, could you bring a cooler full of ice from the ice maker? Carol, you get the bowls. That leaves the napkins and spoons for Winslow and Alison and we're set to go."

Emily said, "I think I'll go call the Weavers to come over and join us." She looked at her grandchildren. "They always came over when my mother and daddy made ice cream in the back yard. Dick made the parties so special with his war stories and magic tricks, like pulling pennies out of my ear or—"

"Can he pull a penny out of my ear?" Alison squealed.

"We'll have to see about that." Emily handed Winslow the napkins; Alison, the spoons. "Now y'all go on outside and help Pop and I'll bring the salt."

A dying custom, Emily thought, watching Jeff adjust the dasher and cover then pack the crushed ice around the can.

"Who wants to be the first turner?" Jeff asked.

"I do," Alison shouted.

"Okay. Winslow, you can be the first sitter." He placed a folded towel over the ice.

"But my bottom'll get cold."

"That's part of the job," Matt teased.

Carol showed Alison how to turn the crank.

"Faster," Brad said. "Fast as you can."

After a few minutes of hard work, Alison's rosy cheeks were getting rosier.

"Time to change places with your sister," Jeff said, adding more ice to maintain the ice level and adding more salt to make the ice melt around the can.

Twenty or thirty minutes later the mixture began to freeze and the crank got too hard for either of the girls to turn.

"It's getting there," Matt said.

"Let me try," Brad grinned. "We didn't do this where I came from."

"Then you don't know what you missed, my dear brother-in-law. Just wait till you taste it."

"Good evening everybody." Sue Weaver was calling from the deck. "Thanks for asking us over."

"Come on down," Jeff called back.

"We don't get invited to many social events anymore and y'all know there's no place we'd rather be than with this fine family," Dick said when they reached the group.

Sue gave Emily one of her encompassing hugs, then stooped over to hug Alison and Winslow.

"I have to get one, too, from all the pretty little ladies," Dick said, also bending down. First Winslow, then Alison got a running start and jumped into his extended arms. "My, my, y'all sure take after you're grandmother. We practically raised her, you know. Did I ever tell you that?"

Carol and Matt looked at each other, but neither bothered to remind the aging man how many times he'd taken credit for helping their mother grow up to be the person she was.

"Will you get a penny out of my ear, Mr. Weaver?" Alison asked. "Pwease."

"Sure thing." Dick reached into his pocket then put his hand up to the little girl's ear. "Here it is." He showed her the penny in the palm of his hand.

"Do it again! Do it again!" she shrieked.

Before Dick had a chance to perform the trick again, Jeff called, "Come and get it!"

Brad and Matt helped him scoop out the ice around the can. Carefully removing the lid, Jeff tried to keep from getting salt in the ice cream. "Who wants to scrape the dasher?" he asked.

"We do." With spoons in their hands, the little girls were ready to go.

"It's de-wish-ous," said Alison, taking the first bite.

"Scrumptious," said Winslow.

And in the dusk of day, representatives of four generations replayed the wholesome traditions: eating homemade, hand-turned peach ice cream; remembering the good ol' days—embellishing its truths; swatting mosquitos; catching lightning bugs and putting them in an old blue Mason jar; and eating more homemade, hand-turned peach ice cream.

Chapter 53

It was their time to be old.

Two people—like the Bible says—joined as one, celebrating a life together. And celebrating the recent news: "We are pleased to inform you that the Psychology Board has found no evidence . . .."

Having just finished a very private dinner of roasted shrimp and oysters, the Kleins were on the upper deck of the beach cottage, rocking in sync, gazing at the cloud-veiled moon slowly rising over the ocean.

"Forty years. That's a long time to live with one woman." Jeff made his updated anniversary comment.

"Maybe for you," Emily said, "but everything turned out just fine, didn't it?" She reached for the hand of her beloved.

"Yes it did," he agreed.

They went on rocking. Rocking and reminiscing until Jeff said, "I think I'll go inside and run one of those old films I found in Dad's basement."

The librarian at the college had showed him how to thread them on an old 16mm projector which he had borrowed for the summer. Turns out, with all the time it had been taking to finish up the school year, and all the time it had been taking to clean up Cleat's messes, he hadn't had any opportunity to use it.

"It'd do my heart good to find something with my mother on it. Will you come watch them with me?"

"Sure. There's nothing else to do before we go to bed."

"And then we can—" He stood, pulling her up with him. They went into the second story foyer and down the steps to the living room. She waited patiently as he set up the projector on the card table.

"'The Wedding,'" Jeff read the label on the first cannister he picked up. "Let's see what's on this one."

While he threaded the antiquated machine, his wife basked in the freeing sensation of having been exonerated by her peers. She was not a bad person who had wanted to make money by implanting false memories of sexual abuse and other crimes in Sandy Witherspoon. She was even thinking about writing a book about her experience as a survivor/therapist when the picture finally reached the wall—hanging upside down.

Again she waited patiently as her husband re-threaded the film.

10-9-8-7-6-5-4-3-2-1—

"The Wedding," in jerky black and white, flashed in front of their eyes:

—*a little boy and a little girl standing side by side facing the camera.*

—*the 'bride' in a long white lacy dress and white shiny shoes with bows on the top. A glimmering headpiece rests over her long curls.*

—*the 'groom' in a jacket, bow tie, and knickers.*

They're standing under an arbor of wisteria vines. A man walks over and stands in front of the children with his back to the camera. He's wearing a white robe over a black skirt, white shoes, and black gloves.

The wall went black for a second, then a different scene appeared:

—*candlelight flickers on a stained-glass window; palm trees all around; painted ocean on the wall.*

—*the little girl is placed on the table.*

"I can't watch anymore," Jeff whispered, reaching for the switch.

"No, don't!" Emily screamed. "I have to watch. I have to see the truth."

He stuck his hand in his pocket and closed his eyes.

—*someone lifts the dress over the little girl's eyes and pulls her panties down.*

—*someone pulls off the little boy's knickers and underwear and places him on top of the little girl.*

"No, don't!" Emily screamed again.

Jeff opened his eyes.

—the little boy is kicking.
—a hand with a missing finger comes down over his buttocks.

"That's enough. You can turn it off now." Emily stood up and walked out to the deck, down the steps, and across the boardwalk. She took off running down the beach toward the pier.

Powered by a lifetime of pent-up rage, Jeff ripped the short film off the reel, entangling it in his fingers, and carried it outside to the patio.

After cooling down a little, he wadded the porn into a ball and slung it down on the still hot grill, the makeshift grill Cleat had rigged so long ago from four concrete blocks and a piece of sheet metal.

The sins of the fathers sizzled, curled up, and melted to obscurity.

He caught up with her just before she reached the end of the pier, surrounding her with his love; holding her strongly and safely—

And she cried . . . and cried . . . and cried, till the night was over.

If the Party could thrust its hand into the past and say of this or that event, *it never happened*—that, surely, was more terrifying than mere torture and death.

George Orwell, *1984*

SOURCES

ACHRE. *Advisory committee on human radiation experiments-final report.* October, 1995. Retrieved June 6, 2003 from http://tis.eh.doe.gov/ohre/roadmap/achre/report.html

Adams, J. (2000). *Childhood ritual abuse: A resource manual for criminal justice and social service.* Odgen, UT: Mr. Light & Associates.

Bainton, R. H. (1950). *Here I stand.* New York: Abingdon-Cokesbury Press.

Ball, T. M. (1999). Monographs: (1) *Dissociative identity disorder: A primer for churches;* (2) *Prayer for inner healing of memories and deliverance: A primer for churches.* The Free Methodist Church, 200 North Fremont Street, Coldwater, MI 49036.

Barker, M. (1989). *The lost prophet: the Book of Enoch and its influence on Christianity.* Nashville, TN: Abingdon Press.

Bataille, G. (1991). *The trial of Gilles de Rais* (R. Robinson, Trans.). Los Angeles: Amok. (Original work published in 1965 by Jean-Jacques Pauvert, Paris).

Bauer, P. J. (1996). What do infants recall of their lives? *American Psychologist, 51*(1), 29-41.

Beardsley, R. M., & Wakefield, H.J. (2002, November). *Voices of survivors of sadistic/ritual abuse: Similarities in reports of healing/recovery from the USA and Canada.* Paper presented at the meeting of the International Society for the Study of Dissociation, Baltimore, MD.

Becker, T. (1999). Ritual abuse: A German cult-counsellors perspective. Presentation at the Symposium on Psychic Trauma and Dissociation, Utrecht, Netherlands. In Empty Memories (Ed.), *Proceedings of the Symposium on Psychic Trauma and Dissociation,* Amsterdam.

Becker, T., & Felsner, P. *Satanismus und Ritueller Mißbrauch.* Retrieved March 1, 2002 from http://www.nemasys.com/rahome/intl-resources/rit.shtml

Benko, S. (1984). *Pagan Rome and the early Christians.* Bloomington, IN: Indiana University Press.

Blackmon, D. (1999, August 17). A long-ago effort to better the species yields ordinary folks. *Wall Street Journal - Eastern Edition,* p. A1.

Blume, E. S. (2000). Sympathy for the devil: "False memories," the media, and the mind controllers. *Treating Abuse Today, 9*(3,4), 8-39; 7-27.

Budiansky, S., Good, E. E., & Gest, T. (1994, January 24). The Cold War experiments: Radiation tests were only one small part of a vast research program that used thousands of Americans as guinea pigs. *U. S. News and World Report,* 32-38.

Bull, D. L. (2001). A phenomenological model for therapeutic exorcism for dissociative identity disorder. *Journal of Psychology and Theology, 29*(2), 131-139.

Burgess, A. (1984). *Child pornography and sex rings.* Lexington, MA: Lexington Books.

Burke, J., Gentleman, A., & Willan, P. (2000, October 1). British link to 'snuff' videos. *Guardian Unlimited.* Retrieved May 23, 2002, from http://www.guardian.co.uk/Archive/Article/0,4273,4070446,00.html

Burns, R. (1995, October 8). 16,000 used in radiation. *Charlotte Observer,* p. 4a.

Cheit, R. *The recovered memory project.* www.RecoveredMemory.org

Chu, J. A., Frey, L. M., Ganzel, B. L., & Matthews, J. A. (1999). Memories of childhood abuse: Dissociation, amnesia, and corroboration. *American Journal of Psychiatry, 156*(5), 749-755.

Coffey, R. (1998). *Unspeakable truths and happy endings: Human cruelty and the new trauma therapy.* Lutherville, MD: The Sidran Press.

Crook, L.S., & Dean, M. C. (1999). "Lost in a shopping mall"— a breach of professional ethics. *Ethics and Behavior, 9*(1), 39-50.

De Young, M. (2002). *The ritual abuse controversy. An annotated bibliography.* Jefferson, NC: McFarland & Co.

Dobson, R. (1998, April 5). Abused lose out over memory scares. *The Independent* (London), p. 2.

Dallam, S. J. (2001). Crises or creation? A systematic examination of "False Memory Syndrome." *Journal of Child Sexual Abuse,* (3/4), 9-36.

Dulles, A. W. (1953, May 8). Brain warfare—Russia's secret weapon. *U. S. News & World Report,* 54-58.

Enquete komission 'Sog. Sekten und Psychogruppen' des Deutschen Bundestages: Endbericht. Bonn, 1998. (Final Report of the Enquete Commission on☐So-called Sects and Psychogroups☐: New Religious and Ideological Communities and Psychogroups in the Federal Republic of Germany).

Erikson, E. H. (1958). *Young man Luther.* New York: W. W. Norton.

Estabrooks, G. H. (1971, April). Hypnosis come of age. *Science Digest,* 44-50.

Feaster, W.R. (1997). *A history of Union County South Carolina.* Greenville, SC: A Press.

Flint, G. A. (2001). *Emotional freedom: Techniques for dealing with emotional and physical distress.* Vernon, BC: NeoSolTerric Enterprises.

Flint, G. A. (2001). *Process healing: Using the subconscious to heal.* Retrieved March 1, 2002, from http://www.process-healing.com

Fraser, G. A. (Ed.) (1997). *The dilemma of ritual abuse.* Washington, DC: American Psychiatric Press.

Frazier, E. (1998, August 20). Therapists cleared in memory suit. *The Charlotte Observer,* pp. C1, C4.

Fröhling, U. (1996). *Vater unser in der Hölle* (Our Father in Hell). Kallmeyer, Seelze.

Fröhling, U., & Huber, M. (1997). Ritual Abuse in Germany: Background of 354 Cases in Treatment. In Becker, T. (1999, October). *Ritual abuse: A German cult-counsellors perspective.* Presentation at the Symposium on Psychic Trauma and Dissociation, Utrecht, Netherlands.

Ganaway, G. K. (1989). Historical versus narrative truth: Clarifying the role of exogenous trauma in the etiology of MPD and its variants. *Dissociation*, 2(4), 205-220.

Gillotte, S. L. *Forensic considerations in ritual trauma cases.* Retrieved March 1, 2002 from http://www.iccrt.org/articles.asp?article=15

Goodspeed, P. (1998, September 6). Cracking secret code of an elite porn 'club'. *The Toronto Star*. Retrieved September 6, 1998 from http://www2.thestar.com

Heijtmajer, H. (1999). Ritual abuse - Questionmark? Presentation at the Symposium on Psychic Trauma and Dissociation, Utrecht, Netherlands. In Empty Memories (Ed.), *Proceedings of the Symposium on Psychic Trauma and Dissociation*, Amsterdam.

Hersha, C., Hersha, L., Griffis, D., & Schwarz, T. (2001). *Secret weapons: Two sisters' terrifying true story of sex, spies and sabotage.* Far Hills, NJ: New Horizon Press.

Hill, S., & Goodwin, J. (1989). Satanism: Similarities between patient accounts and pre-inquisition historical sources. *Dissociation*, 2(1), 39-44.

Hollingsworth, J. (1986). *Unspeakable acts.* New York: Congdon & Weed.

Huber, M. (1995). *Multiple Persönlichkeiten - Überlebende extremer Gewalt.* Frankfurt am Main: Fischer.

International cooperation to tackle child pornography. (2001). *Lancet, 357*(9256), 569.

Jenkins, P. (2001). *Beyond tolerance: Child pornography on the Internet.* New York: New York University Press.

Katchen, M. (1992). The history of satanic religions. In D. K. Sakeim & S. E. Devine (Eds.), *Out of darkness: Exploring Satanism and ritual abuse* (pp. 1-19). New York: Lexington Books.

Katchen, M. (1992). Satanic beliefs and practices. In D. K. Sakeim & S. E. Devine (Eds.), *Out of darkness: Exploring Satanism and ritual abuse.* (pp. 21-43). New York: Lexington Books.

Katz, F. E. (1993). *Ordinary people and extraordinary evil: A report on the beguilings of evil.* Albany, NY: State University of New York Press.

Kent, S. (1997). *Assessment of the satanic abuse allegations in the (name deleted) case.* Retrieved October 25, 2002 from http://www.arts.ualberta.ca/~skent/satanic.html

Kinderporno-ring: Festnahamen in Rom und Moskau. (Child pornography ring: Persons arrested in Rome and Moscow). (September 27, 2000). Retrieved March 1, 2002 from http://www.spiegel.de/panorama/0,1518,95559,00.html

Kluft, R.P., & Fine, C. G. (Eds.). (1993). *Clinical perspectives on multiple personality disorder.* Washington, DC: American Psychiatric Press.

Kluft, R. P. (1986). High-functioning multiple personality patients. *Journal of Nervous and Mental Disease, 174*(12), 722-726.

Lacter, E. (2003). *Mind control; simple to complex.* Retrieved June 10, 2003, from http://truthbeknown2000.tripod.com/Truthbeknown2000/id17.html

Lanning, K. V. (1989, October). Satanic, occult, ritualistic crime: A law enforcement perspective. *Police Chief*, pp. 88-107.

Leavitt, F. (2001). Iatrogenic memory change: Examining the empirical evidence. *American Journal of Forensic Psychology, 19*(2), 21-32.

Lorena, J. & Levy, P. (Eds). (1998). *Breaking Ritual Silence*. Gardnerville, NV: Trout and Sons.

McGonigle, H. (1999). *The law and mind control: A look at the law and government mind control through five cases*. Retrieved March 1, 2002, from http://members.aol.com/smartnews/fivecases.htm

McGowan, D. (2001, July-August). *Special report: The pedophocracy, part I.* Retrieved March 2, 2002, from http:/davesweb.cnchost.com/pedo1.html

Marks, J. (1979). *The search for the "Manchurian candidate": The CIA and mind control*. New York: W. W. Norton.

Miller, A. (1999). *Special issues in treating organized criminal abuse*. Workshop at the Fall Conference of the International Society for the Study of Dissociation, Miami, FL.

Mind control victim awarded $1 million (February 24, 1999). Retrieved March 1, 2002 from http://www.raven1.net/ra1.htm

Moyers, B. D. (1988). *The secret government*. Cabin John, MD: Seven Locks Press.

Napolis, D. *Satanism and ritual abuse archive*. Retrieved June 24, 2003 from http://www.newsmakingnews.com/karencuriojonesarchive.htm

Noblitt, J. R., & Perskin, P. S. (2000). *Cult and ritual abuse: Its history, anthropology, and recent discovery in contemporary America* (rev. ed.). Westport, CT: Praeger.

Noblitt, J. R. & Perskin, P. S. (Eds). (in press). *Ritual abuse in the twenty-first century: Clinical, forensic and social implications*.

Nordland, R., & Bartholet, J. (2001, March 19). The Web's dark secret. *Newsweek*, 44-51.

Owen, A. R. G. (1983). Poltergeists. In *Man, myth, & magic: The illustrated encyclopedia of mythology, religion, and the unknown* (pp. 2223-2228). New York: Marshall Cavendish.

Pasternak, D. (1997, July 7). Wonder weapons: The Pentagon's quest for nonlethal arms is amazing. But is it smart? *U. S. News & World Report*, 38-46.

Raschke, C. A. (1990). *Painted black*. New York: HarperCollins.

Rhoades, G. F. (2002, November). *Sadistic ritual abuse: Overview and research review*. Paper presented at the meeting of the International Society for the Study of Dissociation, Baltimore, MD.

Ross, C. A. (2000). *Bluebird: Deliberate creation of multiple personality by psychiatrists*. Richardson, TX: Manitou Communications.

Rovee-Collier, C. (1997). Dissociations in infant memory: Rethinking the development of implicit and explicit memory. *Psychological Review, 104*(3), 1-32.

Rutz, C. (2001). *A nation betrayed: The chilling true story of secret Cold War experiments performed on our children and other innocent people*. Gross Lake, MI: Fidelity Publishing.

Sakheim, D. K., & Devine, S. E. (1992). *Out of darkness: Exploring Satanism and ritual abuse.* New York: Lexington Books.

Scheflin, A. W., & Opton, E. M. Jr. (1978). *The mind manipulators: A non-fiction account.* New York: Paddington Press.

Scott, S. (2001). *The politics and experience of ritual abuse: Beyond disbelief.* Open University Press.

Seigel, M. (Host). (2000, July 19). *Coast to coast* [Radio broadcast]. Interview with Astronaut Gordon Cooper.

Shengold, L. (1989). *Soul murder: The effects of childhood abuse and deprivation.* New York: Fawcett Columbine.

Simandl, R. J. (1997). Teen involvement in the occult. In G. A. Fraser (Ed.), *The dilemma of ritual abuse: Cautions and guides for therapists (pp. 215-230).* Washington, DC: American Psychiatric Press.

Simon, J. M. (1995). *The highly misleading truth and responsibility in mental health practices act: The "false memory" movement's remedy for a nonexistent problem.* Retrieved September 27, 2002, from http://members.aol.com/conch8/antiTRMP1.html

Sinason, V. (Ed). (1994). *Treating survivors of satanist abuse.* London: Routledge.

S.M.A.R.T. *Ritual Abuse Newsletter.* http://members.aol.com/SMARTNEWS/index2.html

Steele, K. H. (1989). Sitting with the shattered soul. *Pilgrimage: Journal of Personal Exploration and Psychotherapy, 15*(6), 19-25.

Tendler, S. (2002, December 18). 1200 arrested in British paedophile raids. *British News.* Retrieved December 30, 2002 from http://www.timesonline.co.uk/article/0,,2-517566,00.html

Testimony of the witnesses in the preliminary examination of the Lenoir County Prisoners: The secrets of the Ku-Klux-Klan, &c, &c, &c. (1869). New-Berne, NC: Nason & Starns.

van der Hart, O., Boon, S., & Heijtmajer J, O. (1997). Ritual abuse in European countries: A clinician's perspective. In G. A. Fraser (Ed.), *The dilemma of ritual abuse: Cautions and guides for therapists* (pp. 137-163). Washington, DC: American Psychiatric Press.

van Weringh, E. *Online articles related to trauma, dissociation, neglect and the culture of the mind.* Retrieved March 22, 2002, from http://members.rott.chello.nl/emweringh/online_1html

Weinstein, H. M. (1990). *Psychiatry and the CIA: Victims of mind control.* Washington, DC: American Psychiatric Press.

Whitfield, C. L. (1995). *Memory and abuse: Remembering and healing the effects of trauma.* Deerfield Beach, FL: Health Communications.

Woodsum, G. M. (1998). *The ultimate challenge: A revolutionary, sane and sensible response to ritualistic and cult-related abuse.* Laramie, WY: Action Resources.

Yoeli, F. R., & Prattos-Spongalides, T. (2002, November). *The drama, the trauma and the mask of OCD: Life in the shadow of ongoing terror.* Workshop presented at the meeting of the ISSD, Baltimore, MD.